M000120710

Empathic Counseling

Meaning, Context, Ethics, and Skill

Jeanne M. Slattery

Clarion University

Crystal L. Park

University of Connecticut

BROOKS/COLE
CENGAGE Learning™

Australia • Brazil • Japan • Korea • Mexico • Singapore • Spain • United Kingdom • United States

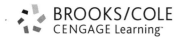
BROOKS/COLE
CENGAGE Learning

Empathic Counseling: Meaning, Context, Ethics, and Skill
First Edition
Jeanne M. Slattery and Crystal L. Park

Publisher/Executive Editor: Linda Schreiber

Acquisitions Editor: Seth Dobrin

Editorial Assistant: Rachel McDonald

Technology Project Manager: Dennis Fitzgerald

Production Manager: Matt Ballantyne

Manufacturing Buyer: Judy Inouye

Manufacturing Manager: Marcia Locke

Marketing Manager: Trent Whatcott

Marketing Assistant: Darlene Macanan

Marketing Communications Manager: Tami Strang

Art Director: Caryl Gorska

Permission Acquisition Manager – Image: Leitha Etheridge-Sims

Rights Acquisition Account Manager – Text: Roberta Broyer

Content Project Management: Pre-PressPMG

Production Service: Pre-PressPMG

Cover Designer: Lisa Buckley

Cover Image: Compositor: Pre-PressPMG

© 2011 Brooks/Cole, Cengage Learning

ALL RIGHTS RESERVED. No part of this work covered by the copyright herein may be reproduced, transmitted, stored, or used in any form or by any means graphic, electronic, or mechanical, including but not limited to photocopying, recording, scanning, digitizing, taping, Web distribution, information networks, or information storage and retrieval systems, except as permitted under Section 107 or 108 of the 1976 United States Copyright Act, without the prior written permission of the publisher.

For product information and technology assistance, contact us at **Cengage Learning Customer & Sales Support, 1-800-354-9706**.

For permission to use material from this text or product, submit all requests online at **www.cengage.com/permissions**. Further permissions questions can be emailed to **permissionrequest@cengage.com**.

Library of Congress Control Number: 2010920861

ISBN-13: 978-0-495-00485-1

ISBN-10: 0-495-00485-5

Brooks/Cole
20 Davis Drive
Belmont, CA 94002
USA

Cengage Learning is a leading provider of customized learning solutions with office locations around the globe, including Singapore, the United Kingdom, Australia, Mexico, Brazil and Japan. Locate your local office at **international.cengage.com/region**.

Cengage Learning products are represented in Canada by Nelson Education, Ltd.

For your course and learning solutions, visit **www.cengage.com**.

Purchase any of our products at your local college store or at our preferred online store **www.CengageBrain.com**.

Printed in the United States of America
1 2 3 4 5 6 7 14 13 12 11 10

For the clients, students, friends, and family who patiently listened to, supported, and guided me, even as I listened to, supported, and guided them.

—JMS

To my teachers.
—CLP

BRIEF CONTENTS

CONTENTS

6 Assessment Strategies for Understanding People in Context   104

7 Clinical Writing   131

LIST OF TABLES

LIST OF FIGURES

PREFACE

Even a cursory look in the local bookstore or on the Internet reveals a plethora of textbooks on counseling skills. All of these books cover the same essential territory and impart the same basic information regarding the elements of counseling skills. In reading through these books, though, we felt that there was something missing. Many try so hard to cover so many bases that they lose their voice: they lack a strong underlying theme or element to guide new clinicians in their development.

We decided to write a book that uses a fundamental aspect of all good clinical work—empathy—as the theme that ties our book together. Empathy, as used here, refers to the understanding, acceptance, and hopefulness that underlies all effective interventions. We approach the various topics within counseling skills from this perspective, basing our discussions on a model of empathy that requires having both a strong framework for understanding other people (and one's own self!) and strong assessment skills for developing an accurate assessment of their worldview.

We believe that it is essential to empathize with our clients' inner worlds and the cultural contexts in which they live; thus, the concepts of worldviews and multicultural identities are used throughout this book to guide the assessment process and help clinicians formulate and implement effective and empathic interventions.

Understanding, of course, is not enough. To be effective, this empathic understanding must be communicated using the fairly simple yet profound set of empathic communication skills that clinicians have honed over the years, such as active listening. Our model of empathy underlies the structure of our book, with sections on developing frameworks of understanding, clinical assessment tools, and empathic communication skills.

REAL-WORLD APPLICABILITY

We focused our discussion of counseling skills around real-world applications and the most challenging tasks that practitioners face throughout their careers. Toward this end, we have incorporated a number of features that facilitate real-world applications:

- It is easy to understand people who are similar to ourselves, but more difficult to empathize with people who hold different worldviews and who make decisions that are counterintuitive to us. To help readers learn how to empathize well, we use considerable case material drawn from memoirs, news reports, videos, and our clinical practices. These cases illustrate the material in each chapter, helping to bring the concepts alive and drawing students to a deeper level of learning. Further, these cases are threaded across chapters, so that students are encouraged to think about people and the process of working with them in complex ways; nonetheless, the skills to do so are broken down into manageable bites that are readily learned.

- To facilitate application of the concepts discussed, we include opening questions, case-related questions, and closing questions for each chapter.

- We help new clinicians see the "whole person," by focusing on the multiple identities and contexts that influence the client; the beliefs, values, and goals that make up their worldview; and their strengths as well as their weaknesses. Contextualized in this way, clients become three-dimensional people and clinicians' case conceptualizations and treatment plans become more sophisticated and helpful.

- Clinical work must be grounded in ethics, and in this book, we discuss the abstract ethical principles underlying good practice. But to make this material more accessible, we also include a chapter late in the book that builds on earlier chapters to get readers to think about the complexities of ethical behavior as it gets played out in the real world. We use this chapter to help readers think about these complexities and strategies to avoid compromising their ethics, effectiveness, or empathy. The *Codes of ethics for the helping professions* (ISBN 0-495-90657-3) is available to be bundled with this book to further support student understanding of and application of ethical issues from the perspective of different professions' codes of ethics.

- Clinical practice is strengthened by its foundation in scientific knowledge. Toward that end, we ground our assertions in the research literature with many citations to the original literature for pursuing more in-depth information on the topics we discuss.

- We emphasize clinical writing, because, in our experience, this task takes up a considerable part of the day, yet most clinicians report being little prepared to do this.

- Our book concludes with a chapter on practitioner self-care. We feel strongly that self-care should be emphasized during training to improve the well-being of practitioners and their effectiveness in helping others.

ETHICS AND PRAGMATICS IN USING CASE MATERIAL

The extended case material in this book is from real people—pulled from published reports in the news, videos, memoirs, and other sources. Some, like Sheila Carluccio, Anna J. Michener, Helen Tinsley-Jones, and Andrea Yates, gave their permission to talk about them in this context. Others gave their permission, but asked that we disguise their identities. Some are dead (Malcolm X, Eric Harris, and Dylan Klebold). These stories are by necessity incomplete, based on what information they—or their families, friends, or acquaintances—have been willing to share with the public. This is much like what happens in therapy, when clients and clinicians, together, tell some stories of their lives, but not others. What they tell is influenced by the context within which their story is told.

We have tried to stay within the ethical aspirations of our profession in how we approached their stories (Kitchener, 1984). Writing and thinking respectfully about the people whose case material is in this book, while avoiding libel, more importantly is consistent with the principles of beneficence and nonmaleficence—doing good while not causing harm. When we solicited case material, we acted in an open and honest manner, asking for permission to use materials in this book, sharing preliminary drafts of what we had written and the context in which it would appear, and making changes to correct errors (autonomy and fidelity). In some cases, people even talked about our interest and empathic understanding as empowering (beneficence). When possible, we also did these things with people who had previously published their memoirs or whose published interviews we used. If these had really been our clients, highlighting the options that they had and have would have promoted their autonomy. Finally, choosing people from a wide variety of contexts and cultural backgrounds, highlighting the contributions of these contexts, and encouraging you to do so, furthers the ideal of social justice.

ACKNOWLEDGMENTS

It's difficult to be complete in attributing influences on this book, because we believe that how we see things was a force that was set into motion from our early childhoods and by many interactions, large and small. Our lunch groups and family and friends have been especially important to this process, sometimes when they were the most irritating. The mother of JMS, Bea Slattery, read drafts of our case studies, provided encouragement, and was very generous in sending newspaper clippings and magazine articles. Friends and colleagues suggested a wide range of fascinating people to include here. Many of their suggestions—Saddam Hussein, Joseph Stalin, Lyndie England—ended up on the cutting-room floor, mostly because of space, but also because of the limited information available on their lives. Nonetheless, these suggestions influenced the development of our ideas.

Anna J. Michener, Helen Tinsley-Jones, and Andrea Yates talked with us about our case material and helped us get it right. Don Finch wrote about his life and generously shared his experience. Others, like Rachael Busch, were willing to let us use things that they wrote for other sources. Unfortunately, space in the book limited what we could use. Others allowed us to disguise events from their lives for case material. To all of the above, thank you.

Our students, friends, and family read drafts of this book. There are too many students to name individually (more than 150), although their careful and encouraging comments are remembered and appreciated. Jamie Aten, Rick Bessetti, Carol Bolland, Lisa Bria, Mary Buchanan, Rachael Busch, Hope Cross, David De la Isla, Craig Esposito, Don Finch, Kathy Fleissner, Marité Rodriguez Haynes, LaDonna Hohman, Debi Jones, Deb Kossman, Diana Kunselman, Julie Locke, Carrie Michieau, Kasundrah Murphy, Niek-o, Ame Pentz, Allison Potter, Sandy Potter, Randy Potter, Kahlid Qureshi, Jean Rumsey, Dave Schlueter, Bea Slattery, Laurie Snyder, Danny Wedding, Jolene Wiesner, and Kristine and Bruce Wilhelm helped me in some way or contributed thoughtful comments and ideas about one or more parts of this book.

We appreciate our editors at Cengage, Marquita Flemming and Seth Dobrin, who influenced the idea for this book, nurtured its growth and direction, and lit a fire under our toes when we would otherwise have stretched our deadlines toward eternity. They were generous in their brainstorming and equally generous when we'd say, No, that isn't how we want to handle this. Throughout, they were good cheerleaders, believing in us—sometimes when we doubted our own direction.

PART I

Empathy and the Mental Health Professional: An Introduction

We believe that empathy is the foundation of all effective therapeutic change. We define empathy broadly, as an affective and cognitive understanding of a person's experience from that person's unique point of view. Effective empathy includes being accepting and hopeful while also recognizing problems and symptoms. In this opening chapter, we introduce our model of building empathy. Building empathy depends on first having a strong framework in which to understand people, then developing assessment skills that lead to an empathic understanding of clients. This strong framework of understanding and strategies for applying those frameworks allows clinicians to build therapeutic relationships that facilitate positive change and express their empathic understanding well. This model is the thread unifying this book. In this first section, we also discuss the various mental health professions, all of which share the common belief that healing and growth occur most easily in the context of a relationship in which one person listens to the other with empathy.

CHAPTER 1

Empathy

WHERE ARE WE GOING?

1. What is empathy? Why is each part of this definition important?

2. What are "common factors"? What are their implications for the fields of counseling and psychotherapy?

3. How do clinicians think about what they do in the course of treatment? What do they believe they are doing?

4. What is the model of building empathy underlying this book?

THE PATH TO EMPATHY

Why did Andrea Yates, a deeply religious woman, methodically drown her five children and then call the police? Why do some people run up debt that they can never hope to pay? Why do some parents overfocus on their children, while others neglect them? Why do some people deliberately injure themselves, make themselves vomit, refuse to venture out from their homes, abuse their children, or engage in behaviors that clearly put them at risk? People who enter counseling and therapy often feel that they are crazy and beyond the understanding of others, even of themselves. They want stable relationships, yet find themselves on a rollercoaster of love, anger, and hate. Their self-induced vomiting and self-injuring revolts them, yet they continue this pattern. Failures in **empathy** and insight—their own and others'—leave clients feeling isolated and alone.

Describing periods of chaos in his own life, Carl Rogers (1980) wrote, "I have been more fortunate than most in finding ... individuals who have been able to hear me and thus to rescue me from the chaos of my feelings" (p. 12). Feeling heard rescues us. The concept of empathy underlies and permeates this book, as we believe that its presence is common to all effective therapeutic encounters. This book can help clinicians hear their clients well and create an atmosphere in which change can occur.

Did You Love Your Children?
Andrea Yates

Andrea Yates (age 36) had five children, four sons and a daughter, under the age of 8. On June 20, 2001, she drowned her children one at a time in the family's bathtub. The following transcript is from her interview with Dr. Phillip Resnick while she was at the Harris County Jail. Earlier in the interview she described herself as a "bad mother" because her children "weren't developing right ... in an academic sense and a righteous sense." Here she describes what she means by this.

Dr. Phillip Resnick 1: You mentioned an aphorism from the Bible about a millstone. Would you say what that is?

Andrea Yates 1: It's better to tie a stone around your neck and throw yourself into the sea ... than to cause ... to cause a little one to stumble.

Resnick 2: Let me make sure I'm getting that. "Better to tie a millstone around your neck and throw yourself in the sea" rather than to do what?

Yates 2: Cause someone to stumble ... stumble.

Resnick 3: Cause someone to stumble. Okay, uh, and when you say "stumble," you mean that, like on the path to righteousness.

Yates 3: Yes. [end Clip 7]

(continues)

Resnick 4: [begin Clip 8] And so you thought that your children, all five of your children, somehow because of what you saw as your defective mothering, were not on the path of righteousness and were stumbling. [Hmm] And did you feel then that it was good for them or bad for them, if you in fact threw them into the sea—or in a bathtub—in a very real sense? What were you trying to accomplish then when you did take your children's lives?

Yates 4: Maybe in their innocent years … God would take them up.

Resnick 5: It would be their innocent years and God would take them up? Is that what you said?

Yates 5: Be with him. Uh huh.

Resnick 6: God would take them up to be with Him in heaven? Is that what you mean? [Uh huh.] All right. And if you had not taken their lives, what did you think would happen to them?

Yates 6: Guess they would have continued stumbling.

Resnick 7: And where would they end up?

Yates 7: Hell. (Andrea Yates Confession, 2001, clips 8 and 9)

- Before continuing, think about Andrea Yates. How would you describe her beliefs about the world and her role in it? What motivates her?
- How would you respond to her given this understanding?

WHAT IS EMPATHY?

What is a weed? A plant whose virtues have not yet been discovered.

–Ralph Waldo Emerson

It can be very difficult to take the point of view of another person, especially someone whose beliefs, values, or goals differ markedly from one's own, but some people are better at this than others. Yet although people differ in empathy, it is not a **trait**, or inherent quality. Rather, empathy is an active set of cognitive and emotional reactions that can be developed across time. Characterizing empathy in this way helps to identify ways of further developing it. Empathy consists of four components: understanding, acceptance, hopefulness, and communication. Further, empathy is only effective when clinicians share it with their clients and their clients recognize it.

Understanding

I do not ask how the wounded person feels. I simply become that wounded person.

–Winston Churchill

People tend to see others whom they know and like in favorable ways, perceiving the best in what they do. They see their mistakes and problems as temporary or quirky aspects of them, or perhaps due to the situations rather than to their own actions. On the other hand, **attributions** for people unknown or disliked often take the form of traits: Those people are more likely to be seen as lazy, inconsiderate, and rude (Gilbert & Malone, 1995; E. E. Jones, 1979). Their behavior seems senseless, irrational, and unmotivated. However, they and their behavior make sense when seen in terms of their own goals, values, and beliefs. Although clinicians may not *agree* with their clients' behavior because they recognize that their clients have other options, they can begin to *understand* it.

In fact, we, the authors, wonder whether any "symptomatic" behavior is purposeless or senseless. Self-injuring behaviors, tantrums, panic attacks, and aggressive acts may appear to happen "out of the blue" and "for no reason," but we propose that these apparently senseless behaviors are motivated by factors outside of awareness—physical or emotional pain, fatigue, situational beliefs, feelings of being overwhelmed, and so on. Recognizing these causes increases empathy, facilitates the **therapeutic relationship**, and can often help one develop effective interventions.

When clients do not feel understood *from their own point of view*, when they feel objectified or dismissed, they are less likely to self-disclose, remain in therapy, or work collaboratively and cooperatively in therapy. When clinicians are able to hear clients from the clients' own viewpoint, the clinicians' work becomes more successful. Clinicians need to hear clients' **worldviews**, recognize their concerns and problems, and—importantly—also hear their strengths.

One essential aspect of empathy is recognizing that different people often view the same situation differently. As will be discussed in Chapter 3, people's values, goals, and beliefs **construct** their experience of the world. These worldviews are influenced by family, community, **culture**, and **context**, but also in turn affect how family, community, culture, and context are perceived (Rigazio-DiGilio, Ivey, Kunkler-Peck, & Grady, 2005).

Empathy is like walking in someone else's shoes—experiencing the world like that person does—and is based on an understanding of that person's unique affective and cognitive inner world. To be empathic, one must be aware of different perspectives on the world and willing to take other perspectives. For example, when someone dies, family and friends may grieve; feel relieved, guilty, hopeless, or alone; or have a sense of calm and of being at peace. A person may have many and apparently contradictory emotions in response to a single event: profound sadness, relief, and guilt about feeling relieved.

This ability to understand another's experience is built by developing curiosity about people and how they see the world, recognizing that there are multiple perspectives, and exposing oneself to multiple perspectives (e.g., by traveling, reading memoirs and psychological fiction, meeting and listening to people from different cultural groups, watching international films, and eating foods and listening to music outside one's normal palate). Simple exposure is not enough, however, but must be combined with a willingness to suspend making judgments in order to listen to another person. In the next case material, Irvin Yalom describes both the difficulty in shifting perspectives and the importance of doing so.

This understanding is both objective and subjective in nature. May (1967) suggested that effective clinical work depends on being able to take a client's point of view, while also remaining objective about his or her worldview, symptoms, problems, and strengths (see Figure 1.1). Effective

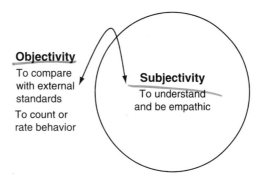

FIGURE **1.1** The balance needed during counseling and while making assessments: to be objective and subjective simultaneously.

counselors can enter suicidal people's experience to empathize with their depressive feelings and simultaneously objectively view their experience from the outside, remaining aware of the severity and course of their depression, the lethality of their suicidal ideation, and the correspondence between the stressor and their response. In this way, empathy is *like* walking in someone else's shoes, although clinicians retain their ability to step out of those shoes to adopt an external viewpoint. Empathy and objectivity are equally important, but many clinicians have difficulty being both empathic and objective simultaneously. Nonetheless, effective clinicians foster both attitudes in their work.

Food for Thought

Let's return to Andrea Yates. Imagine that she was court-referred into treatment with you after the drowning of her children. How would you apply these ideas here?

- Think about your initial description of Ms. Yates. Did you like her? Were you sympathetic to her actions? Did her behavior make sense? Was your initial reaction more objective or subjective—or were you able to balance both perspectives?
- Who is she? *From her point of view*, why did she do the things she did? What beliefs, values, and goals motivated her behavior? How would she describe her motivation?
- How would this new viewpoint change the way you approached her? How would she respond differently to your approach based on your original viewpoint and this new one?

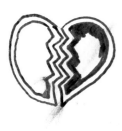

Looking Out His Window

Irvin Yalom

Irvin Yalom was born in 1931 of Russian Jews who had immigrated to the United States. Although he grew up in the ghettos of Washington, DC, he lived and worked in California for most of his life. A psychiatrist, he is best known for his writings on existential psychotherapy and group therapy processes. One thread that he developed in each of these superficially different fields is to help people really listen and connect despite their existential differences. He explores this here:

> Decades ago I saw a patient with breast cancer, who had, throughout adolescence, been locked in a long, bitter struggle with her naysaying father. Yearning for some form of reconciliation, for a new, fresh beginning to their relationship, she looked forward to her father's driving her to college—a time when she would be alone with him for several hours. But the long-anticipated trip proved a disaster: her father behaved true to form by grousing at length about the ugly, garbage-littered creek by the side of the road. She, on the other hand, saw no litter whatsoever in the beautiful, rustic, unspoiled stream. She could find no way to respond and eventually, lapsing into silence, they spent the remainder of the trip looking away from each other.
>
> Later, she made the same trip alone and was astounded to note that there were *two* streams—one on each side of the road. "This time I was the driver," she said sadly, "and the stream I saw through my window on the driver's side was just as ugly and polluted as my father had described it." But by the time she had learned to look out her father's window, it was too late—her father was dead and buried.
>
> That story has remained with me, and on many occasions I have reminded myself and my students, "Look out the other's window. Try to see the world as your patient sees it." The woman who told me this story died a short time later of breast cancer, and I regret that I cannot tell her how useful her story has been over the years, to me, my students, and many patients. (Yalom, 2003, pp. 17–18, italics in original)

1. Have you had the experience of looking out a very different "window" than someone else? How did each of you react? Did your response help the relationship or interfere with it?
2. What did each of you do to signal this failure in understanding?

Acceptance

We cannot change anything until we accept it. Condemnation does not liberate, it oppresses.
–Carl G. Jung

Many people enter therapy because of a shame-invoking event (e.g., being molested, raped, or battered; committing a crime; or questioning their sexual identity). To be empathic, clinicians must be accepting, even providing unconditional positive regard (C. Rogers, 1957/1992). Acceptance is not merely inhibiting actions or criticism. Instead, this sort of acceptance implies listening to a person without underlying judgment or criticism.

Clinicians do not need to accept everything a client says or does, but must find ways to accept the *person*. Judging clients can hook into their fears of being unacceptable or shameful, while listening and accepting can communicate that they are acceptable and free them to change. Acceptance of others is sometimes easier said than done. Taking the time to discover something likeable about them and to recognize that their behavior made sense to them, given their worldview, can be helpful (May, 1967). Understanding and acceptance are related qualities, with understanding fostering acceptance.

Hopefulness

We must accept finite disappointment, but never lose infinite hope.

–Martin Luther King, Jr.

Responding empathically also requires being hopeful about clients and their future. Clinicians may sometimes understand and accept clients but not see a possibility for improvement. A counselor can understand and accept a father's pain and suicidality following his child's death, but an effective one will see his pain as changeable. Hope—both the father's and the counselor's—can be built by recognizing the father's ambivalence about suicide inherent in his choosing to disclose rather than hide his suicidality, remembering that there have been both good times and bad, and acknowledging the healthy aspects of his response (e.g., his ability to connect with his son enough to grieve and with his counselor enough to disclose these feelings). This hopefulness can engage clients and help them to recognize their ability to change.

Hope is not a Pollyannaish optimism but instead implies a real awareness of both the problems that a client is experiencing and the possibility that things can be different. Hopefulness can be built through identifying situational factors and time fluctuations related to periods of improvement. Similarly, having worked with people with similar problems or knowing predictors of successful outcomes for people with similar issues can create hopefulness.

Communication

Clients often enter treatment expecting negative reactions when they disclose their concerns. Given their own feelings of shame, unless the clinician's understanding, acceptance, and hopefulness are shared both verbally and nonverbally, clients may expect that their clinicians will also see them as shameful, bad, and unable to change. A social worker working with a couple who have just learned that they will be unable to attempt another in vitro fertilization, for example, needs to express his or her empathic recognition of their mixed feelings of pain, regret, confusion, and relief. The social worker's empathy needs to be shared both verbally and nonverbally; these verbal and nonverbal communications should be congruent with each other. Furthermore, clients must hear this understanding. In fact, clients' ratings of empathy are better predictors of the strength of the therapeutic relationship and therapeutic outcomes than those of expert observers (D. Y. Lee, Uhlemann, & Haase, 1985).

Many people who enter the counseling fields perceive themselves as "nice" and want to help others. Often they believe that being nice means withholding statements about unflattering aspects of the person; however, some clients will draw inaccurate conclusions about the meaning of ambiguous or nondisclosing behaviors, drawing conclusions consistent with what they already believe.

Doing effective counseling and psychotherapy takes a fair amount of assertiveness. Clinicians may behave nonassertively because they have never had an effective assertive model, because they learned that assertiveness is gender-inappropriate for them, or because they confuse assertiveness and **aggression**. Assertiveness is direct, yet also respectful of the other person. Assertive responses are honest, yet also take into account the person's worldview, stage in treatment, and immediate factors like physical pain or fatigue.   Effective clinicians are able to triage a situation to determine what should be addressed at a particular point in time. For example, a new client may have problems parenting well, be in an emotionally abusive relationship, and be acutely suicidal. Effective clinicians would recognize each of these problems, but respond to the suicidality first and address the other issues once the client is more stable (G. K. Brown, Jeglic, Henriques, & Beck, 2006).

Workers in some fields, especially juvenile justice and substance abuse, often believe that aggressive responses are necessary and therapeutic. However, the research on hostile-confrontational approaches has demonstrated that they are not effective in changing substance abuse or other types of behaviors; people respond better to less confrontational approaches (Beutler, Rocco, Moleiro, & Talebi, 2001; Karno & Longabaugh, 2005). Aggressive responses fail in their empathy or timing and are thus ultimately less respectful and effective.

Food for Thought

Return to your views of Andrea Yates:

- What could you say to Ms. Yates that would express your empathic understanding without missing the larger context (i.e., that drowning her children was wrong)?
- How do your responses meet the four criteria of empathy (i.e., understanding, acceptance, hopefulness, and communication)? If you struggled with one or more of these qualities, what can you do to further develop that quality?
- Which of your three responses would best engage Ms. Yates so that she would willingly work in therapy?

THE COMMON FACTORS

Very early in my work as a therapist, I discovered that simply listening to my client, very attentively, was

Most clients improve as a result of counseling and psychotherapy. A recent summary of the literature concluded that about 75% of clients with most diagnoses (except those diagnosed with bipolar disorder or schizophrenia) improve. The rate of change differs, however. People with some disorders (e.g., panic, phobias) change faster than those with others (e.g., obsessive-compulsive disorder) (Lambert & Archer, 2006).

an important way of being helpful. So, when I was in doubt as to what I should do in some active way, I listened. It seemed surprising to me that such a passive kind of interaction could be so useful.

–Carl Rogers, 1980, p. 137

In the *Consumer Reports* survey of people who had seen a psychiatrist, counselor, psychologist, social worker, or marriage and family therapist, M. E. P. Seligman (1995) observed *disciplinary* differences in effectiveness of treatment, with psychologists, psychiatrists, and social workers equally effective and each better than marriage counselors and long-term medical management by family physicians (see Table 1.1). Practitioners from different disciplines tend to work with different sorts of people and problems, so these disciplinary differences are difficult to interpret. Nonetheless, in treating depression, psychotherapy appears to be equal in effectiveness to antidepressants for all but the most severe depressions (Lambert & Archer, 2006). A recent analysis goes even further, reporting that when both published and unpublished data are considered, antidepressants are no more effective than

TABLE **1.1**

Degrees and Typical Jobs and Job Settings of Common Mental Health Professionals.[1]

	Degrees	Typical jobs
Clinical psychologist	PhD or PsyD	Treats people with psychiatric or behavioral disorders. Significant portion of job may involve performing psychological assessments.
Counseling psychologist	PhD or PsyD	Helps individuals or groups accommodate to change or make lifestyle changes. Often does considerable work with vocational issues.
Counselor	Master's, PhD, PsyD, or EdD	Helps individuals or groups accommodate to change or make lifestyle changes.
Forensic psychologist	Master's, PhD, PsyD, or EdD	Works in legal setting doing competency, custody, identification of mitigating factors in sentencing, assessment of potential for future violence, etc. Often offers treatment of people in legal system.
School counselor	Master's	Generally helps students with vocational issues in a school setting, as well as to help them develop skills to meet academic and personal goals.
Marriage and family therapist	Master's, PhD, PsyD, or EdD	Helps couples and families communicate effectively, resolve problems, develop a healthy structure.
Psychiatric nurse	RN or MSN	Monitors psychiatric medication, consults with other medical professionals, may offer individual or group therapy, often in a medical setting.
Psychiatrist	MD or DO	Usually focuses on biological causes of psychiatric disorders and treats them medically using drugs or electro-convulsive therapy.
Psychoanalyst	Often, but not always, MD or DO	Takes a psychoanalytic approach to treatment, especially looking at unconscious causes to observed symptoms.
School psychologist	Master's, PhD, PsyD, or EdD	Works in school setting to identify and treat emotional or intellectual factors to help students meet their full potential. Consults with teachers, parents, students, and school board.
Social worker	MSW	Although may do individual, family, or group therapy, tends to assume problems have a systemic cause. Focus is often on intervening with the system and larger community.

[1]People in a given field may work in many different settings with different job responsibilities.

placebos, at least for mild to moderate depression (Kirsch et al., 2008). Lambert and Archer concluded that

> psychological interventions have been found to be equal to or to surpass the effects of medication for psychological disorders and should be offered before medications (except with the most severely disturbed patients) because they are less dangerous and less intrusive.... At the very least they should be offered in addition to medication, because they reduce the likelihood of relapse once medications are withdrawn. (p. 115)

Although it is difficult to compare theoretical approaches because they tend to work with different problems and have different goals, different *theoretical* approaches to clinical treatment generally appear to be about equally effective under most conditions (Lambert & Archer, 2006). In fact, as early as 1936, Rosenzweig famously noted the essential equivalence of therapy approaches, concluding, "*Everybody* has won, and *all* must have prizes" (p. 412, italics in original).

In explaining the essential equivalence of therapeutic models, most writers have suggested that although change may be partly attributable to therapeutic interventions, it is almost certainly more due to other factors, including the therapeutic alliance, the clinician's personality, clinician/client match, an opportunity for catharsis, or the receipt of an acceptable explanation of the problem, which have been collectively referred to as the **common factors** (Frank & Frank, 1993). Several of these could be seen as influencing empathy (i.e., therapeutic alliance, the clinician's personality, clinician/client match, and receiving an acceptable explanation). Rosenzweig (1936) concluded with the still-radical suggestion that

> [A] therapist who has an effective personality and who consistently adheres in his [*sic*] treatment to a system of concepts which he has mastered and ... adapted to the problems of the sick personality, then it is of comparatively little consequence what particular method that therapist uses. (pp. 414–415)

In other words, the success of psychoanalysts, behavior therapists, family therapists, and others may not be due to their specific therapeutic interventions, but to the common factors that all therapeutic approaches share.

Researchers have focused on four broad categories of change agents, the first three of which are the common factors (Asay & Lambert, 1999; Hubble, Duncan, & Miller, 1999; Lambert, 1992; Lambert & Archer, 2006; Lambert & Barley, 2001) (see Figure 1.2). These include

a. **Client variables and extratherapeutic events** (40%). Client variables include the symptom type and number, ego strength, psychological mindedness, and motivation for change. Extratherapeutic factors in clients' lives (e.g., family and social support, self-help books, and spiritual support) are believed to account for the large number of people who change without formal treatment.

b. **Therapeutic alliance** (30%). Factors that strengthen the therapeutic alliance are important to many effective treatments; these factors include empathy, warmth, respect, acceptance, and the encouragement of risk-taking.

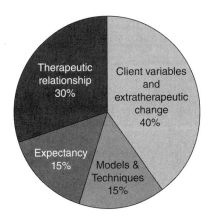

FIGURE **1.2** Percentage of improvement in treatment attributed to common factors.

Note: Modified from Lambert & Barley (2001)

c. **Expectancies for change** (15%). This includes contributions to change that are attributable to a sense of hopefulness and an awareness of being treated. Although sometimes denigrated as placebo effects, expectancies are now seen as active contributors to the change process that clinicians should intentionally foster (Snyder, Michael, & Cheavens, 1999). In fact, Fraser and Solovey (2007) conclude that restoring hope is the ultimate goal of psychotherapy and the common thread of all clinical interventions.

d. **Therapeutic models and techniques** (15%). A relatively small, but important contribution to change has been attributed to therapeutic models (e.g., behavior therapy or psychoanalysis) and interventions (e.g., role plays, empty chairs, flooding). Therapeutic models organize interventions and provide a consistent direction of treatment. They also create expectancies for change and strengthen the therapeutic relationship (Asay & Lambert, 1999; Fraser & Solovey, 2007).

The common factors, discussed at greater length in later chapters, probably influence change in fields as diverse as teaching, religion, and medicine. The therapeutic relationship and expectancies for change are explicitly described at length in Chapters 10 and 11 and are referred to throughout this book. Strategies for assessing client variables are explicitly described in Chapter 6; the ways that these variables can be used to foster treatment are further described in Chapter 12. Finally, the major theoretical models used to organize treatment and to think about clients are briefly described in Chapter 9.

WHAT DO CLINICIANS DO?

Although clinical change may be largely attributable to the common factors, most clinicians believe they are doing specific things to help clients change (Frank & Frank, 1993). Clinicians share a personal commitment to help clients and often work as active partners in the change process, mediating

Today there are hundreds of thousands of clean and sober individuals living productive lives only because, in a moment-of-truth, a counselor was there and made the difference.

–Patrick J.Kennedy

between clients and society as a whole. They listen empathically, creating an atmosphere where changing is safe. Their authority and expertise inspire faith and hope. Clinicians encourage their clients to examine themselves, their lives, and their problems differently; help them better express their emotions; and identify effective strategies for meeting their needs. Clinicians **empower** people, challenge them, engender hope, build strengths, and increase the number of options clients perceive.

Family and friends can be helpful and therapeutic, but counseling and psychotherapy are more purposeful and structured in their approach (B. C. Murphy & Dillon, 2003). Therapeutic interventions are not chosen willy-nilly, but are based on the theory and science of the field (e.g., with an awareness of how an intervention might empower a client or address the avoidance seen with PTSD symptoms). Clinicians often carefully consider the way they dress or decorate their office and the messages these send clients.

Clinicians listen carefully and empathically to people's verbal and nonverbal communication, to what they say or do not say, and to the **content** and **process** of their communications (B. C. Murphy & Dillon, 2003). For example, when asked how her week was, the client Evita's superficially simple statement, "*School* went well today," has many layers that can be heard by the careful listener.

- Why does Evita emphasize the word *school*? Are there other things that did not go well?
- Her breathing became more rapid when she talked about family and she broke eye contact. What does that mean?
- Why did she shift the discussion from family issues to school?

The process observed during a session can often be more useful and informative than the content disclosed.

Although empathic listening requires careful attention to the client, it also involves paying attention to one's own thoughts, feelings, and behavior. What happened as Evita began discussing school? Did this engender interest or boredom? Understanding one's own and others' interests, values, and issues may help identify the meaning of her behavior. A reaction of boredom may reflect her avoidance of any real issues and difficulty connecting with someone else, but it could also reflect the therapist's fatigue, feelings about school, distraction by events in his or her own personal life, or difficulties in connecting with someone else. As is emphasized in Chapters 2, 10, and 14, understanding oneself and one's own reactions will develop one's ability to become a more effective and empathic listener.

The counseling and psychotherapy relationship occurs in a valuing and cultural context. The client's and clinician's cultures and values influence their choices about what they identify as problems and treatment goals, as well as how they agree to meet these goals. Culture and values influence what people choose to do, how they do it, and how they think and feel about it. Most clinicians do not directly solve their clients' problems for them, but rather work to **empower** them to make change. They help clients discover ways of solving problems for themselves that are consistent with clients' values and that their clients will be able to continue using after the counseling or therapy process is complete.

OUR MODEL OF BUILDING EMPATHY

I am a human being, so nothing human is strange to me.

–Terentius

We have described empathy as a multifaceted thread including understanding, acceptance, hope, and communication that underlies a range of therapeutic behaviors and that is an important factor predicting therapeutic success (Lambert & Archer, 2006). Empathy can be learned and may lead to the effectiveness of practitioners from diverse theoretical approaches and in diverse professions, including teaching, religion, and medicine (Frank & Frank, 1993).

Learning to be empathic in clinical settings requires focus on three different kinds of tasks: (a) developing a sufficiently complex framework to understand people; (b) acquiring the skills to make strong, empathic **clinical assessments**, which together create empathy; and (c) building clinical skills to express empathic understandings effectively. Together, these help people make positive change. This model, portrayed in Figure 1.3, is the foundation for our approach to clinical work. We briefly describe the components of the model here and elaborate this model throughout this book.

A Framework for Understanding

People are complicated beings who can be understood in many different ways; however, a strong theoretical and research-based framework makes understanding people easier. Although there are numerous possible frameworks from which to choose, in this book we focus on two types: one more personal and subjective, the other including more external influences. Specifically, in Chapter 3, we describe people as meaning-making beings and examine some of the aspects of worldview that are most salient in clinical settings. Chapter 4 looks at the role of culture and context, especially how clients' multiple cultural identities influence their beliefs, emotions, behavior, problems, and symptoms. Throughout this book, we describe other ways of viewing clients that increase understanding of them, especially theory and research about worldviews and diagnoses (Chapter 9), clients' readiness for change (Chapter 8), and strengths and current successes (Chapters 5 and 12). In Chapter 6 we describe a way of understanding clients holistically—as psychological/physical/cultural/spiritual beings.

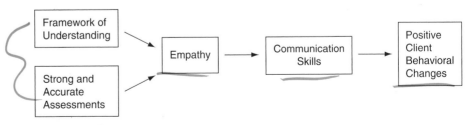

FIGURE **1.3** Our model of building empathy.

Tools for Developing Empathic Understanding

Part 3 of this book focuses on applying the frameworks of understanding (primarily outlined in Part 2) to develop a strong and empathic clinical assessment. Chapter 5 describes the processes of making effective observations, thinking critically, and generating hypotheses that underlie a strong clinical assessment. Chapter 6 outlines four **assessment strategies** to systematically gather information to inform the clinician's diagnostic opinions, conclusions, and treatment recommendations. Chapter 7 discusses the process of communicating clinical observations and assessments, especially in writing. Chapters 8 and 9 demonstrate how clinicians draw on the gathered information (described in Chapters 5–7) to tailor treatment to individual clients.

Clinical Skills for Expressing Empathy and Facilitating Positive Change

Part 4 of this book begins by outlining the relational and structuring skills that clinicians use to engage clients (Chapter 10). Chapter 11 describes the verbal and nonverbal skills that clinicians use to obtain and communicate empathic understanding. Chapter 12 describes ways to address obstacles in treatment and to use strengths and successes to help clients change. Chapter 13 reviews strategies for assessing progress, preventing relapse, and ending treatment well. Chapter 14 discusses the tensions that exist for clinicians striving to be ethical, effective, and empathic when balancing the demands of the real world. Finally, Chapter 15 discusses the importance of regular self-care in maintaining one's effectiveness in working with others and offers many concrete ways to care for oneself.

SUMMARY

Empathy is an affective and cognitive understanding of a person's experience from that person's unique point of view. Effective empathy is accepting and hopeful without being Pollyannaish or ignoring problems and symptoms. Empathy is useless until it is communicated both verbally and nonverbally by the therapist and recognized in turn by the client.

The mental health fields share a common belief that healing and growth occur most easily in the context of a relationship in which one person listens to the other with empathy. In fact, although about 75% of people change during the course of counseling and psychotherapy, a relatively small amount of the change observed is attributable to therapeutic models and interventions (15%). The vast majority of the change that clients make is shared by the common factors: (a) client variables and extratherapeutic events (40%), (b) the therapeutic relationship (30%), and (c) clients' expectancies for change (15%).

We outlined a model of building empathy that is the thread unifying the rest of this book. Specifically, clinicians need a way to think about and understand people (described in Part 2), tools for developing a strong clinical assessment of individual clients (Part 3), and techniques for working effectively with this assessment to help clients make positive changes in their lives (Part 4).

How Do These Issues Apply to Your Life and Work?

Almost everyone has had experiences where they have changed. Think about an important change you have made and what helped you change.

1. What made it easier or more difficult to change? Compare your experience with that of your friends or fellow students. What do you conclude in comparing your story with theirs?
2. If someone—a parent, friend, minister, teacher, or therapist—helped you change, what did he or she do? What characteristics or behaviors seemed particularly helpful? Compare your experience with that of your friends or fellow students. Which of these characteristics would you like to further develop in order to become a better clinician? What steps could you take to make these changes (B. C. Murphy & Dillon, 2003)?
3. How has it felt when someone else really understood you? How has it felt when you were misunderstood, especially about something important?
4. How do you recognize when you are being treated respectfully? Would being treated respectfully in counseling be different than in some other sort of helping relationship in another part of your life? If so, how?
5. If you would like to be more respectful of others, especially in the counseling and psychotherapy process, what changes would you need to make? What steps could you take to make these changes?
6. Although this book emphasizes paying attention to all dimensions of another person—words, vocal cues, nonverbal behavior, dress and grooming, posture, and so on—it necessarily emphasizes the spoken word. What can you do to increase your understanding of someone else's words? What things can you do that go beyond the spoken word?

PART **II**

Building a Framework for Understanding and Contextualizing People

Effective empathy and interventions depend on understanding clients' worldviews and the meanings they draw in response to stressors and trauma in their lives. In this section, we set the stage for this work by first describing the ethical foundations of clinical work and then introducing the central concept of worldviews and the implications of culture on these worldviews. Chapter 2 describes the ethical guidelines and principles that guide strong clinical work. Chapter 3 begins with a definition of worldviews, followed by a description of many aspects of worldviews that may be particularly relevant to clinical settings. Chapter 4 focuses on culture, exploring dimensions such as race, gender, class, religion, and sexual orientation. Potential treatment implications of discrimination, prejudice, and oppression are discussed.

CHAPTER 2

Being an Ethical Clinician

WHERE ARE WE GOING?

1. What are the aspirational principles guiding ethical clinical work?

2. What are the ethical standards guiding treatment? How can clinicians put these standards into practice?

3. How are counseling and psychotherapy different from friendship?

4. What strategies can clinicians use to help them identify where they might run into ethical problems?

5. How do self-knowledge and self-awareness help clinicians maintain ethical treatment?

A Band-Aid for Complex Problems
Dr. Helper

Chapter 1 described empathy as an attitude of hopefulness and unconditional acceptance that is grounded in understanding. Empathy is important to clinical work, but in order to be an effective clinician, one's empathy must be grounded in a strong ethical framework. Without a clear ethical framework, empathy can slip into caretaking that provides a Band-Aid for complex problems, ignoring the competing ethical concerns that frame strong clinical work (Handelsman, Gottlieb, & Knapp, 2005). With a clear ethical framework, treatment becomes respectful, empowering, and compassionate, helping clients meet their long-term treatment goals.

Many clinicians enter the field to help people. Even those clinicians who have committed an ethical violation are likely to have had good intentions and meant to be helpful (Pope & Keith-Spiegel, 2008). This positive intention is seen in the story of Anonymous (2000)—called Dr. Helper here—a psychologist who was "helpful" in response to a deathbed promise to a client. This client asked Dr. Helper to take care of his wife, Edna, and their children. In meeting his perception of this promise, Dr. Helper began seeing Edna as a client, hired her as office staff when she needed work, saw himself as part of her family, bought her jewelry, and eventually started a sexual relationship with her. In nonclinical contexts, these might be appropriately caring responses. In this context, however, Edna eventually felt used, exploited, and abandoned. Dr. Helper's wife divorced him and the Licensure Board censured him. He concluded, "I failed because I didn't know how to limit care" (p. 3).

- What specific problems do you see with Dr. Helper's responses? Why?
- If you had made this deathbed promise, what are some more ethical ways of honoring it? How would you choose among your responses?

THE ASPIRATIONAL PRINCIPLES

Ethics is a code of values which guide our choices and actions and determine the purpose and course of our lives.
—Ayn Rand

Ethical treatment includes both behaving in positive and ethical ways and avoiding harmful acts. The **aspirational principles** of the American Psychological Association's code of ethics (American Psychological Association [APA], 2002), for example, were developed to "guide and inspire psychologists toward the very highest ethical ideals of the profession" (p. 1062). These five principles first described by Kitchener (1984) are that clinicians do good (**beneficence**), avoid harm (**nonmaleficence**), support their clients' ability to think and act freely for themselves (**autonomy**), behave in a faithful, honest, trustworthy manner (**fidelity**), and promote fairness in the community and clinical settings (**social justice**).

Consider Dr. Helper's work with Edna (Anonymous, 2000). His description of this period suggests that he was trying to do good, but it is less clear that he was thinking broadly and working to meet the next three principles: nonmaleficence, autonomy, and fidelity. If he had been acting to avoid doing harm, perhaps he would have steered clear of a series of situations that, as described below, almost certainly would leave Edna feeling exploited. Ethical clinicians consider the long-term consequences of their actions when making decisions, thinking not only about the best possible outcome of their proposed act but also the worst (Pope & Keith-Spiegel, 2008).

Dr. Helper's actions did not seem to be made with the principle of fostering autonomy as a guide. He seemed to believe that *he* should solve Edna's problems and meet her needs as they arose. When she needed a therapist, he agreed to see her, rather than encouraging her to find a therapist. When she needed a job, he hired her. When she was feeling alone, he stepped in as friend, family, and lover. Ethical clinicians encourage their clients to identify strategies for meeting their needs—perhaps with their clinicians' assistance—rather than attempting to meet their needs for them. The latter response may be well received, but it also encourages dependency on both the clinician and the treatment.

Even when writing about this period of his life after the fact, Dr. Helper seemed to have little insight into the motivations that led him to engage in behaviors that most clinicians would identify as very risky. His failure to look at his behavior and question his decisions and motivations led him to behave in ways that were not faithful, honest, and trustworthy—that is, they did not promote fidelity.

As Pope and Keith-Spiegel (2008) conclude, even good people can make ethical mistakes and blunders. Ethical and competent clinicians, however, engage in a decision-making process that decreases the likelihood of these mistakes.

> An important part of our work is questioning ourselves, asking "What if I'm wrong about this? Is there something I'm overlooking? Could there be another way of understanding this situation? Could there be a more creative, more effective way of responding?" (p. 641)

Although anyone can make mistakes, having a well-developed personal moral code, a strong grounding in one's professional ethics, and a good decision-making process for preventing and responding to ethical problems can help one handle ethical dilemmas well. The balance of this chapter will describe strategies for developing these skills.

THE ETHICAL STANDARDS

The aspirational principles outline goals for practitioners of the field. These goals may be difficult to achieve, but they should be used to guide clinicians' behavior. On the other hand, the **ethical standards** set expectations for the field, violations of which can lead to disciplinary censure. Clinicians will face five important ethical issues throughout their careers for which ethical standards must be adhered to: **informed consent, competence, confidentiality,**

Reason guides our attempt to understand the world about us. Both reason and compassion guide our efforts to apply that knowledge ethically, to understand other people, and have ethical relationships with other people.

—**Molleen Matsumara**

dual relationships, and sensitivity to differences. The ethical standards addressing these are briefly described here, but clinicians should read through their profession's code of ethics on a regular basis to understand and apply them more carefully and fully (American Association for Marriage and Family Therapy [AAMFT], 2001; American Counseling Association [ACA], 2005; APA, 2002; National Association of Social Workers [NASW], 2008) (see Appendix A).

Informed Consent

Informed consent is a process whereby clinicians provide clients with sufficient information to make informed decisions about their treatment (Barnett, Wise, Johnson-Greene, & Bucky, 2007). They should be informed about confidentiality, fees, and the clinician's training. Clients have the right to know what other treatments are available, along with their benefits and potential side effects, and to receive a referral to other services when appropriate.

The informed consent process generally starts in the initial session, but continues across time as additional questions emerge. For example, during an initial session, when reviewing the informed consent forms with a client, a clinician might describe his or her general decision-making process about referring clients for medication, and then describe this process more fully in later sessions for clients whose depression does not respond well to psychotherapy alone, because the client may need more information to make a specific decision at that point.

Clients' perceptions of the informed consent process have generally been studied with **pseudoclients** (i.e., research participants in the role of a client during a study). Pseudoclients informed about limits to confidentiality reported being less willing to self-disclose than those who were not told these limits (Nowell & Spruill, 1993). Despite the potential problems that come with informed consent (e.g., decreased willingness to disclose child abuse), in summarizing the evidence, Snyder and Barnett (2006) concluded that the informed consent process fosters the therapeutic alliance, client autonomy, and rational decision making while reducing the potential for exploitation and harm. Pseudoclients informed about the nature of treatment saw their clinicians as more expert and trustworthy than those not asked to give informed consent, and they were also more likely to report being willing to see that clinician again and to recommend that clinician to a friend (Handelsman & Martin, 1992; Sullivan, Martin, & Handelsman, 1993).

Clinical Practice

Marion came to treatment with a phobia about birds that had her increasingly housebound. Based on a review of the literature, Ken decided to use the technique of flooding (i.e., exposing her to a very high level of the feared stimulus) in treatment, although he decided not to tell her what he

(continues)

was going to do first. He concluded, "If I told her, she wouldn't do it!" What do you think of the ethical issues involved in his decision?

*****

Sharlynn was actively suicidal and threatening to take 150 mixed pills. She would not agree to go to the hospital. Dee, her therapist, told Sharlynn what she was going to do at each step as they considered options for keeping her safe. Are there other things that she should have done to remain ethical in this setting?

Competence

Clients will ask their caseworkers, social workers, counselors, and psychologists to do many things, some of which they are competent to do, others for which they do not possess adequate training or expertise. Individual therapists may be asked to give testimony in child custody cases. Adult therapists may be asked to work with children. Caseworkers may be asked to do therapy or provide legal counsel. Social workers in a psychiatric hospital with chronically mentally ill patients may be asked to do vocational counseling.

Competence is multidimensional and includes knowledge and skills as well as the attitudes, values, and judgment necessary to implement them well (Barnett, Doll, Younggren, & Rubin, 2007). Generally, knowledge is gained through formal reading, coursework, or training in an area of specialty; skill is developed through ongoing supervision and consultations. Maintaining competency also requires that clinicians recognize and address psychological issues that can cloud their judgment (e.g., bias, distress, substance use and abuse, and mental and physical illness).

The degree of expertise needed to become competent depends in part on a clinician's initial levels of general clinical competence as well as the uniqueness of the area. A social worker who does individual psychotherapy might be competent to do vocational counseling—depending on the complexity of the vocational issues—but might not be competent to do a custody evaluation. Although competent to do a custody evaluation in English and Spanish, if a clinician fails to recognize the complications of language and culture when evaluating a Mexican immigrant, his or her actions may be less competent. Even if the clinician is skilled in performing custody evaluations with Mexicans and has a good translator, his or her competency to do so might drop during the course of his or her own contentious divorce. Competence is a state that can be achieved, but it must also be maintained and enhanced in the face of a changing field and personal context (Barnett, Doll, et al., 2007). Thus, maintaining competency requires ongoing professional development, self-care, and regular assessments of one's emotional health and level of skill (Barnett, Doll, et al., 2007; Knapp & VandeCreek, 2006).

Why is competence an important issue? When clinicians work without the specific competency to perform specialized tasks (e.g., forensic work, neurological assessments, or family therapy), they offer a lower level of service and, as a result, compromise the client's mental health and the reputation of the profession. Clinicians who do not maintain their level of competence are also more likely to be sued or be the subject of ethical complaints. Behaving ethically and competently is an important risk-management strategy to protect one's reputation and prevent lawsuits (Bennett et al., 2006).

Clinical Practice

Darcy is in the process of going through a divorce. She has been monitoring her stress levels, cut back on accepting referrals to work with couples, and reentered personal therapy, but is still seeing clients and believes herself effective, as does her supervisor. What factors might affect her competence? How would her level of competence be determined?

*****

Nadya is a talented child therapist working with children with autism. She gets so many referrals that she has significant difficulties responding to all of them. In trying to meet this need, she rarely finds time to write her case notes, much less read the newest research on autism, and hasn't been to a **continuing education** workshop in 4 years. Nonetheless, the referrals pour in. What are the issues of competence for Nadya?

Confidentiality

Confidentiality is a very broad right that allows clients to discuss sensitive issues safely without worry that they will be disclosed to someone else. In general, nothing about clients' presence or activity in treatment can be shared without clients' specific permission to do so. State statutes, court rulings, and agency policies, however, limit confidentiality under a variety of situations. Many states mandate that clinicians report child or elder abuse and imminent danger to self or others. Clinicians may receive court subpoenas to disclose confidential information, must discuss treatment issues with their supervisors, and may share information with insurance companies to receive payment.

Sometimes, rules about confidentiality may seem absurd. Family members may know that a client is receiving therapy, but hit a brick wall when they call to see how treatment is going. Unless the client has provided specific permission to release this information, clinicians must respond noncommittally (e.g., "I cannot confirm or deny that she is a client here"). This prohibition protects those people who want to keep their mental health care private, but does not prevent clients from disclosing aspects of their own treatment to others. They own the information and can choose where and how to share it.

Although clinicians may have permission to disclose some information, this permission should be limited to information relevant to the source. For example, it might be relevant to describe interventions that will stabilize the child in school, but be unnecessary and inappropriate to disclose the child's diagnosis. Furthermore, unless the material is specifically related to the difficulties that the child is having in the school, revealing to school personnel that the child's mother is an alcoholic is probably gratuitous and damaging.

Why is confidentiality an important issue? Confidentiality creates a safe environment that helps clients disclose and explore material that they may never have shared before. Legal mandates to report abuse or threats of violence can compromise openness and trust (Nowell & Spruill, 1993). As described earlier, describing these limits on confidentiality during the informed consent process can foster the therapeutic alliance, client autonomy, and rational decision making. Sharing the limits of confidentiality can also reduce client perceptions of being exploited should a disclosure be needed at a later point (Snyder & Barnett, 2006).

Clinical Practice

Liza's social worker, Sophie, talked to Dr. Wu about Liza's status and response to a new antidepressant while he was doing hospital rounds. Dr. Wu asked whether Liza's symptoms stemmed from her history of sexual abuse (in order to guide his prescription). Liza had only given Sophie permission to disclose her symptoms and response to the antidepressant, not to discuss her incest history. What should Sophie do? How could she have handled the consent process differently to prevent problems from developing?

* * * * *

Daria and her 11-year-old son were eating lunch at a local coffee shop when a former client came up to them and began talking about the break-up of his marriage that occurred since they ended treatment. Is this ethical? What should Daria do?

Dual Relationships

Dual relationships occur when clinicians engage in more than one relationship at a time with a client (e.g., becoming the client's friend, employer, teacher, business associate, or sex partner or lover, in addition to being his or her therapist). Any relationship or obligation that exploits clients to further the clinician's personal interests at the expense of the client's—or that appears to do so—is problematic. This other relationship or obligation can cloud the clinician's ability to make objective and sound decisions and can also create expectations in both the clinician and the client that interfere with treatment (Knapp & Slattery, 2004; Slattery, 2005).

Dual relationships differ in their impact on treatment and their degree of clinical risk (Guthiel & Gabbard, 1993). **Boundary violations** (e.g., becoming sexually involved with a client, hiring a client to clean house) can have explosive consequences and should always be avoided. They are associated with increased risk of ethical complaints (Bennett et al., 2006).

Boundary crossings are less risky and can even be acceptable under some circumstances, as when occasionally extending a session's length for a client who is in crisis or self-disclosing material to help clients meet their therapeutic goals (Barnett, Lazarus, Vasquez, Moorehead-Slaughter, & Johnson, 2007).

Boundary crossings can be difficult to avoid in some settings but, like boundary violations, can create unclear expectations, muddy communication processes, and sometimes leave clients feeling exploited. Lamb and Catanzaro (1998) reported that professionals who reported having made some types of boundary crossings (e.g., going to a party that the therapist knows a client also plans to attend, disclosing details of a personal stressor, crying in front of a client, giving the client unused sports or theatre tickets) were more likely to engage in sexual relationships with clients. This suggests that there may be a "slippery slope" in treatment that, once stepped on, increases the probability of unethical acts. Although a number of writers have argued that responding to clients flexibly can strengthen the therapeutic relationship, deviations from professional norms should be thoughtfully considered and discussed with colleagues, supervisors, or clients before the fact or as soon after the fact as possible (Barnett, Lazarus, et al., 2007; Knapp & Slattery, 2004; Slattery, 2005; Zur, 2001).

Why is avoiding dual relationships—especially boundary violations— important? Lamb and Catanzaro (1998) reported that about 50% of professionals who had previously had a sexual relationship with a professor, clinical supervisor, or therapist reported negative consequences from that relationship. For some, the consequences decreased with time, but about twice as many reported that consequences became *more* negative. Whether the second relationship began before, during, or after the therapeutic relationship, dual relationships can be destructive to both parties, as well as to their families, friends, and the profession. The reputations of both that particular clinician and the field as a whole are compromised by boundary violations and inappropriate boundary crossings.

Clinical Practice

Not wanting to be rude, Daria invites her former client, who is clearly shaken while talking about the break-up of his marriage, to join her and her son as they finish lunch. What do you think of Daria's actions? If you see a problem, how could she have handled this more ethically?

* * * * *

Sam lives in a small community where it is traditional for people to give holiday gifts to friends, teachers, and other people for whom they are

(continues)

thankful. He received a child's drawing and a number of plates of cookies. He also received from another client a lovely engraved watch like the one that he has been wanting, but can't afford. Would accepting the watch be ethical? Would accepting the drawings and cookies be ethical? Why or why not? What should he do?

Sensitivity to Differences

Competent, effective clinicians are sensitive to differences in race, culture, class, gender, sexual orientation, religion, and other contextual factors. Such sensitivity improves the assessment, diagnostic, and treatment processes and strengthens the therapeutic alliance. Clinicians sensitive to issues of cultural differences offer services that are user-friendly and user-appropriate; respect differences in values, belief systems, and habits; are sensitive to cultural differences; decorate their offices in a way that reflects their openness to people of other cultures; and consider cultural issues as they develop goals and treatment plans.

Sensitivity to differences is a multidimensional issue. For example, an agency in a Latin neighborhood may preferentially hire Spanish-speaking staff and encourage other staff to develop their language skills and understanding of Latin culture. The waiting room may have magazines, notices, and paperwork in both English and Spanish. The clinician's understanding of Latin culture increases his or her sensitivity to how culturally normative *personalismo* may instead appear to be problems with boundaries (Cooper & Costas, 1994). See Table 3.5. They name and discuss oppression, prejudice, and discrimination as it affects their clients' lives and treatment (Slattery, 2004).

The attitude of cultural sensitivity is a general one rather than one specific to a particular racial or ethnic minority. Some of the many issues to consider regarding sensitivity to differences include: Is the office really handicapped accessible? In addition to a ramp or elevator, is the path between furniture wide enough for wheelchairs? If young children are seen in the clinic, are chairs and decorations child-friendly and child-proofed? Will male clients feel comfortable in a pink, frilly office? Will Jewish clients feel welcome at Hanukah?

Why is being sensitive to differences an important issue? Without this sensitivity, treatment will likely be derailed because clients will believe that their clinicians do not understand them and are unwilling to make the effort to do so (Pope & Keith-Spiegel, 2008). In addition, because of the power differential between clients and clinicians, clinicians who are culturally insensitive may impose culturally oppressive views on their clients that interfere with developing empathy, undermine the therapeutic relationship, and lead clinicians to set inappropriate and sometimes disempowering goals.

Clinical Practice

At his fourth therapy session, Beau discloses that he is gay, although he clearly indicates that this is neither a problem for him nor related to his history of recurrent depressive episodes. Nonetheless, his counselor, Marcee, whose religious and personal beliefs are that homosexuality is a sin, begins to push Beau on this issue. He was offended and made a complaint to her supervisor. What evidence would convince you that Marcee's actions were ethical? Unethical? What should she do at this point in order to behave more ethically, if necessary?

* * * * *

Hank, who only speaks English, hesitantly accepted a client who only speaks Mandarin, although did so because there is no Mandarin-speaking counselor in their community—the nearest one is 125 miles away and his new client does not drive. He has found a translator who is acceptable to his client's family. What else should he consider? Was it ethical to accept this client?

BALANCING CLIENT RIGHTS WITH ETHICAL AND LEGAL REQUIREMENTS

Because our every action has a universal dimension, a potential impact on others' happiness, ethics are necessary as a means to ensure that we do not harm others.

—**The Dalai Lama**

As alluded to earlier in this chapter, clients have rights in the course of treatment. These were articulated in a Consumer Bill of Rights ratified by nine national associations of mental health providers (Cantor, 1998). Many of the rights they described are consistent with ethical behavior previously outlined in this chapter. That is, people receiving mental health care have the right to be treated with dignity and respect, receive competent treatment, and be actively involved in setting the direction of treatment. They have the right to be informed about costs, anticipated risks, and alternative treatments, and to make decisions based on this information. They have the right to have their culture respected. They have the right to keep information about the nature of their treatment confidential and to have disclosures occur only with their permission.

On paper, some of these rights seem clear and unarguable; however, they become more complicated in the real world. This section describes several real-world examples to both outline the potential conflicts that clinicians need to resolve and to further describe the range of ethical and legal considerations that clinicians must consider.

The decision in *Tarasoff v. Regents of the University of California* imposed a duty to warn identifiable victims of a threat. In this case, a client in a university counseling center told his psychologist that he intended to kill his ex-girlfriend. The psychologist took the threat seriously and attempted to hospitalize his client (Bennett et al., 2006). This hospitalization attempt was unsuccessful, and the client dropped out of treatment. The psychologist's supervisors forbade him from breaking confidentiality to warn the intended victim, Tatiana Tarasoff. Unfortunately, the ex-client subsequently killed her. Tatiana's parents sued the psychologist for failing to warn their daughter of the danger. The California Supreme Court concluded that when "a patient poses a serious danger of violence to others, [the therapist] bears a duty to exercise reasonable care to protect the foreseeable victim of that danger" (quoted in Ewing, 2005, p. 112). Protecting an intended victim can be accomplished in a number of ways, including warning him or her; however, addressing the issue in therapy or changing the frequency or focus of treatment may often be enough (Bennett et al., 2006). This duty to warn does not apply in situations where the potential victim is unidentifiable (e.g., a potential new sexual partner of someone with HIV).

Although violence of this magnitude rarely occurs, the *Tarasoff* case raises a number of issues. First, it places limits on confidentiality. In this case, confidentiality is superceded by a serious threat of violence. Second, competent treatment of violent clients requires, among other things, recognizing predictors of violence and the relationship between violence and suicidality, developing a treatment plan based on a careful assessment, and carefully documenting one's assessment and conclusions (Bennett et al., 2006). Third, potential feelings of betrayal may be reduced when the limits to confidentiality are described during the informed consent process and again if threats are made. Finally, the *Tarasoff* ruling suggests that the ethical aspirations of doing good and avoiding harm do not just refer to good and harm for the client, but to the larger community as well.

Similar problems arise in other settings. When should clinicians break confidentiality to tell parents that adolescent clients are engaging in dangerous behaviors? When they are having unprotected sex? Using recreational drugs? How will breaks in confidentiality impact both the therapeutic relationship and the adolescent's developing autonomy and responsibility? How can the clinician use the informed consent process to foster discussions about what information can be disclosed and how disclosures will occur (Behnke, 2007)? How can this dilemma be used to foster the adolescent's autonomy and relationship to parents?

Fostering client autonomy is often balanced by other considerations, including maintaining others' safety and building the therapeutic relationship, which can be damaged by premature disclosures and interventions (Rowe, Frey, Bailey, Fisk, & Davidson, 2001). As seen in the discussion of Andrea Yates in the next box, clients who are involuntarily hospitalized still retain the right to refuse treatment (Schopp, 2001). Unfortunately, allowing psychiatrically unstable people in the court or prison system to refuse treatment has extended their *de facto* imprisonment in some cases well beyond what they would have served for the crime with which they were charged (Annas, 2004; Heilbrun & Kramer, 2005; *Sell v. United States*).

Work with religious homosexuals may bring up similar ethical conflicts about treatment decisions. Homosexuality is no longer identified as a psychiatric disorder by mainstream mental health organizations, and many people argue that it is simply a normal variant of human sexual behavior (Haldeman, 2002). Further, there is significant consensus among mental health professionals that although homosexual *behavior* can be changed, homosexual *orientation* is very resistant to treatment, except perhaps among bisexuals (M. E. P. Seligman, Walker, & Rosenhan, 2006). Haldeman observed that his clients who had previously gone through **conversion therapies** experienced serious adverse consequences as a result of their experience, including increased depression, sexual dysfunction, and difficulties maintaining relationships. Despite these concerns, he defended the right of religious homosexuals to choose treatments consistent with their spiritual beliefs, noting that for many gay men and lesbians, religion is a "central, organizing aspect of identity that the individual cannot relinquish, even if it means sacrificing sexual orientation in the process" (p. 262). How can one be responsive to the published research on sexual orientation (competence); challenge the fears, prejudice, and discrimination that may bring clients into treatment and put them at risk (social justice); and also remain sensitive to the importance of religion in clients' lives (sensitivity to differences)?

How Could They Fail to Protect Our Family from Her?
Andrea Yates

On June 20, 2001, when she was 36, Andrea Yates took each of her five children (ages 7, 5, 3, 2, and 6 months) into their bathroom. There she drowned them in the bathtub, then laid four of the five on their beds, covering them with sheets. Later, her husband, Rusty Yates, said, "We didn't see her as a danger.... How could she have been so ill and the medical community not diagnose her, not treat her, and obviously not protect our family from her?" (quoted in Roche, 2002a, para. 51).

Although Mr. Yates's statements may be self-serving and disingenuous, designed to frame him as an innocent victim of the medical establishment, his question remains an important one. Ms. Yates had a significant psychiatric history: she had a psychotic episode, two hospitalizations, and two suicide attempts following the birth of her youngest son. She had experienced depressions earlier in her life following the break-up of a relationship, after her father's heart attack, and probably after she miscarried in 1998. She reported that she believed she had been bulimic in college.

Although many women are "blue" following childbirth, few are depressed, and even fewer psychotic. Ms. Yates' symptoms, however, were significant and outside normal post-partum responses. When she was hospitalized after her son's birth, she said:

> I had a fear I would hurt somebody ... I thought it better to end my own life and prevent it.... There was a voice, then an image of the knife ... I had a vision in my mind, get a knife, get a knife...I had a vision of this person being stabbed ... the aftereffects" (as quoted in Thompson, 1999, p. 1)

(continues)

Her first vision followed the birth of her oldest son, but she "blew it off" (O'Malley, 2004, p. 38). She reportedly had similar visions about 10 times, although there were discrepancies in the stories she gave across time.

Ms. Yates had a range of symptoms that extended beyond the delusional guilt, obsessive thoughts, and homicidal and suicidal ideation that have been the primary focus of the media. In 1999, her doctors reported that she was "essentially mute," "withdrawn and suspicious," with "severe psychomotor retardation" (Starbranch, 1999, p. 2). She had self-inflicted scratches on her arms and legs and "frequently" picked at her scalp or pulled her hair as "a nervous reaction" (Thompson, 1999, p. 2). She told Dr. Resnick, a psychiatrist for her defense, that she believed that there was a surveillance camera in her home monitoring her bad mothering for months prior to drowning her children. Their television occasionally talked to her and her children:

> Well ... they'd ate some candy one morning and we had the TV on ... cartoon ... and—and just flashed a scene where the comic—the cartoon characters were talking to us... and they were saying, 'Hey, kids, stop eating so much candy.' It was just a flash and then back to the program. (A. Yates, in O'Malley, 2004, p. 155)

She also told Dr. Resnick that she heard Satan's voice, "a deep, growling voice, [that] said my name" (p. 155). Dr. Starbranch referred to her as one of "the five sickest—and most difficult to get out of psychosis—patients that I've ever treated" (Starbranch, in O'Malley, 2004, p. 177).

Ms. Yates' relationship with the psychiatric establishment was mixed at best. After her hospitalizations in 1999, Dr. Starbranch told her that another pregnancy would probably cause an even worse episode of postpartum depression. Nonetheless, Ms. Yates refused Zyprexa when she learned it was an antipsychotic and was intermittent in taking any of her other medications. This reluctance may have been partially related to the fact that she was breastfeeding, and partially to a deep mistrust of psychiatric medicines. She described Haldol, the drug her husband thought worked miracles, as a "truth serum" that caused her to lose control (Roche, 2002b). She was discharged from intensive outpatient treatment and eventually stopped taking her medications and seeing her psychiatrist and social worker.

When she was hospitalized in 2001, Ms. Yates had to be forcibly put into and dragged from the car. In this last hospitalization, her medications were frequently adjusted up and down, leading her husband to speculate that reducing the Effexor caused her psychotic break (R. Yates, 2004). As is often necessary, her new doctor, Dr. Saeed, began treating her before receiving her medical records. When he finally read them, he concluded, "No new info" (Roche, 2002b, p. 49). Although it took 10 days for her to start feeding herself again, and she was essentially mute in the hospital, he concluded that there was no evidence of psychosis and removed her from her antipsychotics because he thought she was experiencing some facial akinesia, an occasional side effect of Haldol.

(continues)

(continued)

Andrea Yates drowned her children 37 days after being released from the hospital, 13 days after last taking Haldol. She had seen her psychiatrist only two days before killing her children.

1. What ethical questions, if any, are raised for you as you read this case material? What, if anything, would you, as a mental health professional treating Ms. Yates, do differently? Why?
2. What rights did Ms. Yates have relative to treatment? What about her family and society? How would you balance these competing rights? How would you make these decisions?
3. How would the aspirational principles outlined by Kitchener (1984) and your profession guide your decision making?

RISK MANAGEMENT

Every clinical intervention incurs some risk of disciplinary complaint or legal action, although sometimes that risk is fairly low. Some actions, however, are inherently risky, including sexual misconduct, nonsexual dual relationships, problems with fees and insurance, child custody, confidentiality and competency (Bennett et al., 2006). Recognizing risk factors and reducing **clinical risk** before a problem develops is an important **risk-management** strategy in an ethical practice.

Bennett and his colleagues (2006) described clinical risk as a function of four types of variables: client, context, intervention, and clinician (see Table 2.1). As this formulation suggests, Dr. Saeed's treatment of Andrea Yates was risky because his actions were below professional standards when he failed to request her previous hospital records and inadequately assessed her risk of harm to self and others (client, context, and nature of

TABLE **2.1**

Factors to Be Considered While Making Assessments of Risk of Ethical Complaints or Legal Action.

a. **Client factors.** The client's diagnosis, especially personality or dissociative disorders, risk to self or others, history of child abuse, history of legal involvement, and wealth.

b. **Nature of intervention.** Especially sexual and nonsexual dual relationships, custody evaluations, breaking confidentiality, problems in competency, and abandonment.

c. **Context.** Especially settings with greater legal exposure (e.g., large group practice or hospital), fewer clinical and legal resources (e.g., solo or small group practices), type of service (e.g., custody evaluation), and when there is a multiple relationship (e.g., friend, relative, or sexual partner).

d. **Clinician factors.** Depends on the clinician's knowledge, skills, emotional resources, and experience at a particular point in time, and the match between these and a particular client.

Note: Modified from Bennett et al., 2006

intervention). Park Dietz's forensic assessment of Ms. Yates was inherently risky because it was a very visible and controversial murder trial (client, context, and nature of intervention); however, his risk was further increased both by clinician factors including his misrepresentation that an episode of the TV show *Law & Order* had inspired the murders (such an episode had not aired) and his lack of knowledge of Texas mental health law (Hays, 2002). Perhaps acute stress levels and his feelings about a mother killing her children contributed to his mistakes, compromised Dr. Dietz's competence in this case, and increased his risk.

Clinicians can do a number of things to decrease their risk of ethical complaint or legal action. They can do a careful assessment of risk factors and make sure that they have the requisite competency and personal and emotional skills to perform a particular intervention or work with a given client. They can examine their context, identify factors that increase their clinical risk and those that decrease that risk, and do things to manage these risk factors in this setting. They can request peer consultations or supervision when they identify potential problems. They can document their decisions and actions carefully, including their rationale for their decisions (Bennett et al., 2006) (see the SOAP note in Table 7.4). They can listen to and respond to their clients respectfully and empathically. As Younggren and Gottlieb (2008) conclude, "Satisfied consumers have no reason to file complaints or lawsuits" (p. 501).

THERAPY IS SIMILAR TO BUT DIFFERENT FROM FRIENDSHIP

The sharing of joy, whether physical, emotional, psychic, or intellectual, forms a bridge between the sharers which can be the basis for understanding much of what is not shared between them, and lessens the threat of their difference.

—**Audre Lorde**

As Audre Lorde's quote implies, some of the tasks of counseling and psychotherapy are similar to friendship. However, friendship is generally not as structured, nor is it generally designed to produce change (Frank & Frank, 1993). Although friendships can be "therapeutic" and therapy can be "friendly," dual relationships with clients are ill-advised and unethical. As discussed earlier, the competing expectations of dual relationships can cause significant problems in treatment (Pope, Sonne, & Holroyd, 1993; Pope & Vasquez, 1998; Slattery, 2005).

Part of the confusion that clients may experience regarding friendship versus the therapeutic relationship is that both provide supportive, intimate, and disclosing environments; however, friendship is a more mutual endeavor (Fehr, 2004), with friends listening to and supporting each other (Fehr, 2004). In treatment, although clinical self-disclosures do occur and can be helpful, client self-disclosures are relatively more frequent and deeper. In fact, too much self-disclosure from clinicians may derail therapy, while high levels of self-disclosure in friendships—as long as it is stage-appropriate—can deepen the friendship bond.

The tasks and goals of friendships and therapy relationships are usually different. People often describe friends as people who help and support them (Fehr, 2004). Friends, however, often believe that they should tell their friends only what they want to hear and avoid sharing anything that would make their friend "feel bad" (Slattery, 2005). Although clients are often initially ashamed and anxious when they self-disclose in therapy, they ultimately gain feelings of safety, pride, and authenticity from doing so (Farber et al., 2004). In fact, client self-disclosures are an important part of therapy. Although friends are usually not supposed to challenge each other, challenge is often an important therapeutic task (Slattery, 2005). Finally, although clinicians should learn and grow in the process of doing therapy (Yalom, 2003), treatment is primarily focused on and conducted for the benefit of the client.

In sum, although counseling and therapy are often friendly, the goal should not be friendship per se, but rather to use the therapeutic relationship to help clients develop other relationships to meet their needs (Slattery, 2005). Helping clients develop other supports fosters client autonomy rather than therapeutic dependence.

STRATEGIES FOR PREVENTING AND RESPONDING TO ETHICAL PROBLEMS

Science cannot resolve moral conflicts, but it can help to more accurately frame the debates about those conflicts.
—Heinz Pagels

No chapter or book can give the reader the answer to all ethical dilemmas. The American Counseling Association (Glosoff & Kocet, 2005), for example, notes that there will often be "reasonable differences of opinion regarding which values, ethical principles, and ethical standards should be applied when faced with ethical dilemmas" (p. 6). As a result, clinicians should have a strategy for responding to ethical dilemmas that will stand up to public scrutiny (Bennett et al., 2006). Having such a strategy is one of the most important risk-management strategies for protecting one's reputation and preventing lawsuits (Bennett et al., 2006). This section outlines several strategies that, together, can help clinicians recognize and prevent ethical problems. Chapter 14 continues this discussion of ethics, delving further into the competing demands that ethical, effective, and empathic practice place on clinicians.

Competent and effective clinicians prevent potential problems proactively, are willing to recognize difficult feelings about clients (e.g., anger, fear, disgust, and sexual attraction), and use these difficult feelings as signals of potential problems. They understand that these feelings can have negative consequences, but also that they can be a therapeutic resource when addressed rapidly and well (Pope & Tabachnik, 1993). Clinicians also pay attention to sets of behaviors and emotions that suggest that they may have moved into nontherapeutic roles, including those of parent, friend, host, guest, or caretaker (Slattery, 2005). For example, a family therapist who regularly disciplines the children during sessions rather than letting the parents do so may have moved into a parental role, which can undermine treatment.

Interactions within one's community present many opportunities to consider and negotiate boundaries. The clinician's challenge is to determine when a boundary crossing is reasonable and meets therapeutic goals and when it is problematic (Gutheil & Gabbard, 1993). Clinicians may attend the same synagogue as their clients, their children and their clients may be on the same sports team, or they may see their clients at the local coffee shop. Many good clinicians work in settings other than the traditional out-patient office, which challenge traditionally defined boundaries of clinical care (Knapp & Slattery, 2004). Some visit client homes or work in schools, prisons, nursing homes, or group homes. The decision to work in these settings may be motivated by illness or transportation barriers, decisions to help clients practice and generalize skills learned in treatment, or attempts to reach out to populations for whom traditional services are less accessible.

Paying attention to behaviors or settings that are at cross-purposes with clinical work can also prevent unethical behavior. Some treatment behaviors are consistently identified as inappropriate by clinicians, including engaging in sexual activity, accepting large gifts, bartering, and borrowing money (Pope, Tabachnik, & Keith-Spiegel, 1988). Some settings, including movie theatres, dark restaurants, and swimming beaches, are associated with expectations that are likely to interfere with treatment. These behaviors and settings may confuse the nature of the relationship—is it professional, or more intimate?

Ethical clinicians also monitor their beliefs about their practice, especially about boundary crossings. Clinicians who believe that what happens outside of therapy has little consequence on treatment can encounter problems (Pope & Keith-Spiegel, 2008). While meant to be kind and respectful, some clients may perceive a clinician's greeting in a public setting as intrusive and a break in confidentiality. One client could see removing a client's coat as kind, while another could see it as seductive. These and other boundary crossings can have different meanings and consequences depending on:

- **Client factors**—clinician's age, race, size, gender, presenting problems and diagnoses, history of abuse, and social skills
- **Clinician factors**—clinician's age, race, size, gender, interactional style, and clinical skill
- **Context factors**—the setting, time of day, nature of the therapeutic relationship, and stressors in the life of either clinician or client

Staying ethical requires remaining aware of the impact of these factors, recognizing clinical risk associated with a given action, and choosing how to act given that assessment (Bennett et al., 2006; Pope & Keith-Spiegel, 2008).

Once a clinician recognizes a problematic situation, Pope and Keith-Spiegel (2008) suggest considering the best and worst possible outcomes, keeping in mind that not all clients will respond in the same way. For example, Dr. Helper's actions had a range of possible outcomes, both positive and negative (Slattery, 2004) (see Table 2.2). Had he considered these potential outcomes and looked at other ways of meeting his therapeutic goals, he might have chosen another approach. Was he really the only person who could have offered Edna a job, who could have served as her support system and family, who could have provided treatment, and who could have become her lover? His decisions led to problems primarily because they were short-term, short-sighted solutions that attempted to meet her needs himself rather than to empower her or help her identify strategies for meeting her needs herself at that time, as well as in the future.

TABLE **2.2**
Costs and Benefits of Dr. Helper's Behaviors.

Costs	Benefits
Providing therapy in exchange for transcription services	
• Edna may feel exploited, especially if their time for therapy and transcription were not equally priced • Edna did not need to learn other ways of solving problems when initial solution was blocked • Edna was not forced to accept responsibility for ways that she blocked other options (e.g., by refusing to pursue *pro bono* therapy)	• Therapy available when it otherwise might not have been • Both Edna and son were stabilized as a result of treatment
Giving jewelry as gift	
• Their relationship was further sexualized by a gift that, in their culture, carries romantic connotations	• Dr. Helper's actions acknowledged her office contributions with a gift that she enjoyed
Entering a sexual relationship	
• Alternative romantic and sexual avenues were intentionally or unintentionally discouraged • Sex and emotional intimacy were confused, compromising both this and future relationships • Because of the confusing factors influencing the relationship, it may have left each more confused about what was therapy and what their romantic relationship • Edna avoided learning ways of interacting with others and meeting her needs that did not depend on sexualizing self and others • Sexualizing their former therapeutic relationship precluded Dr. Helper as a therapist if necessary in the future • Because of preexisting inequities in work and therapy relationships, one or both of them may have felt taken advantage of • Dr. Helper's own family may have felt abandoned as he tried to meet Edna's family's needs	• Both found a romantic and sexual partner who met their needs at that point in time • Their relationship may have served to equalize the power in their relationship (in some ways) and to help Edna recognize her worth

Note: Modified from Slattery's (2004) analysis of Anonymous (2000).

Boundary crossings may have neutral or even positive consequences. When it appears that outcomes may be harmful, however, clinicians should discuss the situation with a supervisor, then openly and nondefensively with their clients (Knapp & Slattery, 2004; Pope & Keith-Spiegel, 2008). Listening to and taking clients' viewpoints seriously has the potential to strengthen the therapeutic relationship even under difficult circumstances.

SELF-KNOWLEDGE AS A GUIDE TO ETHICAL PRACTICE

Know thyself.
— **Plato**

The clinician's personhood is both the vehicle of treatment and a way of monitoring his or her work and the health of his or her practice. As described earlier, competence is a multidimensional variable that includes knowledge and skills as well as the attitudes, values, and judgment necessary to implement them well (Barnett, Doll, et al., 2007). One's level of competency can fluctuate; remaining competent depends on staying aware of one's current skill level and emotional status, recognizing what one can do well at a given point and what one cannot. Presumably, if Dr. Helper had recognized his emotional vulnerability during the period after his client's death, his decision making would have been clearer. Perhaps Dr. Saeed would have recognized the pressures under which he was working and considered how these compromised his ability to make a strong assessment of Andrea Yates and modify it after receiving records from previous treating facilities.

A wise clinician is self-aware and regularly assesses the current state of his or her skills, competencies, attitudes, personal strengths, and weaknesses, especially as they impact clinical practice (Bennett et al., 2006). Because all clinicians have stressful periods, this self-assessment can help clinicians recognize those times and situations ahead of time and prevent or reduce the inevitable problems that they will face. Later in this book (Chapter 14), more explicit suggestions for regular self-assessment are made.

Finally, consistent self-care is an important part of remaining ethical. Clinicians are well-advised to consider their current status and compare this to where they need to be in order to perform optimally. For many clinicians, regular exercise and spiritual practice, time with friends and family, involvement with hobbies, reading, and attending culture events, can be an important part of remaining an ethical clinician. The importance of self-care and specific strategies towards this end are discussed further in Chapter 15.

SUMMARY

As this discussion has suggested, behaving ethically requires an awareness of the ethical standards and the research findings regarding ethical behavior. The aspirational principles describe the goals of ethical work and may never be completely met. These are beneficence, nonmaleficence, autonomy, fidelity, and social justice.

Although the aspirational principles describe goals to reach for in one's work, the ethical standards describe specific behaviors to enact and to avoid. The five standards discussed in this chapter include informed consent, competency, dual relationships, confidentiality, and sensitivity to differences.

Ethical practice should include more than merely applying ethical standards in a rote manner (Handelsman et al., 2005). Other factors should affect and inform a clinician's decisions. These include recognizing and controlling clinical risk; paying attention to emotional responses to clients and motivations for engaging in questionable behaviors or entering atypical settings for treatment; recognizing and responding to legal statutes about confidentiality of clinical information (e.g., the **Health Insurance Portability and Accountability Act [HIPAA]**); state laws mandating reporting of child or elder abuse; court rulings about dangerous behaviors; court rulings about how to respond to imminently dangerous clients; one's personal moral code; one's theoretical approach; agency requirements; and client diagnosis and treatment plan.

Unethical behaviors have broad-ranging short- and long-term consequences. When clinicians behave unethically, their clients and their clients' families and friends may not seek treatment in the future even though they need it or, if they do request treatment, may be skeptical about the services offered. Clinicians may lose their licenses and livelihood after engaging in unethical behavior, even when their intentions were good. Finally, the profession loses credibility when clinicians betray the public trust. Empathic, open, nondefensive communications can decrease the likelihood of occasional missteps (Pope & Keith-Spiegel, 2008).

How Do These Issues Apply to Your Life and Work?

Begin extending your thinking of ethics beyond this book:

1. Write your "ethics autobiography" (Bashe et al., 2007). Think about the reasons why you've chosen to enter the helping professions and what you want to accomplish. What are the personal values and ethics guiding your behavior? What experiences have influenced your own ethical decision making?

2. Pay attention to your reactions to the ethical standards. Do you think they are unnecessary or too strict? Do you feel that you know better about what is important for your clients? What does your self-assessment suggest that you should be doing to develop as an ethical member of your profession?

3. Write an anger, conflict, and violence autobiography (D. Kossmann, personal communication, October 3, 2008), paying attention to your experiences and their meanings in your family and relationships. Use this autobiography to identify forms of anger, conflict, and violence to which you are especially sensitive, your typical responses to these feelings, and factors limiting your ability to respond well. When might your reactions be helpful? How might your reactions cause problems? What do you do to keep yourself safe under these conditions?

4. As you watch movies or read novels depicting counseling or therapy, think about the clinician's behavior. If you believe he or she behaved unethically, what could have been done to behave more ethically? If you think about ethical behavior as stepping off onto a "slippery slope," when could that clinician first have done something differently to behave more ethically?

CHAPTER 3

Different Worldviews;
Different Worlds

WHERE ARE WE GOING?

1. What are worldviews?

2. How are worldviews expressed?

3. How can recognizing worldviews strengthen one's clinical work and the therapeutic alliance?

4. How might failing to recognize one's own beliefs, values, and goals interfere with one's ability to work effectively with clients?

We Talk About Real Life
Doug Muder

Doug Muder (born in the 1950s) is a lay minister who is trying to make sense of his family members' religious views. Their religious views could be seen as either harsh or comforting, rule-bound or open to discussion. He has come to see social class and circumstance as influencing the form of religion his family members have adopted and, through it, their worldview.

> I'm a Unitarian Universalist, but my Dad isn't. My parents seem quite happy in the same conservative branch of Lutheranism in which they raised my sister and me. It teaches the literal truth of the Bible, and its God is real, personal, and powerful. The God I met at home was more liberal than the God of my Lutheran grade school, but not by much. He was, at the very least, secure enough to be amused rather than threatened by my human attempts to be clever. At home, my heretical theological speculations were always matters for discussion rather than reprimand. But nonetheless, God had spoken, and His word was law. If reason and conscience told me something different from what was written in the Bible, then I'd better think things through again. (Muder, 2007, p. 33)

Mr. Muder's father was a factory worker who worked long hours making cattle feed, a smelly and noisy job that ruined his hearing. His was a harsh world. He went to work because he had to in order to put food on the table.

Mr. Muder's sister's world was easier. She went to college and became a professional. She married an engineer whose work involved researching ways to burn coal more cleanly.

> [His brother-in-law's job] was a demanding job, but he believed in it and thought it was important. So he worked long hours and traveled a lot. He was also finance chair of their church, in the same Lutheran synod we grew up in. They were raising money for a new building, and that also seemed important. At the same time his sons, my nephews, were both in elementary school. Ed worried that he wasn't spending enough time with them.
>
> Job, church, family—every part of his life wanted more from him. What to do?
>
> The next morning I went to church with them. The sermon topic was "Resisting Temptation." In my mind I boiled the entire 20-minute sermon down to three words: Don't be bad.
>
> I felt smug that morning because I knew that Ed would have been so much better off in my church. We talk about real life, his real life. He didn't need to be told not to be bad. His issue wasn't Good versus Evil; it was Good versus another Good versus a third kind of Good. (Muder, 2007, p. 36)

Although Mr. Muder believes that his church was more relevant to his brother-in-law's life, he couldn't draw that conclusion for his father. Mr. Muder's religion helped him find purpose, solve the important

(continues)

questions in his life, and make decisions about what sort of Good to pursue. But choosing among several Good paths wasn't the issue for his father: "Because the factory was not a competing Good. It was a necessary Evil" (Muder, 2007, p. 36).

Mr. Muder experienced choices in his life. Many of his fellow professionals encourage their children to find something to do in life that they love:

> Inspiration is the road to success. It's the way out of the maze. Or at least it's one way out, the bright way.... In the working class, the road to success is self-control. That's what you want to teach your children: Resist temptation. Walk the narrow path. Do the hard thing you don't want to do, so that you and the people who are counting on you won't be punished. (Muder, 2007, p. 37)

He worries about the harsh theology of more conservative churches, which "can justify harshness in this world. But the connection between harsh theology and a harsh world goes both ways. If you live in a harsh world, a church with a harsh theology is talking about your life" (Muder, 2007, p. 37). Choices are a luxury that ill-prepare working-class youth for the harsh, very real world that they will face. "Which church is talking about the world you live in? Which message do you want your kids to hear? Which one gives you the mind-set you need to get out?" (p. 37).

1. Mr. Muder is a lay minister in his Unitarian church, while his father and brother-in-law belong to a more conservative Lutheran church. How does Mr. Muder explain these differences to himself? How would his father and brother-in-law perceive him and his religious views? Why?
2. Look at Table 3.1 to begin to consider the impact of your worldview on your work with clients. How might your approach to religion and spirituality influence your work?
3. How would being aware of your religious and spiritual worldview and those of your clients impact your ability to relate empathically to them?

WORLDVIEWS

We are what we think. All that we are arises with our thoughts. With our thoughts we make the world.
(Attributed to the Buddha, as cited in Koltko-Rivera, 2004, p. 3)

Far more occurs in one's experience than can possibly be sensed, understood, or remembered. People actively respond to this overwhelming amount of information by filtering and organizing it through their framework of understanding—their worldview—which includes beliefs, values, and goals (Ivey, Ivey, & Simek-Morgan, 1997; Janoff-Bulman, 1989; Koltko-Rivera, 2004; Slattery, 2004). Worldviews allow people to observe their current reality, imagine alternative realities, interpret the past, anticipate the future, and direct their behavior accordingly. This filtering process means that any two people, including Mr. Muder and his father, can each be in what appears to be the same situation, yet perceive it very differently.

TABLE **3.1**

Consider the Roles of Religion and Spirituality in Your Life and Practice.

1. What kinds of experiences have you had with spirituality and religion throughout your life? Have they been primarily positive? Negative? Mixed?
2. What specific beliefs and values, if any, are most important for you now? How might they be a source of connection or conflict between you and your clients?
3. How do you view human nature? Do you see people as good, evil, or able to become either?
4. Do you believe that people have free will? Can people make their own choices or are their thoughts, feelings, and behaviors determined by outside forces, including God? How might this influence your work with clients?
5. Why, in your opinion, do bad things happen? Do you attribute bad things to God, evil spirits, poor choices, sin, karma, or chance? How might this influence how you see your clients?
6. In what ways do you believe that religion and spirituality can be a source of strength for your clients? In what ways do you believe that they can be a source of weakness?
7. What types of clients or problems involving religion or spirituality do you expect would be the most challenging for you? Which would be the most engaging? Why?

Note: Adapted from Fukuyama & Sevig, 1999

Although they are essential for making sense of the world, worldviews can also limit what one can take in. Ideas and experiences that do not easily fit one's worldview may be forced to fit into preconceived notions or even excluded from awareness altogether. For example, people may be surprised when others do something apparently kind or fail to notice it at all because it does not fit their worldview of how people act. They may be gullible, assuming that everyone has good intentions, and repeatedly talk about problems in their relationships without relating these problems to their own naïveté.

Paying attention to one's own worldview and to those of others is important in many settings, but is especially so for clinical work. Recognizing worldviews and their powerful effects greatly increases one's ability to develop empathy for others. When clinicians understand their clients' worldviews, they find it easier to form strong and positive therapeutic relationships with them and can more readily match interventions to their clients' beliefs, values, goals, and thinking styles (Kim, Ng, & Ahn, 2005).

COMPONENTS OF WORLDVIEW: GLOBAL BELIEFS, VALUES, AND GOALS

We are usually convinced more easily by reasons we have found ourselves than by those which have occurred to others.

—Blaise Pascal

Worldviews comprise one's beliefs about many aspects of the world, along with one's values and goals; worldviews have wide-ranging implications for people's lives. Beliefs regarding control, for example, can affect whether one attempts and persists at a wide variety of tasks (Bandura, 1997). Many beliefs are unconscious or preconscious—that is, they might be available if deliberately focused on, but are rarely brought into awareness. The less available a belief is to conscious awareness, the less likely that that belief can be recognized and challenged.

Values are also important aspects of worldviews. Values refer to the worth that individuals assign to various potential states and are often preconscious, unexamined, and difficult to change (Maio & Olson, 1998; Rokeach & Ball-Rokeach, 1989). Values influence a broad range of human behaviors and choices and prescribe modes of conduct (e.g., being honest, helpful, or polite). Although values cannot be seen directly, they are reflected in one's behavior, words, and thoughts.

Values direct **goals** for the future, which are internal representations of desired processes, events, or outcomes (Austin & Vancouver, 1996). Common life goals include relationships, work, wealth, knowledge, and achievement (Emmons, 2005). Goals are organized hierarchically, with higher-level goals determining middle- and lower-level goals (Vallacher & Wegner, 1987). Mid-level goals receive the most conscious attention and direct typical plans, activities, and behaviors (Austin & Vancouver, 1996).

Worldviews are not static, but change through normal development as well as traumatic experiences. People tend to defend against anxiety provoked by uncertainty and change, preferring **assimilation** of new information into their existing worldview rather than making radical reconceptualizations of their worldviews (**accommodation**; Brennan, 2001; Ginzburg, 2004; Hart, Shaver, & Goldenberg, 2005). Nonetheless, worldviews can shift from mere exposure to new people and ideas. For example, students going away to college for the first time can begin to see themselves as more capable and competent as a result of living more independently, become more tolerant through their interactions with a roommate from a different culture, and grow more liberal after being exposed to new and different viewpoints. On the other hand, trauma tends to trigger large changes in worldview, including feelings of helplessness and despair and losses of meaning and purpose. Trauma can confirm maladaptive assumptions (e.g., "I am worthless and bad things inevitably happen to me."), but can also lead to **posttraumatic growth**, including positive changes in values, priorities, and meaning (e.g., "As a result of this experience, I have become stronger and more compassionate towards others' suffering") (Ai & Park, 2005; C. L. Park, 2004; C. L. Park & Folkman, 1997).

Although worldviews are important to attend to in their own right, inconsistencies and conflicts in worldview are equally important. For any of a number of reasons, behavior can be discrepant with important beliefs, goals, and values. Most people have competing values that become apparent in different contexts (e.g., at work and home) or desire two apparently competing goals (e.g., parenting and achievement). The flashbacks and ruminations associated with posttraumatic stress disorder (PTSD) can be thought about as attempts to resolve contradictory beliefs, for example, "I *should* trust him" and "I cannot trust anyone"(Gray, Maguen, & Litz, 2007). These discrepancies and conflicts can be important to identify and work through in treatment (Slattery & Park, in press a, b).

WORLDVIEWS IN THE CONTEXT OF THERAPY

You never really understand a person until you consider things from his point of view.

—**Harper Lee**

There is no consensus regarding the essential aspects of worldview. Some theorists have suggested that a small set of dimensions, such as benevolence and control, encompasses the critical elements of worldview (e.g., Ibrahim, 1985; Janoff-Bulman, 1989; Slattery, 2004; D. W. Sue & Sue, 2003). Taking the opposite approach, Koltko-Rivera (2004) put forth a model with 42 worldview dimensions, to comprehensively capture the breadth of human experience. Koltko-Rivera's model is far more complete, but not useful in practice. The dimensions discussed below are a compromise between these two extremes. We chose these particular dimensions because of their relevance to the therapeutic process. Case material is presented to provide practice in understanding differing worldviews.

Interpersonal Relationships

There is no such thing as society, only individual men and women and their families.

—**Margaret Thatcher**

Interpersonal relationships—both with friends and family and with the clinician—are often an important focus of treatment. How do clients treat their clinician, office staff, others in the office, and in the balance of their life? Whom do they treat well? How are they treated? Multiple beliefs influence interpersonal relationships, including those regarding attachment style, authority, and individualism/collectivism.

Attachment style. Infants generally respond to a social stressor (that is, having a stranger enter or a caretaker disappear) in one of three ways (Ainsworth, Blehar, Waters, & Wall, 1978). Securely attached children interact well with both caretakers and strangers and are distressed when their caretakers leave, but calm rapidly when they return. Children with an anxious/ambivalent **attachment style** are distressed when their caregiver leaves and are stressed and anxious even when the caregiver returns. Children with an avoidant attachment style are detached, showing little attachment or distress regardless of whether a caregiver or stranger is present.

Childhood attachment styles predict adult attachment styles in romantic relationships (Hazan & Shaver, 1987; Mikulincer, 1998). Securely attached adults are comfortable in relationships and, therefore, can tolerate being apart from their romantic partner. Adults with anxious/ambivalent attachment styles are threatened by separations from their partner and, because they are often perceived as clingy or needy, have rocky relationships. Adults with avoidant attachment styles are uncomfortable trusting or getting close to someone. Their relationships tend to be short-lived and distant. Existential threats (e.g., death, illness, failure, or loss) increase feelings of vulnerability and increase defensive responses, especially among people with anxious attachment styles (Brennan, 2001; Hart et al., 2005). After such threats, people may conclude, "Who would want me? Who is there for me?"

Authority. How does the client expect to relate to the world? Some expect hierarchical relationships, with a clearly defined leader and chain of command, while others want shared and egalitarian interactions with rotating or fluid leadership (Koltko-Rivera, 2004). This dimension differs across both cultures and individuals. Asian Americans, Latin Americans, and Native Americans have often been described as preferring hierarchical relationships, with men having more power and authority than children, and women having more intermediate levels of power (D. W. Sue & Sue, 2003). Individuals within a culture differ on this dimension as well. While Euro Americans often value more assertive and egalitarian approaches, some are also relatively cooperative, compliant with authority figures, and people-pleasing. In the United States, however, people adopting the latter approach are often pejoratively labeled "dependent" (Bornstein, 2005).

Clients differ in their preferences for directiveness in treatment. Those preferring more egalitarian relationships may resent being treated in an authoritarian manner, because they may see authoritarian clinicians as implying that they are incompetent. Others may expect and prefer hierarchical and directive relationships. Asian Americans whose clinicians match and understand their more hierarchical and collectivistic worldview, for example, are more likely to feel understood and develop a more positive therapeutic alliance (Kim et al., 2005). Such clients may perceive clinicians who are not active and directive as incompetent.

Clients' preferences for hierarchical and directive relationships have a potential downside that clinicians must anticipate and address. Clients may be reluctant to disagree with their treating clinicians or may hide problems unless directly asked about them. Clinicians may see this behavior style as passive or resistant when it may, in fact, be culturally normative and respectful (Chen & Davenport, 2005; O'Connor, 2005). Although clinicians should acknowledge that they are the experts about treatment, Chen and Davenport encourage clinicians to communicate to their clients, especially Asian Americans, that they are the experts on their own experience.

For many people, authority is also conflated with other factors—benign benevolence, power, perpetration and trauma, or unearned privilege (L. S. Brown, 2004; R. B. Miller, 2005). These associated meanings of authority should be identified and, when appropriate, challenged in treatment when they cause or maintain problems. This can be a difficult process, however. R. B. Miller, for example, notes that it is tempting to ignore clients' pain and suffering because validating it also means becoming aware of real social inequities and the privileges, authority, and power that clinicians enjoy that their clients may not.

Individualism/collectivism. Imagine: Sara wants to go to college to major in education, but her family needs her help to put food on the table. How is such a conflict between individual and group goals resolved? **Individualism** emphasizes self-actualization, self-reliance, personal rights, personal privacy, competition, achievement orientation, emotional distance from family and group members, and individual pleasure (Oyserman, 1993; Triandis & Gelfand, 1998). Individualists would suggest that Sara should only consider her own needs in her decisions about college and her major, while **collectivism** prioritizes group goals ahead of individual ones and emphasizes interdependence over independence, family connections over emotional distance, and sociability over meeting individual needs. Individualistic cultures emphasize self-reflection, while collectivistic cultures deemphasize it and focus on attending to and maintaining social norms. If Sara had a more collectivist worldview, when making a choice between school and work, she would focus on her family's needs and deemphasize or overlook her own needs and desires.

SOURCES OF INFORMATION

People differ significantly in the ways that they go about understanding the world. Some focus primarily on their own sensory data and others on authority figures, science, or spiritual sources to learn about the world (Slattery, 2004). They may resist or be openly antagonistic to other types of information or explanations. Assessing clients' style of understanding the world can help clinicians find ways of framing clinical interventions (Shafranske, 2005).

For example, the following people describe their depression differently:

Cheryl: I am depressed each fall as the days get shorter. My depression seems to be especially bad each year right around the time that my mother died. (sensory observation)

Justin: Depression is a genetic disorder that seems to run in families and affects catecholamines in the brain. There is significant evidence that drugs increasing the availability of catecholamines decrease depression. What is the evidence for the antidepressant that you're suggesting? (scientific information)

Tosha: My mother says that the women in our family get depressed at menopause. (familial authority)

Marjane: I have been praying for an end to my depression. I will take my Prozac because you tell me to, but the depression will end when it's God's will. (religious authority)

These explanations are not mutually contradictory—Marjane, for example, also listens to medical authorities, although she is skeptical about their advice. Nonetheless, people often rely on some approaches at the expense of others. They may also rely on a particular source of information in some situations, but use another source in situations where it seems more relevant (e.g., a scientist who relies on observations and the scientific method at work, but uses her mother's advice for parenting decisions).

Safety and Benevolence of the World and Other People

The safety and benevolence of the world is often an important aspect of clients' global beliefs (Janoff-Bulman, 1989; Prager & Solomon, 1995). Do they see the world as a safe and benevolent place? Is their world dangerous, with others out to hurt them? Clients who have had a defining experience where they see others as unsafe or out to hurt them often have difficulty trusting others and seeing them as reliable (Thomas, 2005). How people see the world is related to **trust,** their feelings of interpersonal safety.

People may reveal their beliefs about the benevolence of the world through their behavior. How big is their personal space? How far do they sit from others in the waiting room? How do they make eye contact and when do they avoid it? What happens when they are accidentally touched? Observing these behaviors can provide important cues about clients' interpersonal trust and their sense of the world's benevolence.

Why Bad Things Happen

People entering therapy often wonder why bad things happened to them (Janoff-Bulman, 1989). They may become more depressed and pessimistic, conclude that the world has no meaning, or believe that life is capricious. Trauma can shatter previously hopeful and optimistic views of the world, but can also lead to a greater sense of meaning (Prager & Solomon, 1995).

Lerner (1980) described the "**just world theory**," the belief that people get what they deserve and deserve what they get. For example, in talking about her husband, the only survivor of the Sago, WV, mining disaster, Anna McCloy made the following "just world" statement while she waited to discover her husband's fate:

> He's always told me that no matter what, he knew he was in a dangerous job, and if something happened, he said, he would survive *because he had two kids and a wife that he loved and he would take care of.* (Gately, 2006, para. 11, italics added)

Others attribute events to the person's *behavior* rather than to their personality (Janoff-Bulman, 1989). From this viewpoint, events happen because of factors that we either set into motion or that we failed to prevent. Like the just world theory, this worldview leads victims (and their families and friends) to blame themselves (or the victim). This blame is for different reasons, however, more "should have, could have," rather than because they see themselves as bad. This is an important clinical distinction. Attributing problems to behavior rather than personality provides a sense of control and prevents depression (Shapiro, 1989, 1995). It also provides clearer behavioral change targets when planning treatment goals.

When describing what happened in the Sago mining disaster and what they would have to do to get back on track, Mr. Hatfield, CEO of International Coal Group, used some just world attributions (i.e., "good people"), but also focused on the miners' and the company's behavior (i.e., "to do the right thing"):

> We are hardworking people that count on good people to do their job. And we believe we attract skilled miners that want to make this company successful. We want to make this company successful. And so we will do all we can to motivate efforts to that end.
>
> But the people that work for this company and know us, know the management team and know that our intentions are to do the right thing and to protect our people as best we can in what is a fairly dangerous business. (News Conference With CEO of International Coal Group, 2006, para. 62–63)

 Finally, others may believe their fate is due to chance events, that life is random, and that there is no way of making sense of why things happen (Janoff-Bulman, 1989). Hatfield's statement included a sense of that when he commented that it was "a fairly dangerous business." The following comments focus on life's randomness and unpredictability:

Rick Caskey (runs a mining technology program at a community college): There's always things that you don't foresee. You know, methane is odorless, colorless, and tasteless. (Samson, 2006, para. 14)

Mark Popernack (Quecreek mining accident survivor, when talking about the Sago disaster): There's not much we can do right now except pray. (A. Cooper, 2006, para. 138)

People often use their spiritual beliefs to explain why trauma happens, although people of different religious faiths may give different explanations and draw different meanings (C. L. Park, 2005). Negative life events, however, can shatter the meaning-making systems of both religious and nonreligious clients (Brennan, 2001). Religious clients may ask, "Why me, God?" and lose their faith. Nonreligious clients may challenge previously held assumptions about the world and begin searching for meaning, spiritual or otherwise. Trauma can change or foreshorten expectations about the future (Ai & Park, 2005) or, as with Viktor Frankl's (1946/1984) experiences in Auschwitz, deepen a sense of meaning and commitment.

Identity

Men often become what they believe themselves to be. If I believe I cannot do something, it makes me incapable of doing it. But when I believe I can, then I acquire the ability to do it even if I didn't have it in the beginning.
—**Mohandas Gandhi**

Whether clients see the world as a safe place is determined, in part, by how they see themselves and their relationships with others (Hart et al., 2005; Janoff-Bulman, 1989). Clients may believe that people get what they deserve (Lerner, 1980) but also see themselves as good, moral, and worthy, thus relatively safe from hardship. Trauma or significant illness can redefine a client's sense of identity and self-worth (Brennan, 2001). Threats to self-worth can also threaten a person's sense of being loved and cared for and the belief that the world is orderly and predictable (Ai & Park, 2005).

Randal McCloy, the lone survivor in the Sago mining disaster, might conclude that good things happen to him (because he alone survived), that bad things happen (because he was injured), or that he was lucky or unlucky in the disaster and his subsequent treatment. Although some of this interpretation is dependent on his preexisting worldview, it is also influenced by the focus that he and others take in the ensuing months of treatment and recovery.

Approaches to Problems and Problem Solving

Blaming mother is just a negative way of clinging to her still.
—**Nancy Friday**

How people perceive problems influences whether they believe that they can change and how. Do they see a problem? If so, what sort? Do they believe it can change? If so, under what circumstances? What do they believe caused the problem? Something inside themselves? Something outside? Do they believe they can do things to change, or does the change have to come from elsewhere?

Responsibility and control. Perceived control over past and future events has different implications for therapy and can be usefully distinguished. People who believe that they could have prevented something bad (and did not) are more likely to be depressed; people who believe they can control their recovery and prevent future trauma are *less* likely to become depressed (Frazier,

Mortensen, & Steward, 2005; Shapiro, 1989, 1995). D. W. Sue and Sue (2003) differentiated between these two types of control by calling them, respectively, responsibility (for past events) and control (for current or future events).

People can be described as having either an internal or external **locus of responsibility** and an internal or external **locus of control** (D. W. Sue & Sue, 2003). People with an internal locus of responsibility blame themselves or take responsibility for their problems; those with an external locus of responsibility blame others or environmental factors. Rape survivors who blame themselves withdraw from others, which leads to more distress (Frazier et al., 2005). Conversely, people with an internal locus of control believe that they can control recovery and prevent trauma; those with an external locus of control attribute control over future outcomes to others (or society) and recognize little control for themselves.

People with an internal locus of control believe that they are able to control their lives and prevent problems. They are more self-confident and socially engaged and more frequently use **cognitive restructuring** to cope with stressors (Frazier et al., 2005). They are also less likely to be depressed (Shapiro, 1989, 1995). People with an external locus of control are more likely to be depressed and feel helpless (Shapiro, 1989, 1995; D. W. Sue & Sue, 2003). Surviving a trauma in a positive way leads to a greater sense of control. People who have low self-esteem and greater feelings that the world is random experience more distress and more negative outcomes (Ginzburg, 2004).

These two dimensions (responsibility and control) are relatively independent and predict different outcomes when combined (D. W. Sue & Sue, 2003; Slattery, 2004). People with internal loci of control and responsibility (Bootstrappers) hold themselves accountable for the past, but also see themselves as able to change (see Table 3.2). People with an internal locus of control and an external locus of responsibility (Leaders) recognize and change problems, without inappropriately attributing problems to themselves (Goerke, Möller, Schulz-Hardt, Napiersky, & Frey, 2004). They tend to claim successes for themselves. People with an external locus of control and an internal locus of responsibility (Marginalized Self-blamers) blame themselves, but feel helpless

TABLE **3.2**
Connections between Loci of Control and Responsibility.

		Control	
		Internal	External
Responsibility	Internal	Bootstrappers: "It's my fault, but I can change things."	Marginalized self-blamers: "It's all my fault, but I can't do anything to change things."
	External	Leaders: "I didn't do it, it's not my fault, but I can change it."	Flappers: "Life happens and I can't do anything about it."

Note: Based on Slattery, 2004; D. W. Sue & Sue, 2003

to keep themselves safe. People with external loci of control and responsibility (Flappers) see little control, few opportunities for advancement, and little ability to change oppressive rules. They may give up or placate those in power to meet their needs.

Randal McCloy's response after the Sago mining disaster could differ depending on which of these approaches he took. If he responds either as a Leader or Bootstrapper, his psychological adjustment would probably be better than if he responds as a Flapper or Marginalized Self-Blamer.

People differ in their general perceptions of control, but specific control appraisals should vary with and be appropriate to the stressor. For example, people with cancer need to identify positive ways of controlling their health and participating in their treatment, while also at some point coming to terms with the possibility that they may die sooner than they had hoped (Brennan, 2001).

Mutability. People vary in their beliefs about whether a problem can be changed. **Self-efficacy**, one's belief in an ability to change, both increases and decreases with success and failure. Furthermore, self-efficacy can be segmented, so that a woman may believe in her ability to become a better athlete, but believe that her mood swings are genetically caused and unchangeable (Bandura, 1997). Often, word choice signals a person's level of commitment to change (e.g., "I'm not sure I want to do this," "That's it; I'm done using.") and can usefully predict outcomes in substance abuse work (Amrhein, Miller, Yahne, Palmer, & Fulcher, 2003; Prochaska & Norcross, 2001; Thomas, 2005). Self-efficacy is related to adaptive coping, while feelings of helplessness are related to depression (Brennan, 2001).

 Sometimes continuing in the face of failure requires a shift in viewpoint. Rather than being due to a belief that one cannot change, inaction might be due to expectations of negative consequences (Anderson, 2003). Failing to initiate change could be a defensive strategy to protect oneself from regret, anxiety, or other anticipated consequences associated with change. When this is the case, helping clients gather more information, reevaluate their values, goals, and beliefs, and address perceived obstacles can foster change and increase self-efficacy in that realm.

Time Orientation

You can't change the past, but you can ruin the present by worrying about the future.

— Anonymous

Psychological theories vary in their **time orientation**. Psychoanalysis has traditionally focused on childhood events. Gestalt therapy, family therapy, and behavior therapy are much more present-focused and often less interested in the ultimate cause of problems than in what maintains them. Career counseling is often more future-focused, with treatment focusing on present behaviors as a means of meeting future goals.

 Cultures also vary in their time orientation. Buddhist-influenced cultures emphasize living mindfully in the present. Some Eastern cultures honor ancient tradition and ancestors who died centuries earlier. Upper- and upper-middle-class members of Western cultures tend to worry about the past and anxiously plan for the future, while people from lower-class groups often have a foreshortened view of the future and are more fatalistic (Zimbardo & Boyd, 1999).

Relative to Euro Americans, Native Americans, Latin Americans, and Hmong typically see time as more elastic and punctuality as relatively unimportant (Slattery, 2004). Axelson (1993), for example, observes "time-consciousness does not go by the clock in traditional Native American culture ... the right time occurs when one is ready" (p. 71). Euro Americans, on the other hand, more typically see time as a commodity to be saved and spent wisely, earning important dividends in the future. Punctuality is important and tardiness is often seen as a passive aggressive statement about an activity's perceived value. Clinicians and clients holding these two different orientations about time can easily misinterpret each other's actions and become frustrated or angry. For example:

Harris: You're late. Again. It doesn't seem like you really value our time together. I wonder whether you really want to get better.

Dafne: Where do you get that? My car is just so unreliable. I'm here, aren't I?

Harris's interpretation might have been on track, although it certainly was not tactfully expressed. In failing to acknowledge that Dafne does not have the same level of control as Harris, nor the resources and ability to plan ahead, however, he acted out and damaged their relationship. Imagine if he had instead reacted like this:

Harris: You're late again. It seems like you're having a hard time getting here so that we have the full hour together. I wonder what that's about.

Dafne: I *am* having a hard time. My car is just so unreliable. (pause) It's hard thinking about working on what I'm going to do when I get off welfare when, frankly, I just don't see it. I just feel like all I can do is to get by from day to day.

Time orientation can differ on the dimension of productivity ("doing-future") versus spontaneity ("being-present"; Koltko-Rivera, 2004). People with "doing" approaches tend to be more interested in earning worth through productivity while simultaneously being more self-absorbed and self-focused, while those with "being" approaches experience more flow, find tasks more intrinsically interesting, and are more self-aware and absorbed in the task at hand (Csikszentmihalyi, 1990).

Time orientation influences a wide variety of behaviors, including goal setting and achievement, sensation seeking and risk-taking, and guilt and rumination (Zimbardo & Boyd, 1999). Health behaviors, choice and number of sex partners, using safer sex practices, and substance use are all, to some extent, influenced by time orientation. Students from a fatalistic, present-oriented culture might run into problems in school, a setting that rewards people for engaging in sometimes tedious or boring activities for anticipated, but uncertain, positive long-term outcomes (Zimbardo & Boyd, 1999).

As described, our actions derive from past experiences, present appraisals, and expectations about future options. One of these time frames may be emphasized, however (Bandura, 1997; Zimbardo & Boyd, 1999). People might focus on the present, for example, as a way of avoiding the future or because they do not see one. They may tell stories about past and anticipated victimizations or "what might happen if ..." scenarios.

TABLE **3.3**
Successful and Unsuccessful Past, Present and Future Time Orientations.

	Unsuccessful	Successful
Past	Focused on past harm or victimization. May be unable to see the present clearly or anticipate a positive future.	Has a sense of tradition and roots that create a sense of positive identity.
Present	Either engages in hedonistic activities that have a high risk of self-harm or fatalistically withdraws. Is self-focused or self-absorbed. Time drags.	Approaches daily life through genuine joyful or playful interactions. Lives in present rather than postponing satisfaction for future rewards. Loses self-awareness and becomes absorbed in task at hand. Time flies.
Future	Is worried or anxious about the future; puts off present needs in favor of future goals.	Sets goals and plans for the future. Future orientation gives meaning to current work and strivings.

Note: Csikszentmihalyi, 1990; Zimbardo & Boyd; 1999

Most people spend at least some time in each time frame, however. The issue is one of degree, as well as how that time is spent. Table 3.3 describes positive and negative aspects of each time orientation.

VALUES AND GOALS

We can tell our values by looking at our checkbook stubs.

—Gloria Steinem

Hamburger or veggie stir-fry? Shih tzu or golden retriever? Donations to UNICEF or the American Heart Association? Why do people choose one activity or object over another? How do their behaviors reflect their beliefs and goals? Look at these two checkbook ledgers. What conclusions do you draw about their owners? Why? (see Figure 3.1). The next time you stand in a grocery line, look at your groceries. What do they say about you? Then look at the groceries of the person ahead or behind you.

This basic assumption, that people's actions are meaningful rather than random, is common to the mental health fields. Everything that people do reflects what they see as important (values) and what they want to accomplish (goals): How they spend their money, the groceries they buy, how they dress, whether they make eye contact. However, values and goals do not translate perfectly into behavior because of conflicting values and goals; lack of resources, time, skills, or opportunity; and other pressures.

As mentioned earlier, global goals are the basic internal representations of desired outcomes that motivate people in their lives (Emmons, 2005; C. L. Park & Folkman, 1997). How people select goals depends in part on their time orientation (Zimbardo & Boyd, 1999). Some people emphasize being (e.g., living in the moment) rather than doing (e.g., achieving or possessing). Being approaches emphasize inward experience, including emotions, thoughts, personality, or spirituality rather than outward products, including achievements and possessions (Koltko-Rivera, 2004).

			Withdrawal	Deposit	Balance
2542	9/13	Abercrombie & Fitch	$104.93		$53.37
2543	9/13	Wal-Mart (groceries)	$32.13		$21.24
2544	9/13	CVS Drug Store	$13.47		$7.77
	9/13			$453.32	$461.09
2545	9/14	Abercrombie & Fitch	$349.42		$111.67
2546	9/14	Curl Up and Dye	$54.00		$57.67
2547	9/15	Ta-2 U (ladybug!!!)	$99.00		–$41.32
2548	9/15	Wal-Mart (groceries)	$25.32		–$66.65

			Withdrawal	Deposit	Balance
1476	9/13	A & P Groceries	$35.17		$530.37
1477	9/13	Borders (books & music)	$75.28		$455.09
1478	9/13	National Fuel	$36.42		$418.67
	9/13			$1453.32	$1871.99
1479	9/14	Borders (books)	$15.32		$1856.67
1480	9/15	Pittsburgh Rape Crisis	$50.00		$1806.67
1481	9/15	Amer. Red Cross (tornado)	$150.00		$1656.67
1482	9/15	A & P Groceries	$25.32		$1631.35
1483	9/16	First Methodist	$50.00		$1581.35

FIGURE **3.1** What Conclusions Do You Draw About the Owners of These Two Checkbook Ledgers?

Some people tend to pursue goals that are more **intrinsic**—important for their own sake—while others pursue goals that are more **extrinsic**—means for meeting some other sort of need such as belongingness, support, or prestige (Allport & Ross, 1967). Of course, goals can be both intrinsic and extrinsic in nature. For example, reading and writing about philosophy can be intrinsically interesting, yet also put food on the table. Time orientation influences the nature of goals set, because setting and working toward long-term goals requires a future orientation (Zimbardo & Boyd, 1999).

Recognizing Values and Goals

Sometimes values and goals can be discussed directly. However, people are often unable to articulate their values and goals directly. Sometimes, as in the following excerpt, individuals' values and goals can be inferred through their language use, juxtaposition of topics, topics avoided, and nonverbal behaviors (Mozdrzierz, Peluso, & Lisiecki, 2009; A. Rogers, 2001).

Bonnilou: (eyes averted) I can't feel anything but empty toward Ben. I know that staying with him is the wrong thing. I just can't get past the abuse, no matter how much he says he's changed (long pause while wringing her hands) I just don't want to hurt my children....

Jon: It sounds like you're of two minds. You feel used and abused in your marriage, but you also want to do the right thing by your children. It sounds like you don't see how you can be happy—and you've tried to make the marriage work for a long time—and be a good mom.

Bonnilou: (looks up, hands still) Yes. Exactly.

Jon: Right now it feels like you're setting this up as a choice—your happiness or that of your children.

Bonnilou: (looks down) Yes. I don't know what else to do.

Bonnilou's values are revealed in several ways in addition to her choice of words—her hand movements and physical activity, the points at which she makes and breaks eye contact, and her pauses. Values are also communicated by other nonverbal behaviors (e.g., smiles, grimaces, gestures), **paralanguage** (e.g., intonation, cadence, speed, and volume of voice), and actions. Because nonverbal behaviors can have several different meanings, initial hypotheses should be tentative and supported by careful observations. For example, people break eye contact during conversations for at least two reasons—because of embarrassment or shame and because breaking eye contact allows focused thought on difficult ideas (Doherty-Sneddon & Phelps, 2005).

Values and goals are expressed differently in different contexts, in part depending on the perceived relevance of the values to the situation. For example, Bonnilou might be calmer when her husband has been out of town (she is able to focus on her needs, yet also feels like a good mother), but anxious when he is back in town, because he is critical of how her "selfishness" affects their children.

When talking, people may avoid, distract, project, or otherwise distort their experience, depending on their own self-perception, the nature of the listener and the listener's reactions, or the context in which they are speaking (Mozdrzierz et al., 2009; A. G. Rogers, 2001). When discussing personally meaningful issues, people often talk about value conflicts and unsettled aspects of their lives. For example, when Bonnilou complains about her "emptiness" toward her husband, she is both describing a problem and also identifying what she expects and wants in relationships (i.e., warmth and closeness). If she were to fail to see emptiness as a problem, perhaps because that was what all relationships in her family were like, she would not discuss it.

Food for Thought

- What do you value most in your life? What's most important, less important, unimportant to you?
- How well do those values translate into the goals that you pursue? Can you identify ways to make them align more closely?

(continues)

- Approach this question from a different point of view. Imagine that you only had the outcomes or qualities on your list of goals. Would you be satisfied? If not, what else would you need to be happy?
- Does your context influence your values and goals? Are there times when a value may be particularly important and other times when it is less important?

WORLDVIEWS INFORM SITUATIONAL MEANINGS

Worldviews inform the **situational meanings** that people assign to their experiences (C. L. Park & Folkman, 1997). Situational meanings include appraisals of an event as a loss, threat, or challenge, as well as causal attributions for why the event occurred (e.g., God's will, coincidence), determination of the extent to which the events are discrepant with one's global system of meaning, and decisions regarding what can be done to cope with the event. Worldviews and situational meanings differ in the range of their implications, and thus in their effects on treatment. For example, a woman who has been fired from her job might believe that she is to blame and that her job loss will be a devastating blow to her future. Treatment may need to address her self-blame and her tendency to catastrophize about the job loss and its ongoing effects. Others may draw a different situational meaning, focusing on the shaky financial footing of the agency and newfound freedom to pursue more satisfying and lucrative career opportunities.

Worldviews also influence behavior by influencing the interpretation of specific situations. For example, a person who believes that others cannot be trusted might withdraw from others and put on a happy face, while avoiding all but superficial relationships; or that person may attack first, as Reymundo Sanchez (Lil Loco), described below, often did. Understanding clients' worldviews helps to predict their behavior; however, recognizing the role of situational and contextual directives and constraints, as well as one's beliefs about appropriate and effective action in a particular situation, makes predictions more accurate and useful. The man who withdraws may believe that any contact with others will leave him hurt (low trust, low self-efficacy, external locus of control). The woman who puts on a happy face may believe that she can manipulate others to get what she wants and to stay safe (low trust, high self-efficacy, internal locus of control). Lil Loco seemed to believe that he could only stay safe by attacking first (low trust, high self-efficacy, internal locus of control).

Although worldviews may be important determinants of action, particular situations—such as a church service, a family dinner, and a party—pull forth different behaviors. People also perform the *same* behavior for *different* reasons. They can enter therapy because they were court-mandated to do so, because they see it as the most expedient thing to do, or because they truly choose to be there. Effective interventions must be based on a strong assessment of worldview, but also

(a) interactions among relevant aspects of worldview;
(b) the person's perceptions of the applicability of values and goals to a given situation;
(c) beliefs about how to respond in that situation; and
(d) contextual variables influencing the situation.

This is an issue of how, when, and where aspects of worldview are perceived as coming into play.

Sometimes worldviews contain conflicting elements. Clinical work often directly or indirectly addresses conflicts in goals, beliefs, or values. Bonnilou may be unhappy in her marriage but stay because she is afraid of disappointing her family and hurting her children (her family's happiness and children's welfare rather than her own individual happiness). Her husband may be outraged that she wants a divorce because "breaking up a marriage is the influence of the devil" (religious law over individual happiness). Finding ways of identifying and working through these discrepancies in beliefs or conflicts in values or goals is often a central part of treatment.

Exploring these discrepancies and conflicts can help identify a person's values and goals. Why hasn't Bonnilou, in the case above, moved out? Although she may not have the requisite skills and resources to do so, it might equally well be that her goal conflict prevents her from acting on her stated intentions. Clarifying her goals and resolving the inherent conflict can both help her to feel more fully heard and also help her to identify strategies for working through the conflict (Liberman & Chaiken, 1991).

Never Bothered to Consider the Consequences
Reymundo Sanchez

Reymundo Sanchez was born in Puerto Rico in 1963. His father died when Reymundo was four—his mother was 16 when they married, his father was 74 and had children and grandchildren her age. He was told that his father had been a good man (although he certainly questioned his father's motives for marrying such a young girl), but with his father's death, he lost "the advice that only a father could give" (Sanchez, 2000, p. 1).

Soon after his father's death, his mother remarried. At five, while his mother and stepfather honeymooned, Reymundo stayed with his aunt and cousins. He reported being brutally beaten by his aunt and cousins and raped by his oldest cousin Alberto during this period; he believes that the sexual abuse may have continued until his family moved to Chicago when he was seven. There, his mother gave birth to a daughter and, when her second husband disappeared, remarried, giving birth to a son. His life got considerably more difficult with each new child.

> [My stepfather] became an asshole. He would do things like padlock the refrigerator so that only his daughter could drink milk. He would hang a box of

(continues)

crackers from a rope high up on the ceiling so that we couldn't have any. All of his anger was taken out on us. (Sanchez, 2000, p. 5)

He had hoped that his mother would protect him but, at best, his mother stood back from the abuse. As he got older, she also became physically abusive. When his friend Papo called her a bitch for beating him, though, he came to her defense. He later defended his defense of her, saying, "Honor thy mother no matter how much pain and suffering she inflicts on you. That's why no one gets blamed but the kids—a mother's name is sacred" (Sanchez, 2000, p. 22).

When his mother became pregnant again, his stepfather decided to move the family back to Puerto Rico. Reymundo lived there for six months until his mother sent him back to Chicago because she was tired of breaking up fights between her husband and son. There he briefly lived with Hector, his stepbrother, who dealt drugs, but largely left Reymundo alone. However, when Hector moved, Reymundo was homeless and scrambled for a place to stay, sometimes with a girlfriend, sometimes with a surrogate mother (who was occasionally sexual with him), sometimes with the gang, and sometimes on the streets.

Against this background of abuse and neglect, Lil Loco, as he came to be called, both internalized his parents' attitudes about him and looked for ways to feel better. He said:

All the problems of the world were unimportant compared to mine. Feeling sorry for myself also became an excuse for accepting failure. Like my mother, I blamed everything and anything. Nobody felt the pain I felt. Nobody else suffered but me. That way of thinking became imbedded in my mind and became my way of life for a long time. (Sanchez, 2000, p. 33)

Lil Loco learned that there were some things that helped—at least for a while. One of these things was sex. A 35-year-old woman seduced him when he was 13 (only later did he see this as abuse). He observed, "Sex involved touching, kissing, passion. It involved love. I began thinking that I could find all the feelings I was missing in my life in sex" (Sanchez, 2000, p. 30). Drugs—at first only marijuana—also helped:

When I was high I could think about doing evil things and feel good about it. I would imagine killing Pedro and my mother over and over again, and be forgiven.... Marijuana became my way out of the horrible reality that was my life. (Sanchez, 2000, p. 31)

Finally, his membership with a gang gave him a feeling of belonging and respect.

I enjoyed the way crowds in the hallways would part when I walked through. No matter how long the cafeteria line was, I could be first if I wanted to. I could sit in the stairway, smoke a joint, and be warned of any authority figure coming. It never crossed my mind that it was others' fear that made me popular. I never bothered to consider the consequences. (Sanchez, 2000, p. 167)

(continues)

(continued)

Lil Loco was expected to perform hits on other gangs, lauded when he acted bravely and violently, and given special privileges. Signs of weakness or cowardice were punished. He quickly learned what he needed to do in order to stay in the group's best graces.

Initially his gang involvement was mostly positive for him. With time, however, as he was set up to be murdered himself, his friends were killed (and he *was* a loyal friend), and he had nightmares about the murders he had performed, his reaction was more negative. Instead of staying in the gang for positive reasons, he stayed out of fear: "I was too scared to face the world as the person I really was. Being a King gave me a role to play, friends, a lifestyle—everything I wanted. I couldn't walk away from the life" (Sanchez, 2000, p. 181). Besides, there were lots of perks to being a King:

> I learned how easy it was to manipulate people who did coke and took full advantage of it.... I demanded [girls] do things that I saw drug dealers demand from girls in the movies. To come into my apartment they had to agree to disrobe and stay naked, or dress in sexy lingerie as soon as they got there. They had to be prepared to perform any sexual act I desired upon command. Failure to do so would result in the denial of cocaine and possibly an ass whipping. Several girls declined my offer but most readily agreed. Even those who had declined would have sex with me on a one-on-one basis in exchange for coke. The cocaine influence was a powerful one. I loved it. It got me accepted in places I had never dreamed of entering. I got just about every woman I desired and had many Kings willing to lose their lives for me. I was so busy manipulating others that I didn't realize I was also becoming a cocaine junkie. (Sanchez, 2000, p. 256)

1. How would you describe Lil Loco's worldview? What are his core beliefs, values, and goals?
2. How did Lil Loco justify his actions? How are these justifications related to his worldview?
3. How is his worldview related to his early experiences of poverty, physical and sexual abuse, and neglect? Consider how cultural factors like *respeto*, *machismo*, and *familism* influenced the response of Lil Loco to these risk factors (see Table 3.4).
4. If you were assigned to work with Lil Loco and did not speak Spanish, would you see that as an ethical problem? Why or why not? Would it matter that he had learned English and could speak it relatively fluently?
5. If Lil Loco reported having murdered someone of another gang, what would you do? How would your understanding of ethics inform your decision? What if he instead had said that he was *planning* on killing someone?
6. Would there be any conflict between your personal and professional ethical standards with regard to these questions? How would you resolve these questions?

TABLE **3.4**
Latin Cultural Values and Norms.

Collectivism. In contrast with more individualistic cultures, group needs supercede individual needs. In addition, people are sometimes expected to sacrifice their needs for the greater good of the group.

Familism. Reflects strong identification with and attachment to both the nuclear and extended family, and includes feelings of loyalty and reciprocity among family members. This is a special case of collectivism, with people expected to sacrifice individual needs for those of the whole family (e.g., taking a job that will provide better for the family, although being less satisfying for the individual).

Personalismo. Prefers personal relationships over impersonal ones. Expects that knowing someone will be personal rather than primarily based on external factors like occupation or socioeconomic status (e.g., may perceive helper as a family member or friend).

Respeto. Requires that a powerful person or person in authority be treated deferentially or respectfully. Conversely, personal power is derived from being treated respectfully.

Simpatía. Appears to mean sympathy, but better translates as pleasantness and congeniality. It refers to behaviors that promote pleasant, harmonious. and conflict-free relationships (e.g., withholding HIV status to maintain harmony).

Machismo. Emphasizes manly courage and honor. Exaggerated male stereotypical behaviors (i.e., aggressiveness, stubbornness, and inflexibility in interactions with other men and arrogance and sexual aggressiveness in relationships with women) are both expected and valued as signs of power and virility.

Marianisma. Modeled after the Virgin Mary's behavior, *marianisma* idealizes caring for the home and family. Traditional roles are seen as important and valuable. Rather than derogating women, women are often seen as morally superior and needing protection (a manifestation of *respeto*). *Marianisma* can also include an acceptance of fate and of men's *machismo* as the will of God.

Bien/mal educado. Although directly translated as well-educated, in Spanish *bien educado* refers to being brought up well, that is, that a person's parents raised him or her to become a well-behaved, respectful person. Telling parents that their child is *bien educado* is a compliment. Conversely, to say that a child is *mal educado* is saying that the family did not fulfill their responsibility to teach a child to behave well.

BUILDING A THERAPEUTIC ALLIANCE

Clients often hold values, goals, and beliefs that differ from their clinicians'. Their problem behavior generally makes sense to them. Even when clients recognize that their behavior is a problem, it may feel safer to stay in old patterns of problematic thinking and behavior than to attempt changing (Prochaska, 1999; Prochaska & DiClemente, 1982; Prochaska & Norcross, 2001). Nonetheless, clients who see their worldviews as being more similar to their clinicians' worldviews perceive more empathy from and stronger therapeutic alliances with their clinicians (Kim et al., 2005; Lilliengren & Werbart, 2005). Seeing clients from their own unique frame of reference facilitates change.

No one would suggest that clinicians must hold or endorse the same beliefs, values, and goals as their clients. In this regard, it can be helpful to differentiate between respect and uncritical agreement (B. Greene, personal communication, July 29, 2008). Clinicians must be able to respectfully step outside of their belief systems to understand their clients' perspective of their world—not necessarily agree with or support it.

Bonnilou: I am feeling so overwhelmed right now. It's like the world is swirling. I can't imagine that it will ever stop.

Jon: You're feeling overwhelmed and can't imagine that things will ever be different.

Bonnilou: [nods] Right.

Jon: [pause] It feels that way now, but the most consistent part of life is change. [Bonnilou nods, looking at her hands] Things *have* been different, even last week.

Bonnilou: [looks up and makes eye contact] I remember that, but it doesn't feel that it can be different [pause] I trust you, though. I'm willing to believe you.

As seen in this example, a clinician's work often includes helping his or her clients question the status quo and their standard assumptions. This may be more difficult for clinicians who are unaware of, uncomfortable with, or insecure in their own beliefs. These clinicians may push their own beliefs rather than helping clients explore their beliefs and other ways of seeing the world. The ability to keep a stable center, listen to others' views, and help them explore options in the midst of the theory and research in the field is part of what defines professional behavior.

As we discuss throughout this book, people can respond very differently to the same objective situation. While many people open up when they feel deeply understood, others may be threatened by this degree of empathy. Paranoid clients may see empathy as intrusive, while clients with schizoid tendencies may be baffled by their clinician's focus on feelings (L. S. Greenberg, Elliott, Watson, & Bohart, 2001). Understanding their clients' worldviews can help clinicians predict these differences in preferences. Paying attention to clients' verbal and nonverbal responses can suggest when empathic responses are appreciated, off-track, or intrusive.

Food for Thought

What would you do to engage Mr. Muder and his father in therapy? What about Reymundo Sanchez and Andrea Yates? How would your intervention strategies be similar or differ for each of them? Why? Could you remain genuine even if you concluded that you needed to respond differently to match each of their worldviews (Lazarus, 1993)?

SUMMARY

 Worldviews are often difficult to recognize (Ivey et al., 1997; Janoff-Bulman, 1989; Koltko-Rivera, 2004). Furthermore, people actively perceive information to support their beliefs and exclude information that does not fit. Therefore, it is important to recognize some of the ways that people differ in their perceptions of themselves and their world. When people assume that there is one and only one right way of doing things, they push others into a box rather than allow them to find solution that fit them. These are especially important considerations for therapy where, because they are under significant stress, clients may be less articulate than usual about the ways that they see their world. As a result, Chapter 3 has focused on values, goals, and beliefs that are important to the therapy process and considered ways of recognizing these.

Although values, goals, beliefs, and situational meanings are similar in many ways, we have distinguished among them here. Values reflect one's relative ranking of different qualities, activities, or goals, which direct future behavior. Beliefs refer to one's core assumptions about reality. Situational meanings are more discrete than global worldviews and more accessible to awareness. They are also more easily changed. Worldviews comprise a wide range of values, goals, and assumptions that filter one's perceptions of people and the world. They affect a broader range of behaviors and are less flexible and less easily changed than situational beliefs.

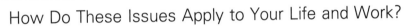

How Do These Issues Apply to Your Life and Work?

1. Describe your worldview, including your values, goals, and beliefs. How is your worldview characterized by both major and minor themes? With what contradictory themes do you struggle?
2. How have you felt when someone failed to acknowledge your own worldview?
3. How is your worldview similar to or different from the worldviews described in this chapter or the previous ones? How might this suggest different intervention strategies for each?
4. How might your worldview affect your work with others? What issues and problems would be most difficult for you to respond to? What might be easier?

CHAPTER **4**

Culture, Prejudice, and Oppression

WHERE ARE WE GOING?

1. What factors shape cultural perceptions, experiences, and worldviews?

2. What does it mean to have multiple cultural identities and in what ways might clients' multiple cultural identities influence clinical work?

3. What are oppression and privilege?

4. What is racial identity and how does it change? Why is it important to pay attention to it?

5. What three factors characterize "multicultural" counseling?

6. How can one become multiculturally competent?

Anybody Black Can Be Treated This Way
Henry Louis Gates

In July 2009, Henry Louis Gates (b. 1950) returned from China where he was doing some filming for a PBS documentary. The door to his house was jammed. After entering the house through a back door, he again attempted to force the front door open.

> All of a sudden, there was a policeman on my porch. And I thought, "This is strange." So I went over to the front porch still holding the phone, and I said "Officer, can I help you?" And he said, "Would you step outside onto the porch." And the way he said it, I knew he wasn't canvassing for the police benevolent association. All the hairs stood up on the back of my neck, and I realized that I was in danger. And I said to him no, out of instinct. I said, "No, I will not." ... He said "I'm here to investigate a 911 call for breaking and entering into this house." And I said "That's ridiculous because this happens to be my house. And I'm a Harvard professor." (Olopade, 2009, para. 9–10)

Dr. Gates was arrested for disorderly conduct and spent four hours in jail before being released.

Dr. Gates, the director of the African and African-American Studies program at Harvard University, was very angry. Although he was upset about being arrested, he was further angered because, "really it's not about me—it's that anybody black can be treated this way, just arbitrarily arrested out of spite" (Olopade, 2009, para. 24). During a press conference, President Obama commented,

> Now, I don't know, not having been there and not seeing all the facts, what role race played in that, but I think it's fair to say, number one, any of us would be pretty angry; number two, that the Cambridge police acted stupidly in arresting somebody when there was already proof that they were in their own home; and, number three, what I think we know, separate and apart from this incident, is that there is a long history in this country of African-Americans and Latinos being stopped by law enforcement disproportionately. And that's just a fact. (Seelye, 2009, para. 11)

Further, President Obama concluded this was "a sign of how race remains a factor in this society" (Seelye, 2009, para. 11). He backpedaled somewhat from these remarks the next day.

The arresting officer's perspective on Dr. Gates' arrest was markedly different from that of Dr. Gates. Sgt. Crowley reported that Dr. Gates was combative from the moment that he arrived on the scene. He described Dr. Gates as saying, "Ya, I'll speak with your mama outside." Sgt. Crowley observed, "I'm still just amazed that somebody of [Dr. Gates's] level of intelligence could stoop to such a level, and berate me, accuse me of being a racist or racial profiling" (K. Thompson & Thompson, 2009, para. 20–21). Sgt. Crowley has taught courses on preventing racial profiling for 5 years and was described by

(continues)

(continued)

the Cambridge Police Commissioner as a "stellar member" of the department, on whose judgment he relies every day: "He was thrust into a crime in progress, and he tried to work his way through the situation" (para. 12).

This incident raises a number of important questions that we will discuss in the following pages:

1. Why did Sgt. Crowley and Professor Gates perceive this arrest so differently?
2. Why might good, well-intentioned people behave in racist ways?
3. What—other than **racism**—could explain the decision to arrest Professor Gates?
4. How would you respond to an African-American client who perceived these actions as racist? How would you respond to one who did *not* see them as racist? Why?

DEFINING AND SEEING CULTURE

Race and other cultural variables (e.g., ethnicity, gender, social class, age, sexual orientation, and spirituality) are important factors to consider when building a contextualized empathy. Members of a **cultural group** generally have a shared identity, with similar values, beliefs, assumptions, goals, patterns of behavior, preferences, and norms. See, for example, Tables 3.5 and 4.3. Although such worldviews may be difficult to identify from within a group (Chavez & Guido-DiBrito, 1999; Cokley, 2002), shared group membership provides a sense of belongingness and mutual understanding (Nelson et al., 2006).

In general, African Americans are relatively more holistic in orientation, emotionally expressive, interdependent, and respectful of the elderly than are Euro Americans (Paniagua, 1998). Common African-American values include spirituality, collectivism, communalism, individuality, and self-knowledge (Cokley, 2005; Oyserman, Coon, & Kemmelmeier, 2002). Euro Americans tend to be relatively more rational, reductionistic, and emotionally restrained. They tend to value self-actualization and autonomy more than African Americans and are generally more youth-oriented (Paniagua, 1998).

People live in a cultural context that is shaped by the typical experiences of their race, ethnicity, religion, gender, class, and other groups with which they identify (see Table 4.1). This context influences both how they perceive themselves and how they are perceived. Sometimes, as seen in Helen Tinsley-Jones' case material later in this chapter, this typical context influences people whose personal experiences are very different from their group's.

Cultures also have unique defining historical events and figures. For example, many Jews' self-concepts and worldviews have been shaped by the Holocaust, the Diaspora, their view of themselves as God's chosen ones yet also outsiders, and their fight for homeland (D. Greenberg & Wiesner, 2004; Prager & Solomon, 1995). The 1992–1995 civil war in Bosnia and the 1999 earthquake in Turkey defined and organized the memories of people living through these catastrophes (N. R. Brown et al., 2009). The history of slavery, ongoing racism and oppression, and the high levels of poverty and community

TABLE **4.1**
Current Status of African Americans in the United States.

Demographics (in 2004)
- 34.7 million African Americans (12.3% of the U.S. population), 54.8% living in the South.
- 32% were below the age of 18, 8% were 65 or older
- 89.3% were employed (vs. 94.9% of Euro Americans)
- The median African-American family income was $30,134
  - 24.5% lived below the poverty rate, 28.3% earned more than $50k (compared to 8.2% and 48.1% of Euro Americans)
  - 20% did not have health insurance
- 48% owned their own home

Education (in 2003)
- 79% of African Americans graduated from high school, 17% from colleges and universities—89% of Euro Americans graduated from high school, 29% from college
- 8% of teens dropped out of high school (6% of Euro Americans, 15% of Hispanics)
- 40% of African Americans attending college were male (46% of Euro Americans, 43% of Hispanics)

Families (in 2004)
- 31.9% of African Americans 15 and older were currently married and living with their spouse; 43% had never married (respectively, 56.1% and 24.9% among Euro Americans)
- 64% of African-American children lived in single parent families (23% of Euro Americans, 35% of Hispanics); 11% live with their grandparents
- 8.2% lived with their grandparents, more of whom had caregiver status and for longer periods than for other races

Crime rates (in 2005)
- African-American males were about eight times as likely to be imprisoned as Euro Americans (3218 vs. 463 per 100k), with Hispanics intermediate (1220)
- Homicide victimization rates were very high (19.7 per 100k)—more than six times higher than for Euro Americans (3.3) and other groups (2.4)
- African Americans were also more likely to commit murder (24.1 per 100K in 2004) than Euro Americans (3.6) or other groups (2.7)

Cause of death (in 2003)
- Homicide was the leading cause of death for 15- to 34-year-old African Americans (32.1% of deaths)
  - Young African-American males (15–35) were murdered more than three times as frequently as young African-American females (38.6% vs. 12.1% of deaths of 15- to 35-year-olds).
- Suicide rates were relatively low (.7%)—about half that of Euro Americans (1.3%), Hispanics (1.6%), and Asian/Pacific Islanders (1.8%), and about a quarter of Native Americans (2.5%)
- Despite African Americans being 13% of the U.S. population in the period between 2000 and 2003, they were 44.8% of cases diagnosed with HIV/AIDS. HIV was the ninth leading cause of death (2.6% of all African-American deaths) and the third leading cause among 25- to 50-year-olds (10.8% of deaths).
  - African-American men were seven times as likely to be diagnosed with HIV/AIDS as Euro American men and three times as likely as Hispanic men

(continues)

TABLE **4.1**

Current Status of African Americans in the United States (Continued)

- African-American women were 19 times as likely to be diagnosed with HIV/AIDS as White women, 5 times as likely as Hispanic women
- Infant mortality rates are very high (13.5 per 1000)—over twice that of Euro Americans (5.7) and Hispanics (5.6), with Native Americans intermediate between these (8.7).
- Infants dying from Sudden Infant Death Syndrome (SIDS) are twice as likely to be African American (108.8 per 100k) as Euro American (50.5). Hispanics (25.6), and Asian/Pacific Islanders (27.7) have much lower rates, while Native Americans have a higher rate (124)

Source: American Council on Education (2006); Bureau of Justice Statistics (2006a, 2006b); Centers for Disease Control and Prevention (2004, 2006), Kids Count Data Center (2009); Mathews & MacDorman (2006); McKinnon, 2003; Simmons & Dye, 2003

dysfunction that are common in many urban neighborhoods influence African Americans whether they are upper-middle class or on public assistance and whether they live in urban or rural areas.

However, people within a given culture may perceive or experience the same defining event differently. In fact, although group differences are important, differences between individuals within a group may be much larger than differences between groups (see Figure 4.1). For example, one study found that many Holocaust survivors (45%) reported that the Holocaust made their own aging and impending death more difficult (Kahana, Harel, & Kahana, 1998). On the other hand, 55% reported that the Holocaust either made no difference or made growing old and dying *easier*.

Group members may share issues and concerns. Boyd-Franklin and her colleagues (Boyd-Franklin, Franklin, & Toussaint, 2000), for example, described special concerns faced while parenting young African-American males, including preparing them to recognize and respond to racism, **prejudice**, and discrimination. In struggling with their sexuality and being excluded from the dominant culture, gay teens have significantly higher rates of suicidality and self-injury (Balsam, Beauchaine, Mickey, & Rothblum, 2005).

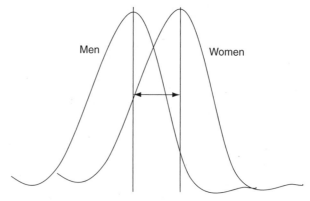

FIGURE **4.1** Two groups may be different from each other *on average*, yet individual members may be much more similar to members of the other group than their own.

Note: About 15% of women are below the mean for men with this hypothetical trait.

Food for Thought

In your observations and reflections about race, ethnicity, gender, class, and other contexts, pay attention to the unique concerns of the groups with which you work. What unique issues do men, women, gifted children, Deaf adults, and so on, face in their lives? In what ways are their experiences similar to each other?

Multiple Cultural Identities

People belong to, identify with, and are influenced by multiple cultures (e.g., ethnicity, race, gender, class, religion, sexual orientation, physical ability, and so on; Cohen, 2009; Fukuyama, 1990; Lam & Sue, 2001; D. W. Sue, Bingham, Porché-Burke, & Vasquez, 1999) (see Figure 4.2). The experience of a White male is often quite different from that of a White female (the former often is less comfortable expressing emotions, more expected to achieve than to nurture, and feels less vulnerable in sexual situations). That of a gay White male can be very different from that of a straight White male (the former often feeling less accepted and safe in daily life). The experience and worldview of a gay, White, male fundamentalist Christian is different from that of a gay, White, male agnostic living in a supportive gay community (the former often having more **internalized homophobia**). As Danny Brem describes here, different contexts also highlight different cultural identities.

> When you live in Holland, certainly if you lead an Orthodox Jewish life, you feel Jewish all the time because you're not able to eat with people in restaurants, for example. And then when you move to Israel, that is not a problem. But then suddenly you feel more Dutch. (D. Brem quoted in Beauchemin, 2006, para. 5)

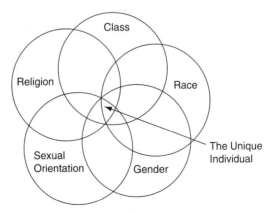

FIGURE **4.2** An individual's worldview is a function of multiple cultures and individual history of experiences and trauma.

Note: Modified from Slattery, 2004.

People's **multiple identities** influence how they perceive the world and how they are perceived by it. Although Professor Gates and Sgt. Crowley were different races, they also had different levels of education and amounts and kinds of power. Which of these factors, if any, contributed to Professor Gates's arrest?

Clients' and clinicians' multiple contexts and identities each influence their statements, behavior, and perceptions of each other. Their contexts affect what is discussed in and omitted from treatment. Although clinicians must learn about other cultures and recognize their clients' multiple identities, they must also recognize their own multiple identities and their values, assumptions, preferences, and worldviews.

Because context is a normal part of the background, it is easily overlooked, especially for the **majority culture** (Pedersen, Crethar, & Carlson, 2008; Slattery, 2004; D. W. Sue, 2004). In the following case, Katy Robinson (2002) struggles with recognizing the values intrinsic to her adoptive and birth cultures. Her experiences and self-perceptions are influenced by race and ethnicity, but also by gender and adoption status.

Learning to See Culture
Katy Robinson

Without contact with another culture, it is easy to feel that there is one right way of doing things, that culture doesn't matter. Kim Ji-yun was adopted from Korea when she was seven, moved to Salt Lake City, and was renamed Katy Robinson. With her adoption, she gained three older brothers and two new parents, becoming, in her words, an "Honorary Irishman" overnight. In her transition to the United States and her new family, she had to give up what it meant to be Korean, including her language (now using English rather than Korean), where she slept (in an American-style bed rather than at the side of her parents' bed), and what she liked to eat (coming to prefer blander, American foods and chocolate rather than fruity desserts).

At age 7, with her *halmoni* (grandmother) and birthmother on another continent and unreachable, she did not have the luxury to hold on to both cultures. At 28, however, she went to Korea to search for her birthparents and *halmoni*, saying to her adoptive mother, "Why didn't you teach me about my Korean heritage? Why didn't you help me keep my name or language?" (K. Robinson, 2002, p. 35).

In the United States she had always felt different, having grown up in an area where she looked different from everyone else. In Korea, she still looked different—her hairstyle, dress, and gestures—and felt equally out of place because she was American rather than Korean in values and viewpoint. She assimilated more easily into the Korean adoptee community, with whom she shared the search for a blood connection and concerns about the adoption process, even though other adoptees were often from

(continues)

Canada or Europe rather than from the United States. She also became more aware of her femaleness as she entered a society where her gender restricted her access to some settings, required some behaviors and prohibited others, and placed her near the bottom of the social hierarchy in most interactions.

No book can completely prepare you for another culture—initially you will be an outsider. Across time, with sensitive listening and observation and lots of mistakes, your understanding of cultural differences may move from judgments that some behaviors are wrong or bad to an understanding that they are simply different. As you spend time in a culture, like a chameleon your voice, gestures, and behaviors may come to be within that group's "language." You may begin to "hear" their behavior and values from their viewpoint rather than only yours. You may learn to communicate with them more effectively. This is part of what Ms. Robinson learned during her year in Korea.

In some ways, both of her families—Korean and American, her birth-parents and adoptive parents—were similar. In both families, her parents were no longer a couple—her adoptive parents divorcing when she was a young adult and her birthparents never marrying. In both families she had difficulties with her fathers, whom she saw as brusque, domineering, and insensitive to her needs. She got along well with her adoptive mother and idealized her birthmother, whom she never found.

However, the two cultures were very different. She learned some Korean habits easily: covering her mouth when laughing, bowing rather than shaking hands, filling her Korean half-brother's glass correctly, and behaving in a self-deprecating manner to protect relational harmony. However, she made mistakes: She gave gifts like chocolate and cake, which would be well-accepted in the United States, but that were embarrassingly inappropriate in Korea. She learned that her U.S.-typical behaviors had different meanings in Korea (e.g., wearing bangs covering her forehead was seen as disrespectful to her husband). She saw things from different viewpoints: She saw her decisions as a personal choice, while her half-brother framed similar decisions in terms of family obligation. She was able to see how discipline, obedience, and diligence were emphasized in the Korean culture and school system, which led to her academic success in the United States.

Other differences frustrated her at every turn as she searched for her birthmother and *halmoni*. Because Ms. Robinson was born during an affair that supplanted her older half-brother's mother, her Korean brother and sister indirectly refused to help her with her search—sometimes telling her outright lies in the process. She was hurt when she discovered that they had lied in telling her that her birthmother was dead, although much later she was able to think about their actions as a way of protecting their own mother's feelings (who had become very upset when faced with information about her ex-husband's affair). As Ms. Robinson became "more Korean," she also was able to understand behaviors that had seemed to be unnecessary subterfuge to the U.S.-born part of her. She was also able to understand why

(continues)

(continued)

her Korean family was indirect in this subterfuge (to maintain harmony) rather than directly refusing to help her.

After Ms. Robinson and her husband had spent almost a year in Korea, her adoptive mother came to visit her. They joined her Korean half-brother for dinner. Ms. Robinson noticed the obvious physical differences (e.g., freckles, round eyes, red hair, jewelry) that set her mother apart from her Korean family, but also her American mannerisms. Her mother was confident, rather than demure and acquiescing. She fed herself first, accepted the best morsels of meat, and did not refill Ms. Robinson's brother's glass. She lounged casually and talked to their translator, rather than to her host. "Didn't she notice the break that caused in the harmonious flow of the group?" (K. Robinson, 2002, p. 266). Ms. Robinson noted, however, with surprise that

> [I]t was not with mounting criticism that I observed these subtle gestures. What I felt was more like a dawning revelation that I had, perhaps, become more Korean during the past year. One culture was not necessarily better than the other, and for the first time I could see that I contained qualities of both. But the differences were fascinating. With my [adoptive] mother, for instance, what you saw was what you got. Every emotion and thought lay open and exposed on her face, ready to slip from her tongue and make instant contact. She embodied the American declaration of individuality: if she had a craving, she satisfied it. If she found herself in the seat of honor, she happily claimed it. My brother, on the other hand, was concerned, foremost, with the harmony of the group at the expense of self-comfort and moments of frivolity. His was a life of self-restraint, as I had come to understand. Gracious and selfless host that he was, one had to guess and pull at the thoughts behind his masked face, subtle gestures and unspoken words. (pp. 266–267)

But, are all Americans like Ms. Robinson's mother? Are all Koreans like her brother? Her brother, as head of his family, had more power than other members of his family and was typically doted on by his mother and wife. His sister was single, planned on never marrying, and turned her income over to their mother, giving the sister an amount of power in their family that was unusual for a woman. Their father, a man who had married twice and fathered at least five children by three women, did not fit in with her brother's family and was as uncomfortable in that setting as they were with him. Her aunt, also 28, also born out of wedlock, lived in Australia for 8 years and flaunted social norms almost to the same degree that Ms. Robinson's brother was bound by them.

1. Think about a situation where you entered a new culture—either for a long period (e.g., studying abroad) or for a shorter one (e.g., watching an international film, eating out, or meeting with a visitor from another country). How did you feel in that setting? Were you comfortable or uncomfortable? Judging or accepting? Would you handle that situation differently now? How?

(continues)

2. Why might it be easier to recognize cultural values as an outsider rather than in one's own culture?
3. Although Ms. Robinson primarily discusses ethnicity, she also alludes to the impacts of her gender and adoption status. How do these contexts influence her?
4. Compare the values and norms described in Table 4.2 with this case example. How do you see these values and norms in this discussion? Do some parts of the example match and others diverge from cultural predictions?

TABLE **4.2**
Asian American Values and Norms.

Collectivism. Focus is on the needs of the group and family rather than the individual (e.g., thus the family name is given first in native language). Group and family obligations are emphasized over individual wishes, thoughts, and feelings. Self-reliance and independence are deemphasized relative to group responsibility and obligation. Individualism is a flagrant social norm violation.

Filial piety. Children are expected to respect their parents, feel obligation to them, and obey their wishes. Parental authority is often difficult to question.

Hierarchical structure. People are expected to defer to rather than challenge authority figures. Authorities often have broad scope and power to make decisions; obedience to and acceptance of decisions are expected. Lower-status individuals are expected to defer to those with more status. Within the family, older individuals and men generally have more power.

Harmony. The emphasis on harmony reflects the emphasis on connections among apparently unrelated events, their interdependence and need for each other. Polar opposites are seen as part of the same entity, with one as unable to exist well without the other.

Interpersonal harmony. Because of the emphasis on the family and group, performing behaviors that maintain the harmony of the group is important. Actions that "save face" foster group harmony, while disclosing problems shames and undermines the group. Announcing one's successes undermines the group; therefore, modesty is valued.

Restraint of strong emotion. Both positive and negative emotions should be restrained. Admitting emotional problems shames the family and should be avoided. Children are not praised directly, although they may be indirectly praised to friends or relatives. Love is not directly shown, although it may be demonstrated by performing actions that benefit family. Impulsive behaviors are discouraged; thinking decisions through is valued. Stress and psychological distress are often expressed through somatic complaints rather than verbally.

Academic achievement. Families expect children to do well and enter careers with high social status. Individual success brings pride to the family and is primarily valued as such.

Note: Summarized from Chen & Davenport, 2005

OPPRESSION AND PRIVILEGE

Counseling is an instrument of oppression designed to transmit a certain set of individualistic cultural values. Traditional counseling has harmed minorities and women. Counseling ... has been the handmaiden of the status quo and as such represents a political statement.

—(D.W. Sue, 1992, p. 6)

Oppression takes many forms, some of which are overt, others more indirect and subtle. For example, in a study reported by D.W. Sue (2004), White men held about 80% of tenured college and university positions, 92% of the Forbes 400 executive/CEO–level positions, 80% of the seats in the House of Representatives and 84% of those in the U.S. Senate, and owned 99% of professional athletic teams. Because White men make up only 33% of the U.S. population, these inequities are assumed to reflect processes limiting access to certain jobs.

Root (1992, cited in L. S. Brown, 2004) refers to more subtle forms of oppression as "insidious traumatization," stressors that are meaningless by themselves but, when summed, are traumatizing. Each of these can be oppressive: seeing members of one's group discriminated against or victimized in a hate crime; overhearing stigmatizing messages, stories, or jokes in the media, from family and friends, or during casual conversations; or observing **institutionalized discrimination** against other group members. These types of incidents can make people feel unsafe or undeserving.

McIntosh (1989) defined **privilege** as "the unearned assets which I can count on cashing in each day, but about which I was 'meant' to remain oblivious" (p. 11). Being denied jobs or housing because of sexual orientation, for example, is **discrimination**, a form of oppression, while being listened to and taken seriously because of group membership alone (rather than intellectual or technical expertise) is a type of privilege. The freedom to walk down the street holding hands with your partner or to buy a greeting card depicting people who look like you are forms of privilege. Professor Gates's arrest might have been related to racist assumptions. His anger when confronted by Sgt. Crowley probably was further increased because the arrest was so different from his typical experience of respect, admiration, and deference associated with his professorial position and reputation.

Recognizing and acknowledging one's own privilege (and oppression) is just as important as acknowledging clients' oppression (and privilege). Recognizing the inequities affecting many clients allows clients and clinicians to make appropriate attributions of external responsibility. It may take considerable courage for many clinicians to admit that there is oppression—that opportunities to work, go to a good school, and live well may be unavailable to some for arbitrary and unfair reasons (D. W. Sue, 2004).

The Impact of Oppression

Oppression has multiple impacts, but one can be seen when there are group differences in values and opinions. In some cases, one set of values and opinions gets suppressed; generally, these suppressed values and opinions belong to the less powerful group or person. As a result, children who are excluded or bullied tend to withdraw from classroom activities, perform poorly academically, and avoid school (Buhs, Ladd, & Herald, 2006). Simply highlighting race or gender during a task with task-related stereotypes (e.g., that African Americans or women are believed to often perform more poorly on that task) causes a drop in performance, even for people with a history of success (Steele, 1997). Notice the ways that Helen Tinsley-Jones loses her "voice" in the next case.

Sometimes the less powerful party does things to equalize the perceived power differential. Children do this by throwing a tantrum or hitting their bigger, older siblings; adults might protest unfair laws, challenge or reject the status quo, damage property, or hurt members of the more powerful group. Rather than abusing power—even unintentionally—multicultural therapies challenge abuses of power by (a) respecting different values and (b) identifying and challenging oppression and unearned privilege (APA, 2003).

Hiding/Not Hiding; Feeling/Not Feeling
Helen Tinsley-Jones

Helen Tinsley-Jones, a psychologist, was born in Germany in 1947 and immigrated to the United States when she was four. Her mother was German, her father African American. As an adult, her race is salient and something that she sees as impacting her relationships with her clients and research subjects. For example, during interviews of licensed psychologists, all of whom were People of Color, several noted that her race influenced their willingness to be open and nondefensive with her. However, she also noted that

> [B]ecause I am a person of color, some of the participants or I might have made certain presumptions about the meanings of some questions and statements. We might have assumed, for example, that by virtue of our shared minority experience, we intuitively knew what each person meant, and, consequently, failed to make additional inquiries. (Tinsley-Jones, 2001, pp. 575–576)

Similar problems can occur in clinical settings, with clinicians and clients inappropriately assuming that they know and understand each other by virtue of their perceived similarities.

> Dr. Tinsley-Jones' race became relevant from an early age:
> I have always (or nearly always) *felt* my race to be as integral to me, to be such a part of who I was/am, as to make its subtraction impossible. I am my color as I am my thoughts. I knew that my color made my safety precarious, and, in response, adopted caution and silence as self-protection. I have known and done this from the moment that I, as a 3-1/2 year old in Germany, stood at the iron gate leading to the courtyard of my family's apartment, and a German (White) boy asked, "Aren't you black?" He said this in German, and in a derogatory manner. Indeed, my brownness is the me through which I have always, at least since the iron gate encounter, viewed the world, through which I have always known some others might judge me negatively. (H. Tinsley-Jones, personal communication, September 29, 2004)

Although she knew it was relevant and important, as a teenager she did not know how to handle her feelings about her race. She wrote:

> While attending high school in rural Massachusetts (read as: all White), I lived what I now know to be a very detached experience. I developed this (now strange to me) ability to act as if nothing were wrong, or as if I didn't really

(continues)

(continued)

stand out. My stance was a true triumph in denial in the service of survival. I made good female friends and excelled academically. I did not do anything to garner negative attention, and the teachers and students acted accordingly. Until the end of my senior year, no one ever even openly acknowledged that I was different because I was of color (except my guidance counselor who managed to help me get a college scholarship reserved for a Negro student).

In the spring of 1964—my senior year—one of my best friends and I, as torchbearers of the nerd bunch, were chosen to give graduation speeches. Now, why would I, after investing so much energy in anonymity, do this? Well, I believe—again, only in retrospect—that I had decided to take a stand for being of color. My graduation topic: civil rights and the Negro. You really must grasp the momentous nature of this event for me. Here I was—a shy kid, who had suppressed/repressed almost every vestige of her color for years; who had not seen her image substantively represented in other students, teachers, or educational materials; who had not been given any opening to be herself without fear of reprisals; and whose parents were complicit in this conspiracy of silence and denial of self. The creation of that speech and its presentation were exercises in necessary pain. In the solitude of my bedroom, I rehearsed my speech until I knew it flawlessly (I had been taught by my father's example that you had to be perfect, or at least overrehearsed, to succeed in a White world). I lay in my bed, eyes staring at the ceiling, stomach tense and filled with butterflies, sleepless, for the handful of days before the event. (The vitriolic telephone call I had received right before the event heightened my intensity. An unidentifiable voice cackled, Nigger, hell and what else, I frankly can't recall.) Then, there I was, standing in front of a packed auditorium of students, faculty, and families, behind the podium. The house lights dimmed, a sea of faces before and below me. A hush. The sound of my voice amplified through the microphone in the large cavernous space. I began, and I finished my speech. Even in the subjectivity of my terror, I knew it had gone well. Genuine applause followed. And, curiously though, I felt alone. And, predictably, the experience went unprocessed, unmetabolized, and was neatly folded and tucked away into the far reaches of my memory. (Tinsley-Jones, 2003, pp. 182–183)

Twenty-seven years later, Dr. Tinsley-Jones decided to tell this story as an opener to a workshop on diversity. In high school, she was able to live this story without being aware of ongoing consequences. Now, however, her story was overwhelming. She choked on the memory, needing to have her husband and grown daughter listen to her and validate her experiences. She repeatedly practiced telling her story, with each time becoming easier. "By the time I stood in front of my workshop audience, a transformation had truly occurred. Pain from the past had been reclaimed; something inside me had gotten repaired" (Tinsley-Jones, 2003, p. 183).

Now, as an adult, she sees race differently:

Allowing myself a wider awareness of racism's impact on myself and on all of us, and speaking out soundly about it—these are things I have not always done. These are more recently acquired, and still are being honed, even as I write this. I must say that my ability to be more aware and more outspoken is something like that upswell in sound that occurs at the

(continues)

beginning of some musical pieces—you first hear a handful of stray and very faint notes wafting to you from a distance, soon followed by a delicate melody. And then the full strength of the song comes upon you, capturing your attention and your heart. The gradually growing, swelling sound of sweet music. My growing ability to speak of race and racism are like that. Although sweet is frequently not the adjective I could apply. Sometimes frightening, but always freeing. (H. Tinsley-Jones, personal communication, September 29, 2004, italics in original)

1. Dr. Tinsley-Jones lived a life that was relatively free of overt racism, especially given the time period in which she grew up. What experiences with racism does she describe, however?
2. What are the advantages of her approach to handling racism? What are the disadvantages?
3. If you were her high school guidance counselor, what would you do to help her better handle being one of only a few African Americans in the school? Why?
4. How does her change in viewpoint about race reflect developmental issues, changing racial identity, and temporal concerns at these points?

RACIAL IDENTITY DEVELOPMENT

I do not understand this squeamishness about the use of gas. I am strongly in favour of using [it] against uncivilised tribes.
—Winston Churchill

All I demand for the black man is, that the white people shall take their heels off his neck, and let him have a chance to rise by his own efforts.
—William Wells Brown

A heavy guilt rests upon us for what the whites of all nations have done to the colored peoples.

Each of these statements reflects a different view of race. Each makes different attributions about other races, sees different causes for those differences, and predicts different actions from them. Churchill objectifies "uncivilised tribes," Brown asks that Whites step back and allow Blacks "to rise by [their] own efforts," while Schweitzer describes "heavy guilt" necessitating atonement. **Racial identity** influences a wide range of behaviors both inside and outside of mental health treatment and should be considered during treatment planning and implementation.

As early as 18 months, children organize their perceptions of the world around gender, using it to guide their choice of toys, activities and clothing (Kohlberg, 1966). Racial identity develops significantly later than gender identity. African-American preschoolers describe themselves using gender or religion rather than race; they accurately describe their skin color, while denying being Black (Kerwin, Ponterotto, Jackson, & Harris, 1993; M. A. Wright, 1998). By adolescence, race is generally central to identity.

Racial identity influences thoughts, emotions, and behaviors. It is not a constant, but shifts due to a variety of factors, including stress and fatigue (Helms & Cook, 1999). Attitudes about race and acceptance of stereotypes change in a predictable developmental sequence that parallels cognitive changes in other realms (cf. Belenky, Clinchy, Goldberger, & Tarule, 1986; Gilligan, 1982; Kohlberg, 1981; Piaget, 1960). In each realm, "higher" thinking is both more abstract and flexible and less dichotomous in nature.

Theories describing the development of racial identity generally focus on (a) awareness of race, (b) attitudes about both one's own race and the

When we do good to them, it is not benevolence—it is atonement.

—Albert Schweitzer

culturally dominant race, and (c) the ability to think synthetically rather than dichotomously (Cokley, 2002; Helms & Cook, 1999; Slattery, 2004; D. W. Sue & Sue, 1999). Four general approaches to racial identity characterize People of Color: acceptance, dissonance, antagonism, and integrative awareness. These approaches are not necessarily unvarying and progressive. Although a person may most frequently be found in one status, status can vary within a single conversation (Helms & Cook, 1999).

1. During the acceptance phase, there is less race consciousness than during other periods. People accept the status quo, including both the negative stereotypes about their own group and the positive ones about other groups.
2. Some People of Color eventually experience a period of dissonance and become aware that resources and treatment are unfairly and unequally distributed on the basis of race. They struggle to understand why some undeserving people get special privileges, why some who are deserving may not get those privileges, and why trusted people or organizations tell them things that seem wrong.
3. At some point they may become antagonistic toward the majority group because of perceived social injustices and inequities. During this period they class people dichotomously according to color, perceiving their own group positively and dismissing and putting down the majority group.
4. People of Color begin to see race less dichotomously during integrative awareness. They are increasingly aware of race and its impact on themselves and others and can maintain positive views of their own and other groups, see members of their own and other groups in complex and complicated ways, and recognize that skin color does not define worth. They can empathize and collaborate with other groups and are less likely to hold either positive or negative group stereotypes.

White racial identity also develops and changes, similarly moving from simple to complex views of race: contact, disintegration, reintegration, pseudo-independence, and independence (Helms & Cook, 1999; Slattery, 2004). Unlike People of Color, Euro Americans initially see themselves and their own race as good, while accepting negative stereotypes about other races.

1. During the contact phase, Euro Americans are unaware that race has an impact; when they do see the impact of race, they only see it superficially.
2. Euro Americans in disintegration, like People of Color in dissonance, begin to discover that life is unfair, but are unable to make sense of apparently incompatible ideals (e.g., evidence of discrimination with ideals of fairness, honesty, and justice).
3. During reintegration, Euro Americans have resolved this struggle, at least for a while, idealizing their own group while denigrating others. Often this requires selectively perceiving or distorting information (e.g., concluding "that is just the way life is"). These explanations and distortions help resolve the anxiety associated with recognizing injustice.
4. Euro Americans begin to see both Euro Americans and People of Color as varying in "goodness" during pseudo-independence, although they fail to recognize either the privileged positions they hold or the oppressive

factors that impact People of Color. They are unable to recognize that Euro Americans have some responsibility for race-related problems and their solution. Positive evaluations depend on a single (Euro American) standard of merit rather than a multiplicity of values.

5. During independence, Euro Americans are increasingly able to recognize racism, think flexibly about their own and other races, and see other people subjectively and as varying rather than as objects in dichotomous categories. They recognize both oppression and privilege and, although they may not become activists, avoid oppressive acts.

The case material for Helen Tinsley-Jones illustrates how her racial identity influenced her actions and choices. She described periods of unawareness, silence, outspoken discussion, and thoughtful awareness about her race. At some points she overtly accepted the status quo—while feeling alone in doing so—but during others she rejected the status quo or accepted a multiplicity of viewpoints.

Working with Racial Identity in Treatment

Being aware of one's own and others' racial identity is important in becoming multiculturally competent. Racial identity may influence clients' assignment to clinicians, as well as the form of interventions they receive. Consider several scenarios:

- A Euro American caseworker acknowledges the historical reality of racism, but dismisses its current reality. Having inappropriately attributed problems solely to her clients, she refuses to help them further because "some people just don't want to be helped!" Her Latina client becomes angry, in return, and refuses further treatment from her or any other caseworkers, saying, "They're all like that!" (Latina client: antagonistic; Euro American caseworker: reintegration)
- An African-American client accepts the negative stereotypes about his race and is self-blaming. His Euro American psychologist is "nice" and is struggling to understand the discrimination that her client faces, but is not confident in her ability to correctly identify these acts as discrimination. (African-American client: conformity; Euro American psychologist: disintegration)
- An African-American woman enters treatment seriously depressed and suicidal. She does not want to work with the African-American man to whom she is assigned, because she does not feel that African Americans can be good counselors. Although she tries to challenge her reactions, she still tends to dismiss everything her counselor says. Her counselor is both very experienced in responding to suicidality and able to work well with people from a variety of races, seeing beyond limited stereotypes. (African-American client: dissonance; African-American counselor: integrative awareness)

As seen in these scenarios, race and racial identity can raise a variety of issues. When is a clinician competent to work with clients of a different race? When should clients be assigned to clinicians of their own race and when to another one? Is it okay to refer a client to another clinician because the client prefers a clinician of another race? How do clinicians' racial identities affect their work with culturally different clients? Can clinicians at earlier stages of racial identity development (e.g., contact or acceptance) work successfully with clients of a different race or culture? Seriously considering these questions is the first step to competent work with clients of other races. These questions can be tricky and should be discussed with colleagues and in ongoing supervision.

Equally important is a continuing journey to learn about and understand other cultures (Slattery, 2004). With greater self-awareness and understanding of other cultural groups, clinicians can respond intentionally rather than impulsively. When appropriate, it can be helpful to validate concerns about race and process them with clients, as in the following example (Thompson & Jenal, 1994).

> I'm wondering whether you are worrying that I, a Black woman, can understand you, a White woman. Whether you think that you've been palmed off on a less experienced counselor. [Yeah...] I have been in the field for ten years and have done a lot of work with people who are suicidal. (pause) I want to work with you, but I also want to make sure that we are working well together. Will you tell me if you feel I'm not understanding you – all of you? (Euro American client: contact; African-American clinician: integrative awareness)

WHAT DOES IT MEAN TO BE A "MULTICULTURAL" THERAPIST?

All mental health counseling [can be] multicultural. If we consider age, lifestyle, socioeconomic status, and gender differences...
—**Paul Pedersen**

Euro American upper-middle-class men have developed most therapeutic models with their own culture-specific values in mind. Most theories of counseling and psychotherapy have focused on **YAVIS** clients (Young, Attractive, Verbal, Intelligent, Successful)—especially insightful, upwardly mobile professionals. **QUOID** clients (Quiet, Ugly, Old, Indigent, Dissimilar culturally), especially racial minorities or people on welfare, often do not fit the mold for which most therapies were designed. Counseling and psychotherapy emphasize rationality, analysis, introspection, insight, individualism, and autonomy rather than intuition, action, collectivism, and interdependence.

In general, ethnic and racial minority clients prefer and respond better to directive, structured, explicit treatment approaches rather than nondirective, unstructured, and ambiguous approaches (D. W. Sue, 1990). They are more likely to prefer more transparent and disclosing therapists. This mismatch in worldviews has consequences. Ethnic minority clients seeing an ethnically dissimilar clinician, for example, have been found to be more likely to terminate early from treatment and to have worse outcomes than those seeing ethnically similar clinicians (Lam & Sue, 2001; S. Sue, 1998). On the other hand, one study found that matching clients and therapists on treatment goals and coping styles predicted better adjustment and more positive client evaluations of treatment (S. Sue, 1998).

D. W. Sue (2004) does not attribute the problems in treating ethnic minority clients to clinicians' racism, sexism, and homophobia. He believes that his colleagues are "well-intentioned and truly believe in equal access and opportunity," but that they also have "great difficulty freeing themselves from their cultural conditioning.... They are, in essence, trapped in a Euro American worldview that only allows them to see the world from one perspective"

(p. 762). The approaches described throughout this book are designed to help clinicians view their clients from multiple perspectives.

Therapeutic Relationships across Cultures

Greene (1985) describes four approaches to being "fair" in treatment with people of a different cultural background. Some clinicians try to ignore cultural differences: "People are people," "We're all the same under our skin," "I don't look at color; I look at the person." Trying to be colorblind is probably well-intentioned, but in denying differences, clinicians fail to acknowledge the very real role culture has on people's behavior (APA, 2003; Greene, 1985). Furthermore, it can cause clinicians to apply assessments and interventions without considering culture or racism and prejudice—the client's, the clinician's or the culture's—and how each of these may influence behavior (Greene, 1985; Pedersen et al., 2008).

Greene (1985) discusses three other approaches that clinicians adopt in attempting to be responsive to cultural issues. Clinicians who adopt a paternalistic viewpoint attribute all problems to race or culture and, because they assume that their clients are incapable of solving their own problems, solve their problems for them. Although also well-intended, this approach fails to encourage responsibility or help clients recognize the control that they do have and encourages dependency. Other clinicians adopt a stance of unquestioning acceptance. They accept their clients' perspective on problems and encourage them to act on their feelings without considering others' perspectives and rights or taking responsibility for their contributions to problems. The most ethical approach to working with people of another culture is one of acknowledgment and respectful challenge—acknowledging the impacts of culture, prejudice, and discrimination while challenging clients to exercise appropriate control over their life and problems (Greene, 1985).

Food for Thought

Observe your own and others' responses to culture-related issues for several days. In addition to outright racism, do you see examples of Greene's (1985) four other approaches? How did you feel when you saw someone using one of these other approaches? How did the person respond?

BECOMING CULTURALLY COMPETENT

Most people initially see their values, beliefs, habits, and assumptions as normative, even as the "right" way of doing things. Becoming culturally competent requires a paradigm shift in perception—from an **essentialist** to a **constructivist** viewpoint. Culturally competent clinicians recognize that

I come from the East, most of you [here] are Westerners. If I look at you superficially, we are different, and if I put my emphasis on that level, we grow more distant. If I look on you as my own kind, as human beings like myself, with one nose, two eyes, and so forth, then automatically that distance is gone. We are the same human flesh. I want happiness; you also want happiness. From that mutual recognition, we can build respect and real trust of each other. From that can come cooperation and harmony.

—The Dalai Lama (in Craig, 2002)

knowledge is socially constructed. There is no absolute reality; instead knowledge is formed as a result of habit, experience, and perceptual processes. Furthermore, they recognize that although people are similar in many ways, no two are exactly alike; they have had somewhat different experiences and contexts that shape their world, influencing what they see and how they see it (Pedersen et al., 2008). Therefore, "all interactions are cross-cultural … all of our life experiences are perceived and shaped from within our own cultural perspectives" (APA, 2003, p. 382).

In sum, multicultural clinicians recognize and accept differences in cultural values, beliefs, assumptions, and preferences (APA, 2003; Stuart, 2004). They identify attitudes and beliefs that can negatively impact their perceptions of and interactions with clients of other cultures. They develop multicultural sensitivity, knowledge, and understanding. They use culturally appropriate skills and techniques in their clinical practice.

Food for Thought

Consider the roles of ethnicity, race, and context in your life and practice (adapted from Fukuyama & Sevig, 1999).

1. What kinds of experiences have you had with your own and other ethnicities, races, and contexts throughout your life? Have they been primarily positive? Negative? Mixed?
2. What specific cultural beliefs and values, if any, are most important for you now? How might they be a source of connection or conflict between you and your clients?
3. In what ways do you believe your clients' ethnicity, race, and context can be a source of strength? In what ways do you believe they can be a source of weakness?
4. What types of clients or problems involving ethnicity, race, and other contextual issues do you expect would be the most challenging for you? Which would be most interesting? Why?

The Cognitive Skills of a Multicultural Clinician

S. Sue (1998) also emphasized the active cognitive processes involved in multicultural competence. He concluded that culturally competent therapists must also be scientific-minded and able to apply their understanding of cultures flexibly. Being aware of cultural values, beliefs, assumptions, and preferences; using a scientific mindset; and flexibly applying one's knowledge are central to working effectively with culturally different clients, and are important when developing empathic understanding in any clinical work.

Culturally competent clinicians are **scientific-minded**. They are aware of research on group differences, using it to guide assessments and therapy, while remaining sensitive to individual differences (S. Sue, 1998). Culturally competent clinicians test their hypotheses. They might approach a new client as Randi does:

Randi: My new client is an African-American woman. I wonder how her racial identity will impact her ability to work with me, a middle-class White woman. Will she be comfortable with psychotherapy, especially the values inherent in my typical approach?

Because she has recently begun losing her eyesight and seems to have concerns related to this, we should also consider the breadth and depth of her support system, special transportation needs, and other potential vision-related opportunities and obstacles. I need to recognize that my guesses about potential issues are just hypotheses that must be tested over time and that these should lead to changes in my behavior.

Culturally competent clinicians are knowledgeable about cultural differences and their implications for treatment. They understand their own worldviews, are knowledgeable about the cultural groups with which they work, and possess intervention techniques and strategies that are uniquely suited to working with clients from different cultural groups (S. Sue, 1998).

Knowing these things, Randi might think about her new client like this:

Randi: Although I am more collectivistic in orientation than many Euro Americans, I am probably less collectivistic than she is. I probably also value logic and reductionistic thinking more. I am pretty emotionally reserved and have more difficulty expressing feelings than many African Americans do, which might affect my ability to be assertive with her, especially if we have problems in understanding each other.

Of course, not all members of a group are alike. Culturally competent clinicians are able to engage in **dynamic sizing** (S. Sue, 1998). They can flexibly apply knowledge of cultural values, worldviews and behaviors to individual clients, recognizing cultural patterns while avoiding stereotypes. It is helpful neither to believe that nothing is due to culture nor to attribute everything to it; both beliefs interfere with the development of empathy.

Culturally competent clinicians are also able to make appropriate generalizations from their own experiences. They can understand a gay man's reaction to being discriminated against based on their own experiences with discrimination. They are also aware that being discriminated against on the basis of race might feel different to being discriminated against because of sexual orientation. Culturally competent clinicians might respond as Randi does:

Randi: What stereotypes and impressions do I have about this particular client and her cultures? To what degree is she typical of other working-class African-American women? Of people who are losing their eyesight? In what ways is her experience unique? How do my own experiences help me understand hers? What problems are there in generalizing from my experience?

Although these ideas—awareness of cultural differences, scientific mindedness, and dynamic sizing—are ideals to strive for, how do clinicians start moving toward them? A number of authors (APA, 2003; Stuart, 2004; S. Sue, 1998) have described strategies for developing cultural competence. These cognitive, affective, and behavioral strategies are outlined in Table 4.3.

TABLE **4.3**

Suggestions for Developing Multicultural Competence.

1. Acknowledge and control personal biases by becoming aware of personal values, beliefs, and assumptions, evaluating their sources and validity.
2. Think about people using a complex set of cultural categories, aware that differences in cultural values, beliefs, assumptions, habits, and preferences may be important to the course of treatment.
3. Become skilled in listening to each person's unique cultural outlook.
4. Listen sensitively to cultural differences without applying categories rigidly.
5. Develop strategies for identifying the salience of clients' cultural identities.
6. Develop strategies for identifying a person's acceptance of culturally relevant themes.
7. Critically evaluate culturally relevant research before applying it to clinical practice.
8. Use culturally appropriate assessment techniques.
9. Contextualize findings from assessments using an understanding of cultural values, beliefs, behaviors and oppressive attitudes.
10. Consider clients' cultures and worldviews in selecting therapists, interventions, and treatment goals.
11. Respect clients' values, beliefs, habits, and preferences, while influencing them as appropriate.

Note: Modified from APA, 2003; Stuart, 2004; S. Sue, 1998

SUMMARY

Rather than focusing on the unique needs of racial and ethnic minority groups, this chapter has emphasized the ways that all people are racial and cultural beings with multiple cultural identities (e.g., race, ethnicity, gender, social class, religion, sexual orientation, etc.). Each cultural identity influences values, goals, habits, preferences, beliefs, and the ways people perceive the world and are perceived by others. Paying attention to culture helps clinicians contextualize clients' experiences, recognize the meanings they draw, and listen empathically.

Clinicians can generate hypotheses about the impacts of culture by considering a variety of sources. These include examining research on typical worldviews, customs, expectations, and challenges. The group's historical context and typical group experiences—even when different from a client's own—also influence how clients see themselves and are seen by others, the meanings they create in response to a stressor, and their coping strategies.

Because people have multiple cultural identities, it can be difficult to see culture on an individual level. This difficulty also comes from the significant within-group variability that can hide even moderately large group differences. However, as Katy Robinson (2002) noted, it can be easier to identify group and cultural differences in a culture different from one's own.

Like other aspects of identity, racial identity changes as part of a normal developmental process. Generally, identity goes from an acceptance of positive and negative stereotypes and dependence on dichotomous thinking to more complex and flexible thinking that recognizes that "goodness" is independent of skin color. Racial identity is important to the therapy process; in particular, it influences the acceptance of therapists and their ideas and contributes to premature terminations from therapy, especially when the assigned therapist is a poor match with the client's racial identity.

Multicultural therapies pay attention to issues of oppression and privilege—respectively, the ways life is less than fair or the role of unfair advantages. Identifying oppression and challenging privilege can be strategies for building a strong therapeutic alliance, for recognizing inequities in life, and for promoting both individual and community change. In addition to discussing oppression and privilege, most multicultural approaches emphasize using empowering interventions within an egalitarian relationship.

Becoming multiculturally competent is a process. S. Sue (1998) talks about this process as requiring scientific mindedness, cultural competence, and dynamic sizing. That is, culturally competent therapists test their hypotheses about clients rather than assume inflexible stereotypes; and they are aware of cultural differences, but consider the degree to which stereotypes apply to individual clients. Becoming culturally competent requires recognizing the role of culture in one's own life, as well as considering and respecting how it affects clients' lives; attending to differences in values and goals; and using culturally appropriate assessment tools and therapeutic approaches (APA, 2003; Stuart, 2004).

How Do These Issues Apply to Your Life and Work?

1. Most people experience some kinds of both oppression and privilege. In what ways is your life privileged? What are you less able to do, feel, say, or be as a result of your group memberships? What do you believe you should do, feel, or be as a result of your group memberships?
2. Think about a time in your life when you felt like you were on the outside. How did you feel? How was your functioning impacted—positively or negatively? What consequences could you anticipate if you felt this way much of the time?
3. What similarities are there between experiences in your life and the reactions of Ms. Robinson and Dr. Tinsley-Jones? How could you use these similarities to understand yourself—or someone else—better?
4. Using the ideas in Table 4.3, as well as the rest of this chapter, develop a plan for expanding your own multicultural competencies.

PART ███ III

Developing Contextualized and Empathic Assessments

This section of the book focuses on developing the tools and strategies necessary for developing strong contextualized and empathic clinical assessments. Chapter 5 describes the observational and critical thinking strategies that are foundational to the assessment process. Four assessment strategies are described in Chapter 6 that help contextualize the clinical assessment. Chapter 7 describes effective clinical writing, which is both a strategy for communicating an empathic clinical assessment and also a way to further develop empathy. The last two chapters of this section demonstrate how clinicians draw on the ideas in Chapters 5–7 to develop individualized approaches to treatment. Chapter 8 demonstrates how to tailor treatment to clients based on referral questions, stage of change theory, and careful selection of goals. Chapter 9 describes the case conceptualization process, which is influenced by referral questions, the assessment process, clients' goals, theory, and research. This chapter ends with a discussion of how to use case conceptualizations to create useful and individualized treatment plans.

CHAPTER 5

Careful Observations and Critical Thinking in Developing Empathic Assessments

WHERE ARE WE GOING?

1. How do observations and inferences differ?

2. How does worldview influence perceptions and assessments?

3. What social psychological processes bias the assessment process?

4. How can critical thinking be seen in clinical work?

5. How does context influence assessments?

6. Why is recognizing strengths important to developing a strong assessment?

7. Why should assessments recognize both strengths and weaknesses?

Why Court Disaster?

Eminem

Eminem (b. 1972), a White rap musician, has often said and done things that seem designed to offend. When asked why he would say such things, he gives several different sorts of answers. He explains, "I come from Detroit, where it's rough, and I'm not a smooth talker" (Gabriella, 2001, para. 15). He also says that words like "faggot" don't have the same meaning to him as they might to others. "It just means you're being a fag. You're being an asshole or whatever.... Battling with somebody, you do anything you can to strip their manhood away" (Gabriella, 2001, para. 13).

Eminem wonders why what he says seems to be taken out of context and has a different connotation than what it might mean when someone else says the same thing. "You know, I call it being honest, but some sick asshole who does sick things on the sly and doesn't talk about it is cool?" (Gabriella, 2001, para. 17).

> All I'm saying is, if I say the word faggot on my album, it's taken as if I'm speaking directly to gay people and I'm homophobic and a bad influence on kids. But if you watch *American Pie*, the same word is in there, and that's cool with everyone. Why is it all right for them to say it, but if I say it on a record it's not OK? (Bozza, 2002, para. 51)

Although his lyrics and language are often violent, misogynistic, and homophobic, he has also done and said things that would challenge simple characterizations. Eminem has started a charitable foundation serving disadvantaged youth in his hometown and, sung with Elton John (who is openly bisexual), and describes himself as a loving and devoted father to his daughter (Lane, 2004). Elton John (2005) concluded, "Eminem has the balls to say what he feels and to make offensive things funny. That's very necessary today in America, with people being muzzled and irony becoming a lost art" (p. 90).

1. How did you feel about Eminem as you read this piece? How might these feelings influence your work with him? What might help you work effectively with him as a client?
2. What do you know about Eminem and his worldview based on the above excerpts from his interview and this short history? What evidence supports your conclusions?
3. People sometimes say things that are not true. Eminem says that he is being honest when he is swearing. How else could you explain the things he says? How would you know whether he is being honest?
4. Eminem was raised in inner-city Detroit, in a working-class family. How do his statements and actions reflect that upbringing and his social class? See Table 5.1.
5. Did your picture of Eminem change as you read about other parts of his life? How did you make sense of these apparent contradictions?

TABLE **5.1**
Social Class Differences among Euro Americans.

Lower socio-economic status	Upper-Middle socio-economic status
Parenting—Method and goals Raise children with a "hard" individualism. Children must be "toughened up" to maintain their identity and values in an uncertain world. Children are teased, contradicted, and exposed to negative events and emotions.	Raise children with a "soft" individualism, Children are "delicate flowers" who must be allowed to discover themselves and blossom in a welcoming world.
Children are encouraged to become self-reliant, self-disciplined, honest, fair, and reliable.	Children are encouraged to self-actualize, express themselves, and are given choices.
Values Value honesty, fairness, reliability, adjusting to contingencies, and resisting social influence.	Especially value growth, control, and productivity.
Economic and political opportunities Generally earn less money, have fewer and more dangerous housing options, less geographic mobility, poorer health outcomes, and less leisure time.	Often earn more money, have more housing options, safer living conditions, more geographic mobility, better health outcomes, and more leisure time.
Have more feelings of powerlessness, greater sense of constraint and external locus of control, and lower self-efficacy. Emphasize self-control and are more accepting when they do not get what they want.	Expect greater ability to control their world and become more frustrated when they cannot do so. Expect that getting what they want should be possible and easy.
Nature of work Work is often more physical. Intellectual work and education are less valued.	Work often depends on intellectual skills and may be invisible to the casual observer. Intellectual skills, per se, are valued.
Communication All communication, including anger, is expected to be direct and forthright.	Talking directly about conflict and problems creates problems and disrupts the social fabric. Anger should be disguised, repressed, or indirect.

Note: Based on L. M. Brown, 1998; Nelson, Englar-Carlson, Tierney, & Hau, 2006; Snibbe & Markus, 2005.

WORLDVIEWS IN ACTION: HOW ASSUMPTIONS AND VALUES AFFECT CLINICAL PRACTICE

We don't see things as they are, we see them as we are.

—Anaïs Nin

Most people believe that they can understand others, yet the social psychological literature clearly demonstrates that people tend to make consistent and predictable errors. This chapter provides the tools for effectively using the frameworks developed in the previous chapters. In particular, this chapter emphasizes looking for other explanations for observations, recognizing the role of context, and seeing strengths as well as weaknesses.

Accurately and carefully observing behavior before drawing inferences is an important first step to being a good observer and effective clinician. However, strong work depends on being aware of and testing **assumptions** about others and the world. These untested beliefs are often invisible and outside awareness. Clinicians may believe that clients behave with others the way they behave during a counseling session, that their behavior is reflective of underlying personality traits, or that they cannot be trusted to tell the truth. They may believe that children of divorcing parents are best placed with their mothers, that men are not insightful or interpersonally interested, or that change is always happening, both in and out of therapy.

Recognizing assumptions and their consequences is important to the therapy process. Some assumptions have positive consequences. For example, the belief that people have strengths that can be used to resolve problems can help a clinician identify intervention strategies. Other assumptions—for example, that court-referred clients do not want to change—while sometimes accurate, may interfere with the therapeutic alliance and the change process.

Clinicians' values vary widely and influence both their perceptions and goals (Liszcz & Yarhouse, 2005; Pitts & Wallace, 2005). When clinicians believe that education and achievement are important, they are more likely to perceive people who have not continued their education or who are not employed out of the home as lazy or irresponsible. On the other hand, people who had families instead of attending college may question time "wasted" on achievement rather than spent with the people who matter most. Clinicians who value active and curious children may respond negatively to quieter children, perhaps seeing them as passive. On the other hand, clinicians who expect children to be "well-behaved" may see an active child as hyperactive.

Clinicians' values have a direct impact on the treatment process (Liszcz & Yarhouse, 2005; Norcross & Wogan, 1987). Clients' and clinicians' values and beliefs influence choice of therapeutic approach, problem definition and goals, and even clients' ability to change (Bolter, Levenson, & Alvarez, 1990; Ford & Hendrick, 2003; Liszcz & Yarhouse, 2005). Clinical assessments of the nature and causes of problems have considerable associated power. Concluding that a child is oppositional has different treatment implications than believing that her parents engage in power struggles with her. Rather than painting others' behavior with a broad brush, it can be productive to wonder when a child is oppositional and with whom, observing when parents set up power struggles and when they are able to bypass them.

Food for Thought

Consider your assumptions about people who talk the way that Eminem did. Would your assumptions help or interfere with treatment?

SOCIAL PSYCHOLOGICAL PROCESSES INFLUENCING CLINICAL JUDGMENTS

What happens when good people are put into an evil place? Do they triumph or does the situation dominate their past history and morality?

—Philip Zimbardo

The problems people have during decision making have been well described in nonclinical settings; there is no reason to believe that they disappear during the assessment and treatment processes (Meehl, 1954). In fact, unless clinicians recognize and challenge factors that bias their judgment, these factors will interfere with their assessments.

This bias can be seen with a short example. Even before Ryan, a man with a history of significant heroin abuse, enters the office, the process of **expectancy confirmation** may already be operating: The clinician may look for characteristics consistent with her schema about heroin addicts and overlook behaviors that are inconsistent with it, including his commitment to family, his love of animals and the outdoors, and his desire to help others (Trope & Thompson, 1997). **Confirmatory biases** may cause the clinician to *recall* behaviors consistent with her biases (Hirt, McDonald, & Erikson, 1995). For example, when discussing Ryan during a case conference, traits consistent with stereotypes are recalled and reported (e.g., he is currently unemployed and significantly ambivalent about treatment), while others are ignored (e.g., that he has not missed a session and has completed six of seven homework assignments). When several people discuss him in case conference, divergent opinions tend to disappear due to **groupthink**, each person conforming his or her opinion to the group consensus (Janis, 1997).

The case conceptualization of Ryan is also influenced by **trait negativity bias**, which causes clinicians and other observers to weigh mistakes, symptoms, and problems more heavily than positive coping strategies, successes, and effective functioning (Ito, Larsen, Smith, & Cacioppo. 1998). In practice this may mean that Ryan will report a bad week because he had a **slip**, overlooking the fact that for much of the week he handled his cravings well.

When clinicians see Ryan's heroin use as reflective of his addictive personality, rather than as a coping mechanism to handle stress or as something that he does around friends who also use drugs, they have engaged in the **fundamental attribution error**, the tendency to see others' behavior as due to internal traits, while overlooking or minimizing the contribution of external and situational factors (Ross, 1977). What is striking about this process is that although people underestimate the role of context for others' behavior, they tend to make situational attributions for their own problematic behavior (e.g., "I wasn't feeling well when I took that test. That's why I did poorly."). However, when clinicians overestimate the role of traits in clients' behavior and fail to see the roles of situations and context, they miss opportunities for change.

Finally, Banaji and her colleagues have repeatedly demonstrated that people may behave in a biased way, even when they believe they are not prejudiced (Banaji, Hardin, & Rothman, 1993; Blair & Banaji, 1996; J. Park & Banaji, 2000). Good intentions are not enough; being vigilant to counter **implicit biases** can help.

Food for Thought

Return to the opening description of Eminem. Do you see any of these factors in your reactions to him? Where?

CRITICAL THINKING

The first step toward success is taken when you refuse to be a captive of the environment in which you first find yourself.

—Mark Caine

In short, making strong assessments depends on vigilant awareness of and **critical thinking** about the factors biasing perceptions. Most people fail to question their expectations and biases, accepting initial perceptions as reality. They often seek simple, black-and-white answers to explain complex and difficult problems. Rather than testing expectations and beliefs, they often seek confirmation of them. Perhaps this is one reason that so many bad things seem to happen on the same day. For example, people often notice a series of frustrations and setbacks (e.g., lost wallet, flat tire, forgotten appointment). Partly in response to seeking patterns, a person may notice only these bad occurrences and fail to notice the good things that happened around the same time. Further, the causal nature among the setbacks may not be recognized (e.g., being stressed from the flat tire or lost wallet caused distraction, leading to the forgotten appointment).

Critical thinking involves making strong and systematic **observations**. It means recognizing alternative explanations for why people behave as they do and looking for data that helps discriminate among these explanations. It requires becoming aware of biases and challenging their **validity**. It also demands becoming aware of the role of context and culture in observations.

Good and careful observations are important tools for developing a strong, empathic understanding of others. Observations are sensory-based bits of information that can be seen, heard, felt, smelled, or tasted. Each of the following is an observation:

Danny slowly said, "She doesn't want me anymore," his statement marked by two hesitations and one stutter. His cheeks were flushed, his hands cold. His posture was closed and his head down. He made little eye contact while talking.

In contrast to observations, **inferences** are the meaningful interpretations of observations and are influenced by one's worldviews and biases. Although people agree about sensory observations, even reasonable people can disagree about the inferences drawn from a set of observations, because multiple inferences can be used to explain any single observation. For example, why are Danny's cheeks flushed? They could be flushed because he is embarrassed, angry, hot, recently sunburned, having an allergic reaction to some food, or hypertensive. Alternatively, his face could be red because that is his normal coloration. Well-collected observations and inferences about them lead to **clinical assessments** about the causes, maintenance, and treatment of problems and symptoms.

Clients—and their family members, friends, and referral sources—will offer explanations of their behavior; some explanations will be accurate, others inaccurate. While considering these explanations, think about the motives and assumptions of the source. Is the explanation extreme? Is it reasonable? Is it supported by evidence? Good assessments require being open to these explanations, without excluding others prematurely. Good assessments also require being open to alternative explanations. Are there mitigating factors? Exceptions in the behavior? What is the positive intent in the behavior?

CHOOSING AMONG ALTERNATIVE EXPLANATIONS

Consider the T-shirts in Figure 5.1. What would you guess about the person wearing each T-shirt? What other explanations are there? How could you choose among these hypotheses?

Several behavioral strategies lead to stronger clinical assessments. As we have discussed, effective clinicians make good observations in multiple situations and recognize the factors that potentially bias their perceptions. Effective clinicians recognize the tentative nature of their inferences and test their hypotheses rather than jumping to conclusions (S. Sue, 1998). Effective clinicians would do more than read the words on these T-shirts to gain an empathic understanding of their clients; they would also pay attention to other things (e.g., grooming, other items of clothing, and speech patterns) to identify whether the T-shirts directly reflect their wearers' values, are an ironic statement about cultural mores, or were the only clean clothing in the wearer's roommate's closet.

Some inferences initially look like observations. Many people, upon meeting Danny, might say that he was depressed, believing this to be a simple observation. Although he might be depressed, when clinicians draw this inference without identifying and excluding other explanations for his behavior, their assessment could both misdirect treatment and bypass other, more accurate explanations of his behavior.

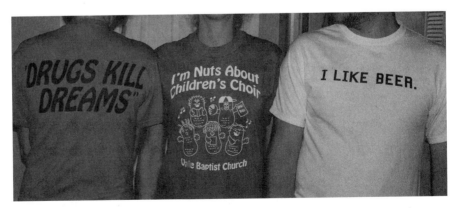

FIGURE **5.1** What hypotheses do you draw about the people wearing these T-shirts?

The validity of assessments is increased when a broad range of observations is obtained: from different days, situations, or kinds of measures. The clinician's confidence in the validity of his or her diagnosis is increased when Danny is interviewed on several different days, observed both in the office and in his second-grade classroom, and understood through his mother's responses to a questionnaire about his sleep, eating habits, friendships, and behavior in the home. His lethargy during an assessment could stem from the fight he had with his mother earlier in the day; be a side effect of the medicine that he was recently placed on; be related to his perception of the clinician's goals for the interview (e.g., out of home placement); or be caused by a lack of sleep.

COUNTERING OBSERVER BIASES

Taken out of context I must seem so strange.

—Ani DiFranco

One of the paradoxes of making observations is that simply paying attention to a person or group changes their behavior (Labov, 1997). The **observer's paradox** is a particular case of the systemic nature of all interactions, which are both affected by and affect observers and their contexts.

Clinicians' contexts influence what they observe and how they interpret it. For example, if Danny's social worker had had an argument immediately before their session, he or she might have difficulty paying attention to his statements or perceive innocent remarks as threatening. Because clinicians are also part of their clients' context, his or her size, appearance, dress, grooming, and interpersonal style may cause Danny to respond differently towards him or her than he does to others.

Children with attention-deficit/hyperactivity disorder (**ADHD**) may behave differently in two different settings; two observers may perceive the same behavior very differently. Because clinical observations can introduce bias, Pitts and Wallace (2003) suggest viewing children's behavior in a culture- and context-sensitive manner. Their process, although developed for African-American children who might have ADHD, is appropriate for any population and behavior:

(1) *Description*: Identify and carefully describe the problem.
(2) *Frequency*: Compare the frequency of the problem with baselines appropriate for the general population and for the specific population (e.g., 9-year-old African-American boys).
(3) *Intensity*: Compare the intensity of the observed behavior with cultural norms and established baseline.
(4) *Environmental setting*: Note the environment in which the behavior was observed or in which it was reported to have occurred. Then determine whether the behavior can be explained by environmental or biological factors, including hunger, stress, or abuse.
(5) *Recognition of biases*: Minimize the roles of reporter values, judgment, and biases by recognizing and accounting for these biasing factors. Counter the subjectivity associated with labeling behavior a problem by observing the costs and benefits associated with the "problem behavior" accruing to all involved parties.

Think about these issues for the Lee family in the case below, who were charged with medical neglect and lost custody of their daughter Lia for several months (Fadiman, 1997).

Her Parents' Favorite
Lia Lee

Lia Lee (b. 1981) was the youngest of 14 children born to Hmong immigrants in Merced, California. Seven others were still living when she was born; six had died before they came to the United States. Lia was a healthy infant, weighing 8 pounds, 7 ounces at birth. When she was 3 months old, Lia had the first of what would be numerous, eventually uncontrollable, seizures (Fadiman, 1997).

Lia's parents, like most Hmong, were loving parents who took a child-centered approach to parenting. They especially loved Lia. Anne Fadiman, a journalist who listened carefully to the Lees over a 9-year period, said that it was clear that "Lia was her parents' favorite, the child they considered the most beautiful, the one who was most extravagantly hugged and kissed, the one who was dressed in the most exquisite garments" (1997, p. 23). This might have been due to a number of different reasons—perhaps because she was the youngest child, perhaps because she was ill, perhaps because she was ill with epilepsy.

Epilepsy has unique connotations for the Hmong, who both recognize it as a serious illness and also see it as an illness with special distinctions. The Hmong believe that people who have seizures can perceive things that others do not, which will allow them to enter trances more readily. That they have also been ill gives them an "intuitive sympathy for the suffering of others and lends them emotional credibility as healers" (Fadiman, 1997, p. 21). Thus, having a seizure reveals the person's calling to be a *txiv neeb*, a "person with a healing spirit" (p. 21).

In the first four and a half years of her life, Lia Lee was admitted to the hospital 17 times and made more than 100 visits to the emergency room or pediatric clinic. Her prescriptions were changed 23 times during this period, changing the combination of medications, doses, and frequency of administration. Some medications were given daily, regardless of how she was feeling (i.e., vitamins and anticonvulsants), others when she was symptomatic and were to be taken until the prescription was completed (i.e., antibiotics), still others were to be taken only when she ran a fever. While this regimen might be difficult for most parents, it was more difficult for the Lees, who were illiterate in both English and Hmong, and who could not read the markings on thermometers, medicine droppers, and measuring spoons.

When Lia continued to have seizures after having been prescribed an antiseizure medication, her doctor tested her blood levels and determined

(continues)

(continued)

that Lia had subtherapeutic levels. When her blood levels continued to be low after the higher dose was prescribed, her doctor, Dr. Peggy Philp, wondered whether she was having seizures in spite of adequate levels of the medicine or because the dose was still too low. Lia's mother said that she was giving her medicine as prescribed. Was she confused, telling the doctors what they wanted to hear, or lying?

Her doctors concluded that the Lees were not giving Lia her medicine as prescribed and sent a public health nurse with a Hmong interpreter to the Lee home. Effie Bunch, one of these nurses, concluded that

> I don't think the mom and dad ever truly understood the connection between a seizure and what it did to the brain. And I don't know how else you get through to them that they have to give the meds. My general impression was that they really felt we were all an intrusion and that if they could just do what they thought best for their child, that child would be fine. They were courteous and they were obstinate. They told us what we wanted to hear. (as quoted in Fadiman, 1997, pp. 48–49)

Lia's doctors saw the Lees as noncompliant with their daughter's medication regimen and treatment and as seriously endangering her life. Therefore, when Lia was almost 3 years old, Dr. Neil Ernst filed a report with Child Protective Services, in order to get her placed in a foster home where her medication could be administered as prescribed. Perhaps because of language and cultural differences between the Lees and their doctors, perhaps because they only saw Lia when she was ill, they underestimated both the Lees' parenting ability and Lia's intellectual ability.

> The doctors only saw her when she was sick and never in her home environment. When we saw her, sometimes she was a windup toy because of the phenobarbital and sometimes she was post-seizure and looked like a little ball of dough in the corner, but sometimes she was just bright and cute and actively playing, happy, gay, climbing, crawling, on her mother's back, laughing and chattering and what have you. (E. Bunch, as quoted in Fadiman, 1997, p. 55)

1. How would you describe the Lees' behavior with regard to taking care of their daughter?
2. Relative to baselines for the general population and the Hmong, would you describe the Lee family's behavior as problematic? If so, how?
3. What values and biases might Lia's doctors hold that would influence how they viewed the Lees' parenting and their treatment of Lia's epilepsy?
4. How might Lia's doctors' values and behaviors influence the Lees' behavior? How do your values and biases influence your reactions to this story? How did the Lees' values influence their parenting and interactions with Lia's physicians?

RECOGNIZING STRENGTHS AND EXCEPTIONS TO PROBLEMS

Strength does not come from winning. Your struggles develop your strengths. When you go through hardships and decide not to surrender, that is strength.

—Arnold Schwarzenegger

As seen in the case of the Lee family, pejorative descriptions of people both reflect and create problems in the therapeutic alliance (Linehan, 1993). Becoming aware of and challenging derogatory descriptions of clients, and recognizing clients' strengths as well as their weaknesses, can strengthen empathic connections with them.

Diagnoses and pejorative attributions about behavior have negative consequences. Benjet, Azar, and Kuersten-Hogan (2003), in their summary of the literature, concluded that being diagnosed with a significant mental illness interferes with equal access to jobs and housing. People with a significant mental illness are more likely to lose custody of their children, even when the diagnosis is unrelated to ability to parent, inability to profit from parenting interventions, or even the presence of ongoing problems.

The person receiving clinical assessments and diagnosis may also be negatively impacted as a result of a **self-fulfilling prophecy**, where others' perceptions and expectations shape a person's self-perceptions and behavior (Merton, 1948). This process can work in negative ways, as when a man is diagnosed with bipolar disorder and concludes that he cannot do anything to control his moods ("It's biological and I can't do anything about it"). This phenomenon has been observed in a variety of settings, including classrooms, courtrooms, and physicians' offices (Rosenthal, 2002).

Problems are important to recognize, describe, count, and contextualize, but strengths and exceptions to problems are equally important. Identifying exceptions to problems can **reframe** a situation and provide a foundation for change. For example, the Lees' social worker might ask, when do the Lees give Lia her medicine? When don't they? What's different about these two sets of circumstances? Are they more likely to give some sorts of medicines than others (e.g., those with particular side-effect profiles or that are more acceptable to their cultural and spiritual beliefs)?

One way of identifying exceptions to problems is to have clients complete a **functional analysis**, often identified using the acronym ABC. Clients can observe what is happening when the behavior occurs (Antecedent), describe the behavior (Behavior), and identify all consequences of the behavior (Consequences). Although clients should be asked to record when there is a problem, they should also record when there could have been a problem but it did not occur. See Table 5.2. For example, what distinguishes between instances when Lia is given her medicine and when she is not?

Recognizing real strengths builds hope and self-esteem, identifies resources for solving problems, and builds the therapeutic alliance (Slattery, 2004). Clients feel heard and understood and the clinician is more likely to respond compassionately, caringly, and empathically. However, good assessments and treatment require hearing people from their own point of view while also being objective about their symptoms, strengths, and weaknesses.

TABLE **5.2**
A Hypothetical Functional Analysis for the Lees' Administration of Medicine to Lia.

Antecedents	Behavior	Consequences
Lia is being given five medications, three times a day for two, twice a day for three.		
8 A.M. Lia woke up in a good mood.	Gave medication with breakfast.	She laughed and spat out medicine. Gave her one of the three that she spat out. Felt mean giving medicine when she does not want to take it. No seizure this morning.
12 P.M. At sister's apartment. Forgot to bring medicine. Sister disapproves of Western medications	Did not give medicine.	Relieved that sister does not hassle me about giving medicine. No seizure this afternoon.
7 P.M. Lia's brother was tired and feverish. Everyone went to bed early.	Gave both noon and evening medicines.	Slept well and woke late. No seizure.
8:30 A.M. Lia overslept. Had doctor's appointment at 10 A.M. Could not find one medicine.	Gave other medicines on shelf.	She laughed and spat them out. Do not have any extra pills and cannot afford to refill prescriptions.

Food for Thought

Consider the Lee family's interactions with the medical system. Who was objective and unable to empathize? Who was able to empathize without being objective? Was anyone able to balance both? What could they do to develop a stronger empathic understanding of this family? As you read the following case, consider whether Dylan Harris's and Eric Klebold's probation officers were able to balance both their strengths and weaknesses while developing their assessments and writing their reports and to what degree.

Seeing Strengths *and* Weaknesses
Dylan Harris and Eric Klebold

Clients often paint their world in black and white, perhaps expecting that clinicians want to hear this. Clinicians and clients tend to focus on problems in their efforts to resolve them, while overlooking strengths. However, no person is totally good or bad. Focusing on problems and weaknesses to the

(continues)

exclusion of strengths interferes with empathy and creates a weaker assessment of the person, devoid of clients' strengths and natural success strategies. It forms a one-sided clinical assessment that creates distance rather than understanding and connection.

The reports written by Dylan Harris and Eric Klebold's probation officers illustrate the difficulty of seeing things that go against one's own biases. Dylan (age 17) and Eric (age 18) had been arrested for breaking into a commercial van and stealing electronics; both were on probation. They felt lonely, alienated, and disrespected by peers, who would throw them into lockers and call them names. In 1997, Dylan wrote in his journal, "I swear— like I'm an outcast, and everyone is conspiring against me…" (Abelson, Frey, & Gregg, 2004, p. 314). He repeatedly wrote about being depressed and wanting a gun so that he could kill himself.

Both Dylan and Eric were reportedly members of the Trenchcoat Mafia, a group of loners who felt different and ostracized at school. As members of this group, they talked about getting back at the jocks and minorities who put them down. Eric had threatened a fellow student with a gun and described how to make bombs on his web page. Both were enamored of Nazi culture: the Columbine Massacre, where they killed 12 other students and a teacher before killing themselves, occurred on Adolph Hitler's birthday.

They were also described as coming from good families. Eric's father was a recently retired Air Force officer, Dylan's a geologist. Both were excellent students; Dylan was able to quote Shakespeare easily and was in the gifted and talented program at his grade school. Eric was described as a leader, Dylan a follower. Both played Little League when younger and enjoyed the video game Doom. Dylan operated the lights and sets for high school play productions, was involved in video productions there, and helped maintain his school's computer as well as building his own.

What did their probation officers conclude in their reports? About Dylan Klebold, the officer wrote, "Dylan is a bright young man who has a great deal of potential… He is intelligent enough to make any dream a reality but he needs to understand hard work is part of it" (Glick et al., 1999, p. 26). And for Eric Harris, "Eric is a very bright young man who is likely to succeed in life… He is intelligent enough to achieve lofty goals as long as he stays on task and remains motivated" (Glick et al., 1999, p. 26). The difficulty with these reports is that they were written before the Massacre, when information that in retrospect appears to indicate the danger they posed had not been identified.

Clinicians need to recognize clients' strengths and exceptions to their problems. However, recognizing strengths does not mean overlooking weaknesses and problems. Eric wrote in his journal, "It's my fault! Not my parents, not my brothers, not my friends, not my favorite bands, not computer games, not the media, it's mine." For Mother's Day, he quoted Shakespeare in the following note in his journal, "Good wombs have born [sic] bad sons" (Senior, 1999, para. 9).

(continues)

(continued)

1. What factors may have contributed to the probation officers' underestimates of Dylan and Eric's potential for violence? Why?
2. How does their potential for violence match the factors described in Table 5.3?
3. How could you have approached Dylan and Eric so that you could see their strengths, while also being aware of their propensity for violence?
4. Recently, Cullen (2009) reported that Dylan and Eric were *not* part of the Trenchcoat Mafia, had not been bullied by fellow students, and had not targeted jocks and minorities. How does this development influence your perception of them, as well as the usefulness of secondhand reports at the time of a crisis?

TABLE **5.3**

Factors Predicting Relative Safety from School Violence.

- School system promotes positive school environment rather than focusing on punitive approaches
- Students feel close to others in school system and connected to school
- Students trust the school administration
- Students believe that rules are enforced fairly and consistently
- Students have strong, positive attachment to family
- Surrounding community has low levels of gun-related violence

Note: From Mulvey & Cauffman, 2001.

SUMMARY

Making good observations is a difficult process, complicated by many factors. Many people confuse observations (sensory data) with inferences, the conclusions people draw about observations. It is important to recognize that inferences are influenced by many factors, including the values and assumptions of one's worldview. Assessments are clinical judgments, based on a number of observations and the inferences drawn from them.

In many nonclinical settings, people jump to conclusions rather than thinking critically. In professional work, assessments are strengthened by questioning expectations and biases and considering other hypotheses. Being open to complex answers to difficult problems and testing hypotheses rather than only seeking confirmation for them further strengthens the assessment process.

People's judgments are biased by a series of factors that interfere with critical thinking and the development of an empathic understanding. People engage in expectancy confirmations, the tendency to *look* for what they believe, and operate by confirmatory biases, the tendency to *recall* observations that confirm beliefs, both of which compromise the accuracy and usefulness of observations. Negative behaviors are more likely to be observed, particularly when observers are primed to look for symptoms and problems (trait negativity bias). Because of such processes, behaviors are seen as reflective of internal and persistent traits rather than environmental or transient factors (fundamental attribution error). Furthermore, even when people report being bias free, they often have implicit biases against some groups that affect their inferences and behavior.

There is no such thing as pure, unadulterated observations: observers both affect that which they observe and are affected by their observations (observer's paradox). Clients are also influenced by their own expectancies (self-fulfilling prophecy). Although working in groups can bring in new points of view, groups can engage in groupthink, with diverging opinions disappearing in favor of the group consensus. Challenging this tendency in treatment increases critical thinking and retains openness to other viewpoints and options.

In addition to being aware of these factors in treatment, clinicians can approach their observations systematically. Rather than describing behavior globally and vaguely, a practice that is susceptible to bias, Pitts and Wallace (2003) suggest carefully describing behavior, observing its frequency and intensity and the setting in which it occurs, and acknowledging and challenging biases. Finally, recognizing strengths and exceptions to problems is important to developing an empathic understanding of clients, although recognizing strengths should not exclude recognizing weaknesses.

How Do These Issues Apply to Your Life and Work?

This chapter has focused on the observer in the assessment and treatment process and how these influence the conclusions drawn.

1. Pay attention to your style of observations. What do you generally pay attention to? What do you tend to overlook?
2. Pay attention to how you draw inferences about others. Are your inferences useful, respectful, and based on a range of information, or do you tend to jump to conclusions that are primarily positive or negative in tone? Do you tend to draw a single type of conclusion (e.g., that you cannot trust others)? If so, what kind? How can you increase your confidence about your interpretations (S. Sue, 1998)?
3. Pay attention to the assumptions that underlie how you view the world and your decisions. What types of assumptions do you tend to make? Do they tend to be useful and accurate? Are they assumptions that will be helpful in therapy? When? How?

CHAPTER 6

Assessment Strategies for Understanding People in Context

WHERE ARE WE GOING?

1. Why should clinicians attend to context during assessments and treatment?

2. How can psychosocial histories, family genograms, timelines, and mental status evaluations be used to effectively understand clients?

3. How do one's sources influence the information collected?

4. What can clinicians do to create a less-biased assessment process?

Stupid and Crazy?

Raymond J. Corsini

While working as a psychologist in a prison, Dr. Corsini performed what he described as "the most successful and elegant psychotherapy" he had ever performed (Dumont & Corsini, 2010, p. 10). Before leaving prison, the man made an appointment with Dr. Corsini to thank him.

> When I left your office about two years ago, I felt like I was walking on air. When I went into the prison yard, everything looked different, even the air smelled different. I was a new person. Instead of going over to the group I usually hung out with—they were a bunch of thieves—I went over to another group of square Johns [prison jargon for noncriminal types]. I changed from a cushy job in the kitchen to the machine shop, where I could learn a trade. I started going to the prison high school and I now have a high school diploma. I took a correspondence course in drafting and I have a drafting job when I leave Thursday. I started back to church even though I had given up my religion many years ago. I started writing to my family and they have come up to see me and they remember you in their prayers. I now have hope. I know who and what I am. I know I will succeed in life. I plan to go to college. You have freed me. I used to think you bug doctors [prison slang for psychologists and psychiatrists] were for the birds, but now I know better. Thanks for changing my life. (Dumont & Corsini, 2010, p. 10)

Dr. Corsini was puzzled. How had he changed this man's life? He did not remember this man and he did not do therapy. What had he done? The man continued to tell him that

> [H]e had always thought of himself as "stupid" and "crazy"—terms that had been applied to him many times—by his family, his teachers, and his friends. In school, he had always gotten poor grades, which confirmed his belief in his mental subnormality. His friends did not approve of the way he thought and called him crazy.... But when I said, "You have a high IQ," he had an "aha!" experience that explained everything. In a flash, he understood why he could solve crossword puzzles better than any of his friends. He now knew why he read long novels rather than comic books, why he preferred to play chess rather than checkers, why he liked symphonies as well as jazz. With great and sudden intensity he realized ... that he was really normal and bright and not crazy or stupid. (Dumont & Corsini, 2010, p. 11)

1. How did Dr. Corsini's assessment contribute to this man's changed view of himself? What about it was important?
2. Could just anyone say this so effectively? What made Dr. Corsini's simple statement so effective?

RECOGNIZING CONTEXT

There's never a figure without ground.

—Kay King

Effective interventions depend on a strong clinical assessment of clients, empathically recognizing them in the context of their lives. This chapter outlines four assessment strategies that are easily conducted during initial sessions. This contextualized understanding is essential for the empathy underlying effective treatment and positive behavioral change.

Context influences and sometimes distorts one's perception of events, even of visual stimuli, as illustrated in Figure 6.1. A hard day at work might be challenging and invigorating to someone who feels well, but frustrating to someone who is ill. While working on sexual assault issues in treatment, a client who received sexually suggestive comments on the job might be overwhelmed, although a year earlier she might have felt validated and beautiful by the same comments—and 3 years later she might be able to make attributions to help her handle this situation well.

People are embedded in an overlapping and complex set of contexts, only some of which they are aware. They may consistently recognize and identify with some contexts (e.g., religion, culture, or trauma), yet be unaware of highly influential contextual influences. For example, a woman may recognize the impact of being a lesbian from an evangelical Christian family that rejects her, but fail to identify how her mother's chronic illness impacts her own sense of urgency about resolving family issues.

Assessing people in a three-dimensional manner is an essential part of treatment, without which clinicians may fail to be empathic, make inaccurate clinical assessments, or be outright judgmental. As Corsini's (1984) example demonstrates, it can also help clients have new experiences and change. Although this section outlines four strategies for assessing people and their context, there are, of course, other approaches. Yalom (2003), for example, asks clients to describe the course of a "typical day" in detail, in order to assess the pace and nature of their lives, as well as other details that may be so mundane that they would otherwise go unreported. A. G. Rogers (2006) asks her clients to draw a river depicting their lives. In the rivers' turns, they

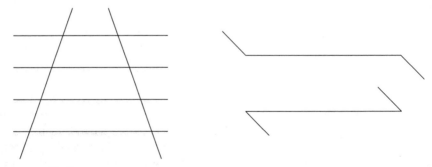

FIGURE **6.1** Two visual illusions.

Notice the ways that context influences perception. The horizontal lines are each the same length.

describe the events that have had major impacts on their lives (e.g., deaths, sexual abuse, changing homes).

DEVELOPING THREE-DIMENSIONAL ASSESSMENTS

All assessment is a perpetual work in progress.

—Linda Suske

In this section, we examine four strategies that highlight context and that help identify issues that might be concerns for a client. These strategies are the psychosocial history (Park & Slattery, 2009; Slattery & Park, in press a), family genogram (McGoldrick, Gerson, & Shellenberger, 1999), timeline, and mental status evaluations. These strategies gather clusters of events—or their absence—to identify factors that contribute to or ameliorate presenting problems, serve as obstacles, or facilitate change.

Psychosocial History

A **psychosocial history** is a collection of current and historical information about client behavior and functioning in a wide range of realms. Psychosocial histories gather information with a high potential for impacting treatment, including relative strengths and weaknesses, obstacles to change, available resources and social supports, and client meanings. This information-gathering process helps clinicians understand their clients as three-dimensional beings, move beyond their biases and typical ways of looking at people, and develop empathy for them. Psychosocial histories can help clinicians draw a differential diagnosis, identify treatment goals and possible interventions, and assess prognosis. They help identify hypotheses about how these factors might contribute to the presenting problem and symptoms.

Rather than asking questions in a rote manner (e.g., "What is your current use of drugs and alcohol?"), most clinicians gather information for a psychosocial history in the course of an interview. They typically start with more general prompts (e.g., "Tell me why you're here today"), then move to specific questions addressing areas not spontaneously addressed earlier in the interview (e.g., "What do you do when you're stressed?"). Table 6.1 includes topics that are common to many agencies (e.g., symptoms, family background and functioning, familial history of psychiatric problems, drug and alcohol use, trauma history) and those that are more particular to our model (e.g., client's attributions about a life stressor, sense of life meaning and purpose, obstacles to change, therapeutic alliance). While learning how to assess and write a psychosocial history, clinicians should focus less on the categories, which may change across settings, and more on developing a general strategy for gathering broad, yet detailed, information about a client.

As you read the next case material, imagine that Malcolm Little (the young Malcolm X) had been referred to you by his caseworker at age 14, when he first began running into problems at school and in his community. The caseworker's referral might include questions about why Malcolm was running into problems and whether an out-of-home placement was appropriate. The information in the following case material is incomplete—as it will be any time when seeing a client for the first time—but provides useful ideas to pursue further.

TABLE **6.1**

Questions to Address during the Assessment Phase and throughout Therapy.

The problem

Presenting problem or symptoms

What symptoms does the client report? How severe are they? How chronic? When did they begin? How much are they interfering with functioning? Are they specific to certain situations or do they occur across situations? What are his or her beliefs about what is wrong? About the appropriate treatment for his or her symptoms? Does he or she expect to get better?

Because clients often have difficulty reporting "bad" symptoms, be careful to assess major concerns, especially about suicide, rather than expecting clients to freely disclose them. Ask, *What else?*

Precipitating event and other recent events

Why is the client having problems now? Why is he or she entering treatment now?

What negative or positive events have occurred recently at home, work, and school, and in important relationships? What ongoing stressors? Are reactions proportionate or disproportionate to the stressor?

Personal and family history of psychological disorders

Has the client or family experienced either similar symptoms or different ones at some time in the past? How were problems handled? What was helpful? Specifically assess whether suicide was considered as a way to cope with problems.

If either the client or family received formal treatment in the past, how might this affect current treatments? Were previous therapists respectful? Hopeful? Effective? Empowering? From the client's viewpoint, is current therapy an extension of previous work or work on totally new and unrelated issues?

Current context

Physical condition and medication use

How is the client's physical health? Can any medical conditions or medicines account for the symptoms reported? Have these potential explanations been ruled out? Has the client been compliant with medications and treatment in the past? In what health-promoting (or health–undermining) practices is the person currently engaging?

Drug and alcohol use

Is the client taking any recreational substances that could cause symptoms? Is he or she taking any street drugs that could interact with medications prescribed to treat symptoms? What is the familial history of substance use and abuse?

Intellectual and cognitive functioning

What are his or her intellectual strengths and deficits? Could symptoms be caused by cognitive deficits?

Coping style

Is he or she engaging in generally adaptive or maladaptive coping strategies? When is he or she most successful in coping with the problem? What works? Are coping strategies generally short-term or long-term solutions? How do these coping strategies fit with spiritual and religious goals?

Self-concept

What are his or her beliefs about himself or herself (e.g., *I'm helpless with regard to the winds of fate*)? What beliefs about self or problems in the past are particularly helpful? Does he or she have a generally strong or weak sense of self-efficacy?

Sociocultural background

In what culture was the client raised? If an immigrant, how long has he or she been in this country? Why did he or she come to this country? What are his or her connections to his or her homeland? What is his or her

TABLE **6.1**
Questions to Address during the Assessment Phase and throughout Therapy (Continued)

level of acculturation? What other group identifications (e.g., race, affectional orientation, gender, age, physical abilities, etc.) are most important?

How does his or her cultural background or group influence symptoms and reactions to symptoms? Could the behavior be "normal" in his or her culture and not in the clinician's (or vice versa)? Could differences in group identification influence the nature and quality of your relationship?

Spirituality and religion

What (if any) religious affiliation does he or she report? Is religion important to him or her? In what ways? How do spiritual and religious beliefs, values, goals, behaviors, and resources influence current functioning? Do they provide a supportive network? Are beliefs culture-typical or -atypical? How does the nature of the beliefs influence feelings of support and acceptance in the community?

Trauma history

Does the client describe a history of trauma in the home, community, school, or work settings? How did he or she perceive it? What reactions did others have to it?

Resources and barriers

Individual resources

What does he or she do particularly well or feel good about? How can these attributes (e.g., persistence, loyalty, optimism, intelligence) be resources for treatment? How might they undermine it?

Social resources (family and friends)

What is the nature and composition of client's current family, family of origin and, if applicable, birthfamily? How supportive are the client's family and friends? Are they sufficient in both quantity and quality to meet the client's needs? Do they increase or decrease the client's stress levels? Do they empower or undermine him or her? What messages about self do family and friends provide? What other issues are occurring in the family (e.g., job losses, illness, frequent moves, etc.)?

Relational style

What relationship style characterizes most of the client's relationships? Open? Trusting? Suspicious? Manipulative? What are the client's general views of others? What is the therapeutic relationship like? Can the client be honest about symptoms, actions, side effects and concerns? Can he or she honestly disclose the level of compliance with recommendations? Does he or she feel comfortable correcting any misassumptions made in the course of treatment?

School/work

In what setting does the client attend school? Where does he or she work? Is school/work perceived as challenging? Supportive? Meaningful? Frustrating? Does it increase or decrease the client's stress levels? Does it empower or undermine him or her?

Mentors and models

What real, historical, or metaphorical figures serve as pillars of support or spiritual guides? How have they handled similar problems? Note: Some models may be primarily negative in tone. What are the positive aspects of these "negative" models?

Sense—and sources—of meaning

What sense of meaning does the client have and from where? Is life meaningful? Chaotic? Unpredictable? What is his or her worldview? From where is meaning drawn? Does he or she have a strong sense of

(continues)

TABLE **6.1**
Questions to Address during the Assessment Phase and throughout Therapy (Continued)

purpose or mission in life? A strong sense of direction? How "on track" does the client perceive his or her life to be regarding ultimate sources of meaning and purpose?

Community resources

What agencies (if any) are involved? How supportive are they? How well do they work together? Are they at loggerheads, undermining each other's recommendations, or do they generally share information in an open and collaborative manner?

Community contributions

How does the client contribute to the community? Does this contribution feel useful and meaningful to him or her? Are contributions acknowledged by important people in his or her support system? Are they related to and do they feed spiritual goals?

Obstacles and opportunities to change process

What might serve as potential obstacles or aids to the change process? These can be financial, educational, social, intellectual, spiritual, etc. What does he or she believe will (or might) happen when change occurs (e.g., marriage will dissolve, family will work together more effectively, will lose financial support, will be excommunicated from the Church, etc.)?

Note: Modified from Park & Slattery, 2008; Slattery, 2004; Slattery & Park, in press.

The Young Malcolm
Malcolm X

Malcolm Little was born into a society full of problems and into a family that expected him to do something about whatever he faced. Numerous threads contributed to his activism: the surrounding violence, color and race consciousness, and poverty, in particular, but also the family's mobility and search for self-sufficiency.

Born in 1925, Malcolm was Rev. Earl and Louise Little's fourth of their seven children together and his father's seventh. Malcolm was born in Omaha, Nebraska. While his mother was pregnant with him, their home was threatened by the Ku Klux Klan. His parents waited until Malcolm was born, then moved to Milwaukee, Wisconsin. Shortly after his younger brother's birth they moved to Lansing, Michigan, a place where his parents hoped for greater financial independence. His remaining four siblings were born there. His youngest brother was born 7 years after Mr. Little's death.

In 1929, his family was threatened again, this time by the Black Legion. The previous attack had broken their windows; this time their home was burned to the ground. The police and fire departments were called to the fire but they just stood watching the devastation. The Little family then moved outside of East Lansing, Michigan, where they could be largely self-sufficient.

(continues)

His father, a Baptist minister, was a follower of Marcus Garvey, who argued that "freedom, independence and self-respect could never be achieved by the Negro in America, and that therefore the Negro should leave America to the white man and return to his African land of origin" (Malcolm X & Haley, 1964/1999, p. 2). Malcolm attributed his father's Black separatist attitudes to the violence his family suffered. Four of Malcolm's uncles were killed by White men, one in a lynching. Malcolm's father was also reportedly murdered by White men. Malcolm X later said, "It has always been my belief that I, too, will die by violence. I have done all I can to be prepared" (Malcolm X & Haley, 1964/1999, p. 2).

Race and the racism that permeated his environment were formative factors in Malcolm's development. His family was very aware of color differences; he suspected that his father favored him, because he "was his lightest child. Most Negro parents in those days would almost instinctively treat any lighter children better than they did the darker ones" (Malcolm X & Haley, 1964/1999, p. 4). Because of his father's favoritism, Malcolm also traveled with his father to the meetings of Garvey's followers. He described feeling that Blacks at these meetings were "more intense, more intelligent and down to earth" in this setting than in other places where he saw them and "made me feel the same way" (Malcolm X & Haley, 1964/1999, p. 6). This intensity and naturalness were qualities that he valued in himself and others in his adulthood.

In contrast to Malcolm's father, his mother was born in Grenada and looked White. Her mother had been raped by a White man. Malcolm believed that his mother, as a result, favored her darker children.

> I remember that she would tell me to get out of the house and "Let the sun shine on you so you can get some color." She went out of her way never to let me become afflicted with a sense of color-superiority. I am sure that she treated me this way partly because of how she came to be light herself. (Malcolm X & Haley, 1964/1999, p. 8)

Mrs. Little was a force to be reckoned with, holding high standards for their children and making sure that they were well-educated. Her oldest son, Wilfred, described their childhood like this:

> [W]hen we were doing our homework, there was always a dictionary on the table, and when we mispronounced a word my mother made us look it up and learn both to spell and to pronounce it correctly. By reading that Marryshow paper day after day, we developed reading and writing skills superior to those of our white classmates. By reading Garvey's paper and Marryshow's paper, we got an education in international affairs and learned what Black people were doing for their own betterment all over the world. (Carew, 1998, p. 21)

While much of the violence that Malcolm saw was overt—including violence between his parents and toward their children—other violence was often subtle and more pervasive. Police and firefighters did not respond when their family home was attacked. The insurance companies paid off the smaller, but not the larger, of his father's life insurance policies after

(continues)

(continued)

his murder. The welfare system undermined, then split up, Malcolm's family after his father's death. Regarding this last, he wrote:

> I knew I wouldn't be back to see my mother [in the state hospital] again because it could make me a very vicious and dangerous person—knowing how they had looked at us as numbers and as a case in their book, not as human beings. [My mother] was a statistic that didn't have to be, that existed because of a society's failure, hypocrisy, greed, and lack of mercy or compassion.... I have no mercy or compassion in me for a society that will crush people, and then penalize them for not being able to stand up under the weight. (Malcolm X & Haley, 1964/1999, p. 22)

He learned to identify both kinds of violence, recognizing that subtle violence was as destructive as its more overt sibling.

In Malcolm X's childhood stories, Whites were at best a benign presence, generally helpful when he excelled by their rules—as he did in school—and when he did not rock the boat. When he spoke out, when he tried to take more than they thought he should have, they quickly backed off or moved him to a safer distance. For example, when he was 13, a teacher asked what he wanted to be when he grew up. He said he wanted to be a lawyer.

> Mr. Ostrowski looked surprised, I remember, and leaned back in his chair and clasped his hands behind his head. He kind of half-smiled and said, "Malcolm, one of life's first needs is for us to be realistic. Don't misunderstand me, now. We all here like you, you know that. But you've got to be realistic about being a nigger. A lawyer—that's no realistic goal for a nigger. You need to think about something you *can* be. You're good with your hands—making things. Everybody admires your carpentry shop work. Why don't you plan on carpentry? People like you as a person—you'd get all kinds of work."
>
> The more I thought afterwards about what he said, the more uneasy it made me. It just kept treading around in my mind.
>
> What made it really begin to disturb me was Mr. Ostrowski's advice to others in my class—all of them white.... They all reported that Mr. Ostrowski had encouraged what they had wanted. Yet nearly none of them had earned marks equal to mine.... But apparently I was still not intelligent enough, in their eyes, to become whatever *I* wanted to be.
>
> It was then that I started to change—inside. (Malcolm X & Haley, 1964/1999, p. 38, italics in original)

Religion was important to both of his parents—his father was a Baptist preacher, his mother a Seventh Day Adventist. However, "Even at that young age, I couldn't believe in the Christian concept of Jesus as someone divine. And no religious person... could tell me anything. I had very little respect for most people who represented religion." (Malcolm X & Haley, 1964/1999, p. 5).

Malcolm's native skills in many different areas—academics, social skills, dancing, carpentry, hunting—gave Malcolm a leg up. But several

(continues)

other things also influenced him. He had two very powerful and assertive role models: his father and his half-sister Ella. His father believed that things could be different for Blacks and worked to make it happen. Ella was "the first really proud black woman I had ever seen in my life" (Malcolm X & Haley, 1964/1999, p. 34). Although he didn't follow her upper middle-class path, she showed him that one could aim high, be successful, and reach out to help other Blacks. From his quiet brother, Wilfred, who often went hungry as a result of his lack of assertiveness, he learned that "if you want something, you had better make some noise" (p. 8). And, he also concluded, "that anytime you find someone more successful than you are, especially when you're both engaged in the same business—you know they're doing something that you aren't" (p. 21).

1. What questions would you want to ask to further flesh out your understanding of Malcolm? How would you go about asking them?
2. If you tended to focus on problems as you read his story, go back and identify strengths. Why might this be useful in your work with him?
3. The numbers in Table 4.1 are for the *current* status of African Americans, rather than for their status when Malcolm was a child, which were far worse. Nonetheless, what does this say about the conditions under which African Americans frequently live—or the context against which they may be judged or which they may react to? Why might these be important to pay attention to when working with him?

As seen in the case material and in the psychosocial history in Table 6.2, Malcolm's story is complicated, including both considerable violence and family problems (e.g., parental arguments and domestic violence, murders, poverty, his early fighting and thieving), but also numerous strengths (e.g., good health, academic success, an assertive and gregarious nature, strong work ethic, and strong spiritual background). It would be easy to overlook either the weaknesses or strengths; systematically gathering them encourages a more complete clinical assessment. Other issues of note:

- Malcolm has considerable supports, but many of these seem conflictual in nature. What does this mean in terms of how he sees and interacts with others? What does this mean about what he will expect to find in treatment and how he will respond?
- Malcolm reports numerous racist events (e.g., his family members' murders, his family home being burned, his family's color bias) that influence how he sees the world. Failing to pay attention to race and racism in treatment would probably undermine the therapeutic relationship.
- Despite numerous stressors that would crush others, if anything, Malcolm seems to have been strengthened by these stressors. He seems to both recognize injustice and believe that he can do something about rectifying it. He is someone with considerable self-efficacy and an internal locus of control who admires assertive action in others. Taking a passive or neutral stance in treatment would likely be ineffective. Because he was

TABLE **6.2**
A Psychosocial History of Malcolm Little in 1940, Age 15.[1]

	Objective description	Client's global and situational meanings	Hypotheses about treatment
The problem			
Presenting problem or symptoms	Caught stealing food and other items occasionally, engaging in small mischief (e.g., tipping outhouses), and fighting with his brother and other teens.	Feels justified in these actions, both supporting family and opposing a system he sees as racist.	Does not see himself as source of problems and may be unmotivated to change.
Precipitating event and other recent events	His father died in a train accident 10 years earlier; the courts ruled his death a suicide, although the family discounts this. He reports that his parents were both abusive of each other and of their children, although his father was not abusive to him. In the last 4 years his siblings were split up and put into foster care. His mother was placed in a psychiatric hospital 2 years ago. The family has not had enough food to eat following his father's alleged murder.	Sees life circumstances as unfair and, frequently racist.	Joining may necessitate recognizing and naming racism in his life.
Personal and family history of psychological problems	Denies a history of psychological symptoms, attributing problems to the racist society he lives in. Reported, however, that his mother had been recently placed in a psychiatric hospital as a result of a "nervous breakdown."	Angry at the system that forced his mother's hospitalization. Attributed his mother's hospitalization to psychosocial stressors, especially pervasive racism.	Aligning with his meaning of these events, at least initially, may be necessary to join.
Current Context			
Physical condition and medication use	Is strong and in good health. Good basketball player. No health problems reported. No medications reported.	Values his health, which he sees as outward manifestation of his personal vitality.	These strengths influence his self-concept and are strengths that can be harnessed in treatment.

---

[1] The information included here is consistent with Malcolm X and Haley (1964/1999); however, because Malcolm X's accounts are retrospective, selective, and incomplete, this material is included for its educational rather than its historical value.

TABLE **6.2**
A Psychosocial History for Malcolm Little in 1940, Age 15 (Continued)

	Objective description	Client's global and situational meanings	Hypotheses about treatment
Drug/alcohol use	None reported for client or family.	No problem.	
Intellectual/cognitive functioning	Reports being one of the top students in his class. Thinks abstractly, both recognizing what is and also what could be.	Feels smart and competent and sees this as a means for meeting personal goals.	More strengths to harness in treatment.
Coping style	Reports identifying problems, recognizing their societal causes, and protesting these loudly.	Sees this coping style as normal and healthy.	More strengths. Treatment should be active and address societal injustices.
Self-concept	Sees self as "intuitive" like his mother, and as capable of addressing or circumventing problems.	Values his style of approaching the world.	His self-efficacy can foster change. Treatment should be active and intuitive rather than rational.
Sociocultural background	Is African American in a frankly racist society. His parents have had two houses threatened, one burned to the ground. Five of his uncles and his father were murdered in race-related violence. Attended Marcus Garvey's group as a young child with his father and felt that the members of this Black separatist group were "more intense, more intelligent, and down to earth" than other Blacks.	Sees world as racist and unfair, with normal means to success being blocked. Sees the activist and separatist approach of Marcus Garvey as offering an avenue for success.	Race and issues of social justice must be addressed in treatment. Describes several positive African-American models. White workers, especially those failing to acknowledge and challenge racism, will have difficulty creating an effective therapeutic alliance.
Spirituality and religion	Was raised in a family with strong religious beliefs. His father was a Baptist minister. His mother is a Seventh Day Adventist and has been criticized for refusing "unclean foods," given their obvious poverty. He reports not believing that Christ was divine or respecting most religious leaders.	Feels disillusioned about much organized religion.	Although he feels disillusioned about organized religions, religion has been both a family strength and a unique part of their family identity. This may be a resource to access in treatment.

(continues)

TABLE **6.2**
A Psychosocial History for Malcolm Little in 1940, Age 15 (Continued)

	Objective description	Client's global and situational meanings	Hypotheses about treatment
Trauma history	His father was reportedly murdered when he was five; his uncles were also murdered. Insurance companies and the community were perceived as unresponsive and disbelieving. His parents were violent toward each other and sometimes toward their children.	This history of race-related violence has alienated him from mainstream (White) community and created an expectation that he will die young as the result of violence.	This sense of alienation and hopelessness might undermine the therapeutic relationship and may be a significant barrier to change. What does he see himself as able to change?
Resources and Barriers			
Individual resources	Has strong reading and writing skills, and is a strong problem solver. Is a good debater, hard working, and assertive. Is a good carpenter, gardener, and hunter. Recognizes that he can learn from anyone, including people who are more successful than he is.	Sees these individual strengths as attributes that will make him successful in almost any situation.	Has considerable self-efficacy and high aspirations that can be helpful in treatment. These can partially counterbalance his feelings of hopelessness about racial injustice.
Social resources (family and friends)	Client is the seventh of 11 children (fourth in his father's second marriage). Despite numerous stressors, his family has considerable strengths. His parents were strong models who worked hard to create a sustainable life in the face of racism. His father strongly supported him, while his mother challenged him. He and his siblings fight with each other, but are also loyal and supportive. Since his father's alleged murder, the family has been very poor and without food; some children have been placed in foster care.	Values the social support within his family and attributes recent problems to racism and the ways that the system has undermined his family.	Wants the welfare system and treatment to support rather than undermine family.

TABLE **6.2**
A Psychosocial History for Malcolm Little in 1940, Age 15 (Continued)

	Objective description	Client's global and situational meanings	Hypotheses about treatment
Relational style	Dominant, gregarious, and argumentative. He is intuitive and able to read others well. He is able to get them to like and help him.	Feels good about his social skills. Believes that reading others is a way of meeting his individual goals.	His social skills might create a difficult therapeutic relationship, but could also be a significant strength in other parts of his life.
Work/school	Is near the top of his class in school; however, when he announced that he wanted to be a lawyer when he grew up, a favorite teacher instead encouraged him to be "realistic" and become a carpenter.	Sees teacher's evaluation of his future as unfair and as a major impetus to his recognition of racism.	Needs to find some way of resolving this discrepancy between his abilities and his treatment by society.
Mentors and models	Sees both his father and oldest sister as proud and capable and had strong, positive relationships with both. His mother emphasized the importance of learning and hard work, which he respected. On the other hand, he saw his brother Wilfred going hungry because he was both quiet and unassertive. He learned that you've got to "make some noise" to get what you want.	Sees people as getting ahead by being strong, proud, capable, assertive, and smart. These qualities were valued in his family, although not within the racist society in which he lives—at least when these lead him to excel or become "uppity."	These mentors and models indicate social resources, but also attributes that he wants to develop. They can be accessed when he looks for positive ways to resolve problems.
Sense—and sources—of meaning in life	Is both acutely aware that the world is racist, color-conscious, and unfair, but also believes that if one makes "some noise," things can be changed. Although surrounded by violence throughout his childhood, he believed that his mind was a more important agent of change than violence alone. Believes that he will also die a violent death.	Recognizes the importance of being smart, but also of "making noise" to make a difference. Does not see a positive personal outcome to his struggles.	Focus is individual, familial, and societal. Framing treatment goals only individually would miss an important part of his story.

(continues)

TABLE **6.2**
A Psychosocial History for Malcolm Little in 1940, Age 15 (Continued)

	Objective description	Client's global and situational meanings	Hypotheses about treatment
Community resources	Families in the community have been buying food from client and his siblings, as well as sharing food with the family. The welfare system is actively monitoring the family since his mother was hospitalized; they are considering placing her younger children in foster care.	Is ambivalent about his neighbors' support and very negative about the welfare system's involvement in his family.	Wants supportive relationships, not those that he sees as undermining his family or himself.
Community contributions	None reported, although he is actively supportive of family and neighbors.	Feels strong and capable. Sees this as normative.	A strength to harness in treatment.
Obstacles and opportunities in change process	Is bright, capable, with strong sense of self-efficacy. Has been undermined or treated as a "pet" by authority figures.	Distrusts most Whites and authority figures. Does not see himself as having a problem, attributing problems to societal factors.	Should consider racial identity in assigning clinician. Choose goals that he is willing to work toward, while acknowledging societal contributions to problems. Acknowledge and access considerable strengths in treatment.

referred as a result of minor mischief and thieving, perhaps treatment should focus on helping him identify positive ways of responding to stressors and oppression.

• Although there are considerable stressors and conflict within his family, Malcolm also reports considerable support and numerous positive models. As a result, perhaps treatment should identify ways of making these supports more effective for him.

Often the write-up of a psychosocial history follows a standard format that includes the first two columns from Table 6.2, although generally using headings and brief paragraphs. We include two additional columns: the meanings that clients draw in response to factors described in the psychosocial history and hypotheses about the impact of these events on treatment (Slattery & Park, in press). Although these last two columns are not normally included in psychosocial histories, they illustrate the kind of thinking in which a reflective clinician might engage while gathering or reading a psychosocial history, the sort of thinking that builds empathy.

Family Genogram

The **family genogram** (McGoldrick et al., 1999) is a visual means of generating hypotheses about familial factors that may contribute to the problem or serve as resources to treatment. Simple genograms generally include genealogical material, but they also show relationships, patterns of mental health diagnoses or substance abuse, and major events in a family history. Most genograms include basic information about number of marriages and children, birth order, and deaths (see Figure 6.2). Genograms can also include information on disorders running in the family (e.g., alcoholism and depression), alliances, the nature of relational interactions (e.g., cut-offs and enmeshments), and living situations. Slattery (2004) described using genograms to track family strengths. Their use is only limited by the imagination.

One way of using genograms is to keep track of complicated family information; this would certainly be advantageous for a clinician working with Malcolm Little (see Figure 6.3). Another, more important use of genograms, however, is to generate hypotheses about family relationships. For example, family events have unique meaning, and familial patterns may be carried forward to impact future generations (either be repeated or reacted to). While the meaning of family events and patterns may differ across clients, some issues are common across people. Triangles often reflect and cause problems in communication; enmeshed families often have difficulties with privacy and boundaries. Some questions and hypotheses that could be drawn based on the patterns in Malcolm Little's genogram include the following:

- How might being his father's fourth child in his second marriage, seventh of 11 children total, have influenced Malcolm? What about the relatively close spacing of children in his parents' marriage—seven children in 9 years?
- Malcolm reported that his skin color created and, perhaps, undermined alliances in his family. How was this influenced by his grandmother's rape? How did his skin color and people's reactions to it influence how he saw himself and his relationships with others?
- How did his father's and uncles' murders by White men—and his grandmother's rape—influence Malcolm's self-concept, activism, and attitudes about race?
- There appears to be an important triangle between Malcolm and his parents—what was its impact on his family status? How might that influence his later relationships?
- How can the alliances in the family be used to support Malcolm during this vulnerable period?

Because family genograms are a standard part of family therapy and have been well-described elsewhere (McGoldrick et al., 1999), they will not receive detailed coverage here. Nonetheless, as seen in this brief description

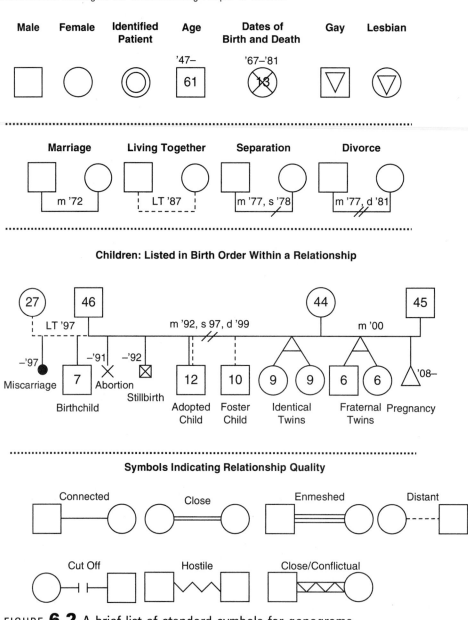

FIGURE **6.2** A brief list of standard symbols for genograms.

Note: Modified from McGoldrick (1999).

of Malcolm Little's family genogram, they help clinicians keep track of complicated extended families and are an important tool for generating hypotheses about clients' symptoms and problems. They can be very useful for helping clients gain insight into their family's patterns.

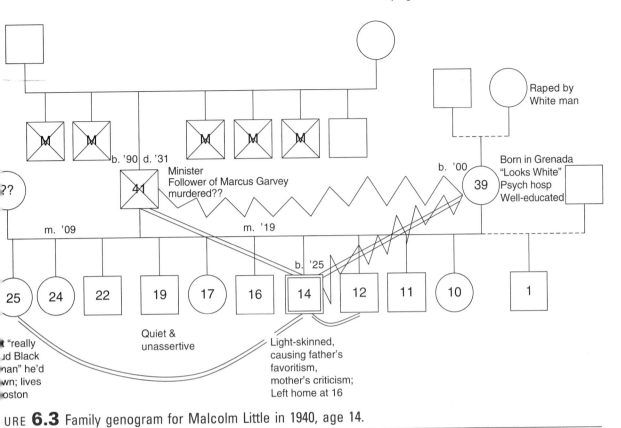

URE 6.3 Family genogram for Malcolm Little in 1940, age 14.

Timeline

People exist in a family and systemic context; however, they also exist in a temporal context. A **timeline** is a useful strategy for describing clients' temporal and historical context, and can be especially useful with people who have complicated histories or for whom the relationships among events are unclear.

A timeline is a record from birth to the present describing all major events for clients and their immediate family. It is a handy organizing system for information and highlights the temporal contiguity of events. Timelines generally include the kinds of information gathered during a family genogram, including dates of births, deaths, marriages, divorces, and so on in the immediate family. In addition, timelines record both the mundane (e.g., a voluntary job change) and the unusual (e.g., being charged with statutory rape).

One way of looking at a timeline is as a kind of informal version of the Social Readjustment Rating Scale (SRRS, Holmes & Rahe, 1967). However, instead of simply listing stressors in the last year, as the SRRS does, a timeline looks at stressors and major events *from the client's idiosyncratic point of view* over the lifespan. That is, while flying may not be a stressor for most people, being told that one has to fly across country as a regular and ongoing part of one's job could be a major stressor for someone who is phobic about flying. Furthermore, timelines afford the opportunity to look at clustering of stressors as well as reactions to them. Losing a job is almost always a stressor, but its meaning may be amplified during a year when a child has been diagnosed with cancer, one's partner has asked for a divorce, and the mortgage has gone into default. In addition, the person who experiences four major stressors in a relatively quiet life may perceive these stressors differently than the person who has had major stressors throughout life.

Generally this assessment process also notes reactions to these stressors, including depression, suicide attempts, ulcers, and increased drinking. How does the person respond to stressors? Do relatively trivial stressors overwhelm the client or can clusters of stressors be handled well? Has this pattern of reactions changed across time, with the person seeming to become either more easily overwhelmed or hardier and more stress-resistant? What sorts of stressors seem to overwhelm the client (e.g., job-related, interpersonal, familial)? Is there any sort of theme to these stressors (e.g., personal threat, loss of control, perceived abandonment)?

A number of the themes raised in the timeline echo those seen in Malcolm Little's psychosocial history and genogram (see Table 6.3).

- Malcolm reports his parents had a number of children in rapid succession, again echoing the questions raised by the genogram about the availability of physical and emotional resources in the family.
- He had a number of significant traumas throughout his life including five murders, two house fires, his mother's psychological decline, and his placement in foster care. To what extent are the concerns raised by the referring agency related to trauma?
- The family's level of functioning appeared to decline in the years following his father's murder—to what extent was this related to grief and to what extent poverty?

Each of these hypotheses suggests that the problem is treatable, although in different ways.

This timeline is useful in organizing information from Malcolm's life, but it provides an incomplete picture of his experience. Rather than being a defeated and traumatized child, Malcolm is bright, astute, and assertive. How did he get that way? Although his psychosocial history begins to answer this question, his timeline should also incorporate these strengths in order to provide a three-dimensional clinical assessment that will engage him in therapy. Adding the information in Table 6.4 begins to round out this story.

Mental Status Evaluation

An important part of most assessments is a description of mental status. The client's mental status in numerous areas including mood, affect, cognition, and impulsivity is normally assessed in the course of other assessments or during treatment. Along with other assessments, a **mental status evaluation** creates a three-dimensional description of the client's psychological status during the assessment. Such evaluations are helpful to the process of differential diagnosis, and can help a clinician conclude whether social isolation, for example, is related to depressive processes, developing psychotic processes, or an autistic spectrum disorder.

TABLE **6.3**
A Timeline of Malcolm Little's Recent Family History and His Early Life.[2]

1890—Earl Little was born in Reynolds, Georgia.

1900—Louise Norton was born in Grenada.

1909—Earl Little married Daisy Mason, his first wife.

1914—Ella was born.

1915—Mary was born.

1917—Earl was born.

1919—Earl Little married his second wife, Louise Norton, in Montreal.

1920—Wilfred was born.

1922—Hilda was born.

1923—Philbert was born.

1924—Family and home threatened by the KKK while Mrs. Little was pregnant with Malcolm.

1925—Malcolm was born.

1926—Moved to Milwaukee, WI.

1927—Reginald was born.

1928—Family moved to Lansing, MI, hoping for financial independence.

Wesley was born.

1929—Yvonne was born.

Home was threatened and burned to the ground while fire department watched.

Family moved outside of East Lansing, MI.

1931—Earl Little was run over by a streetcar and died; he was rumored to have been murdered by a White supremacist group. Two of the family's three insurance policies refused to pay, claiming that Mr. Little had committed suicide. Family had difficulty putting food on the table.

1936—Mrs. Little was courted by a "large, dark man from Lansing."

1937—Mrs. Little's relationship ended—perhaps because of the number of mouths to feed. Mrs. Little began to decline: "the beginning of the end of reality for my mother."

Family was "destroyed" by state, which began placing children in foster care.

1938—Robert was born. Malcolm was expelled from school.

Mrs. Little was declared legally insane and committed to a state hospital.

Note: Drawn from Malcolm X & Haley, 1964/1999; Twenty-first Century Books, 2008.

Unlike similar-sounding assessments, including the **Mini-Mental State Exam** (Folstein, Folstein, & McHugh, 1975), descriptions of mental status include both client strengths and weaknesses. The specific content of the mental status evaluation varies considerably depending on the evaluation setting and

----

[2] Dates from official sources describing Malcolm X's life are inconsistent and contradictory. Information included here is not presented for its historical accuracy—although we believe it to be consistent with available historical records—but to describe how one might use biographical information to understand a person.

TABLE **6.4**
Strength-Based Additions to Malcolm Little's Timeline.

1929—Family moved outside of East Lansing, MI, hoping to become self-sufficient, and built home.
1929–1931—Traveled with father to the meetings of Garvey's followers. Described believing that Blacks at these meetings were "more intense, more intelligent and down to earth."
1931–1938—Attended school and was recognized as one of the smartest and most talented children by both adults and children, Whites and Blacks.

Note: Drawn from Malcolm X & Haley, 1964/1999; Twenty-first Century Books, 2008.

the population assessed (e.g., an adult in an Alzheimer's wing of a nursing home or a preschool assessment of a child suspected to have autism), but generally includes the following areas.

- **Appearance.** The client's age, race, sex, relational status, dress, grooming, gait, posture, level of activity, and coordination.
- **Interviewer/client relationship.** The client's interpersonal skills and the rapport between client and interviewer are described as well as the clinician's perception of the interview's validity. A weak relationship between interviewer and client can cause the client to withhold or disguise information, which introduces bias in interpreting other indicators.
- **Affect and mood.** Mood refers to the client's "emotional atmosphere," which is internal, subjective, and relatively more sustained and which may vary across time. Mood is often inferred from the client's verbal tone and subjective report. **Affect** refers to the client's observable emotion. Descriptions of affect usually include level of reactivity (i.e., flat, blunted, restricted, normal, broad, labile) and the congruency between affective expression and verbal content. In addition to describing current status, indicators of anxiety or affective disorders are noted (e.g., eye contact, posture, nervous mannerisms).
- **Speech and language use.** The volume, speed, fluency, length, and articulation quality of responses, their appropriateness to the situation, and the clarity of answers are assessed. Unusual speech components (e.g., echolalia, overgeneralization, poor word use) are identified.
- **Cognition and memory.** Includes alertness, attention, concentration, and orientation (to person, place, time, and purpose of interview), long and short-term memory, general intellectual level and fund of knowledge, abstract thought, and the ability to perform simple tasks (e.g., arithmetic, reading and repeating sentences, ability to understand and perform tasks, and copy or generate figures).
- **Disorders in thinking.** Problems in fluently expressing thoughts in speech include irrelevant detail, unnecessarily repeated words and phrases, interrupted thinking (thought blocking), and loose, illogical connections. Disease processes may be reflected in behavioral indications or verbal reports of hallucinations, delusions, obsessions, dissociative processes, derealization, depersonalization, and confusion about one's identity. Thoughts of suicide or homicide are described as well as indicators of level of dangerousness.
- **Insight and judgment.** Insight refers to an awareness of the presenting problem and its nature, severity, and need for treatment, while judgment

refers to the ability to identify reasonable and appropriate responses to commonsense problems. Judgment is often identified by looking at a client's pattern of coping with problems, including whether coping efforts tend to increase or decrease problems.

Do Malcolm's actions reflect sociopathy? Mental retardation? Depression? Poor social skills and social awareness? Cultural alienation? Notice how the write-up of a mental status evaluation for Malcolm Little provides a new perspective on his behaviors that, with previously gathered information, helps to draw a differential diagnosis (see Table 6.5).

TABLE **6.5**

Mental Status Section of a Report That Might Have Been Written for Malcolm Little in 1940, When He Was 15.[3]

Malcolm Little is a tall, thin, 15-year-old African-American boy, who appears older than his stated age. He was well-groomed and neatly dressed in a dapper green suit, of which he appeared proud. His gait was athletic and exuberant, his gestures loose. He was charming and affable and responded openly to questions, suggesting that the observations made would be valid. He is currently in the eighth grade, where he reports he is excelling. His mother has recently been placed in Kalamazoo State Mental Hospital after a nervous breakdown; his father was reportedly murdered in racial violence when he was 5. Michigan Department of Human Services is considering placing Malcolm in foster care after a series of small thefts and petty mischief in school and the community.

Malcolm's affect was broad and generally matched the content of the interview. He neither appeared depressed nor anxious, and reported no symptoms of either. He leaned forward, and maintained good eye contact and a relaxed open posture throughout the interview. He displayed no nervous habits except tossing a small ball that he had brought to the interview and playing with small objects on the desk. Despite his apparent relaxation, several times he seemed to become vigilant and less disclosing verbally and in his facial expressions, especially in response to questions about the welfare system's involvements with his family.

Malcolm reported no hallucinations or delusions; no evidence of these or any sort of dissociative or other disease process was observed. He reported no history of suicidal or homicidal ideation and, although he had a number of visible scratches, scrapes, and bruises, reported no history of self-injurious behavior, instead attributing injuries to a recent hunting expedition through underbrush.

Malcolm is a bright, abstract thinker who responded nimbly to questions. Rather than responding only to the direct questions asked, he was able to respond cogently to the underlying question and identify patterns in his life. His speech was within normal limits in rate, tone, and modulation, varying in volume to emphasize his points. He used an unusually large vocabulary, with well-developed sentences, carefully chosen words evincing a history of wide and thoughtful reading, and a sophisticated use of alliteration and puns. He was assertive and outspoken, his speech clearly and forcefully articulated with few stutters or interruptions.

Malcolm was observant and socially curious, noticing small details and drawing good insights into his and others' behaviors. He appeared self-confident and interacted comfortably with adults. However, his recent thievery and petty mischief is impulsive and narcissistic in tone, and demonstrates poor judgment. He admitted to having committed the thefts with which he was accused, justifying his acts based both on his family's current poverty and the ways that his family has been mistreated.

---

[3] The information included here is consistent with Malcolm X and Haley (1964/1999); however, because Malcolm X's accounts are retrospective, selective, and incomplete, this material is included for its educational rather than its historical value.

Although a mental status evaluation can be very useful in identifying the presence of problems and pinpointing their nature, it can be subjective in nature based on the worldviews of interviewer as well as interviewee. Being aware of this subjectivity and its impact on the validity of the interview is important, especially for assessments of clients raised in an ethnic community, another country, or those for whom the interview language was not their first language. Even when clinicians and clients share a language and country of origin, nonverbal behaviors and colloquial language can have very different meanings for each party. As a result, written reports of mental status evaluations include both inferences and the observations leading to them. This allows the reader to evaluate the data used to draw conclusions and determine whether other interpretations of the interview data might be more valid.

TAKING MULTIPLE PERSPECTIVES

It does not do to leave a live dragon out of your calculations.

—J. R. R. Tolkien

Strong clinical assessments take advantage of multiple sources in order to gain multiple perspectives on clients and avoid rigid cognitive sets. When doing a clinical assessment of an oppositional child, a behavioral observation of the child, an interview with the parents, parent ratings (e.g., the Child Behavior Checklist; Achenbach & Rescorla, 2004), and consults with teachers are standard protocol in many settings.

Rather than only looking for a single view of clients, it is important to gather multiple perspectives. Empathic, effective clinicians listen to clients, but also observe their behavior—in their offices, waiting rooms, and other settings. They often talk to family members and contact other agencies involved in the case (e.g., Juvenile Probation, Child Protective Services, psychiatrists, and physicians). Clinicians can also have their clients make observations of the frequency, severity, antecedents, and consequences of their behavior.

In order to produce fair and unbiased clinical assessments when gathering material from multiple sources, clinicians should consider the following questions. What other perspectives of behaviors, problems, and symptoms can be taken? Which respondents report more problems and which fewer? What is different about those settings or respondents? What things do some sources omit? Are these differences related to differences in the observer's worldview and context? Are they related to differences in the settings in which the observer sees the client?

Food for Thought

In Andrea Yates's case (see Chapter 2), there are numerous original source materials available on the web. Although these sources have been summarized in or have influenced the case description in Chapter 2, draw your own conclusions by reading the original sources. Pay attention to the writer's viewpoint and biases.

(continues)

Associated Press. (2002, February 21). Transcript of Andrea Yates' confession. *Houston Chronicle.* Retrieved from http://www.chron.com/cs/CDA/story.hts/special/drownings/1266294#top
Overwhelming at times, but gives a good indication of her state of mind at the time of her confession.

Denno, D. W. (2003). Appendix 1. Timeline of Andrea Yates' life and trial. *Duke Journal of Gender Law and Policy, 10,* 61–84. Retrieved from http://www.law.duke.edu/journals/journaltoc?journal=djglp&toc=gentoc10n1.htm
A comprehensive summary of information contributing to Ms. Yates' state of mind at the time of the murders.

Religious Tracts by Michael Woroniecki. (2008, November 13). Retrieved from http://www.flickr.com/photos/86593188@N00/3028898336/sizes/1/in/set-72157609022093567
Copies of Michael Woroniecki's newsletter Perilous Times, *including sections introduced at Ms. Yates's trial.*

Yates, R. (n.d.). Welcome. Retrieved from http://www.yateskids.org.
Rusty Yates's site includes a variety of original materials, including photos and videotapes of his children and family, as well as a link to materials about his wife's case.

- What do you conclude after reading these materials? If your viewpoint shifted as you read additional sources, how did it shift? What influenced you?
- What biases did each writer have? How did these influence his or her presentation of the facts or conclusions?
- Given that everyone has biases, how can you listen to or read sources so as to reduce bias in your clinical assessments?

PULLING ASSESSMENT STRATEGIES TOGETHER

For every complex question there is a simple answer—and it's wrong.
—**H.L. Mencken**

The process of assessing clients and generating hypotheses discussed in Chapters 5 and 6 is an important way of building a careful and contextualized understanding of a client. We have described systematically gathering behavioral observations and information obtained during formal assessment strategies, drawing inferences and hypotheses from these strategies, then organizing these various types of information into an overall clinical assessment to guide treatment. When conducted well, this integrated assessment creates a three-dimensional picture of a client that moves the clinician beyond symptoms and problems to an empathic and contextualized understanding of a person. This empathy and contextualized understanding is essential for engaging clients, developing treatment goals and interventions, recognizing factors that increase or diminish problems, motivating change, anticipating barriers and obstacles to change, and harnessing strengths for treatment.

As the examples in this book demonstrate, there is often a web of interrelated factors that influence a person's behavior and current status. For example, abuse does not directly cause problems in current functioning; outcomes are moderated by the meanings people draw from the abuse, social support, intellectual and social strengths, previous level of functioning, and previous trauma history. A strong assessment pays attention to these factors to identify strengths and vulnerabilities and to generate effective treatment strategies.

Food for Thought

Writing up assessment reports well is an important skill that is described in more detail in Chapter 7. Table 6.6 presents an excerpt from a report addressing the referral questions that might have led Malcolm into treatment. While reading this excerpt, evaluate its strengths and weaknesses, then compare your reactions with the recommendations outlined in Chapter 7. Then, return to earlier cases (e.g., Andrea Yates and Lil Loco in Chapters 2 and 3, respectively), to practice using these assessment strategies and writing reports summarizing your clinical assessments of them.

TABLE **6.6**

Sections of an Evaluation Report for Malcolm Little.[4] Information leading to the summary and recommendations are omitted in this example, but are presented in rough form in earlier tables and figures.

Jenevieve J. Swanson, Ph.D.

Clinical Psychologist, Licensed in Michigan

1431 Maple Street

Kalamazoo, MI

Psychological Evaluation

Name: Malcolm Little

Date of birth: 5/19/1925

Date of assessment: 6/14/1940

Date of report: 6/16/1940

Reason for Referral: Malcolm Little was referred by Michigan Department of Human Services as a result of a series of small thefts and petty mischief in the community. They requested an assessment to determine why he is running into problems in school and the community and a recommendation as to whether an out-of-home placement is appropriate.

Ms. Little was made aware of the nature and purpose of this examination. First, that it was being performed at the request of Michigan Department of Human Services to identify what services would be necessary to stabilize her son and whether an out-of-home placement would be appropriate and necessary. Second, that a report based on this interview, third-party consultations, and completed assessments would be compiled for Michigan Department of Human Services and that this report would be used for the purpose of making recommendations regarding possible treatment. Given this, Ms. Little agreed to participate in this assessment.

Evaluation Procedures:

Interview with Malcolm Little (1.0 hr)

Interview with Mrs. Louise Little at Kalamazoo State Mental Hospital, gathering family genogram, psychosocial history, and timeline (2.0 hrs)

---

[4]Although this information is consistent with historical data, this material was not based on an original evaluation. Information included here is not presented for its historical accuracy, but to describe how one might perform an assessment and write about its products.

TABLE **6.6**
Sections of an Evaluation Report for Malcolm Little. Information leading to the summary and recommendations are omitted in this example, but are presented in rough form in earlier tables and figures (Continued)

Teacher Consult, Mr. Ostrowski (.25 hr)

Review of summary of client records, Michigan Department of Human Services

...

Summary and Recommendations: Malcolm Little is a 15-year-old African-American male with significant intellectual, physical, and social strengths. He has recently been acting out in school and engaging in petty thievery and mischief in the community.

Malcolm is the fourth of Mrs. Little's seven children. Both Malcolm and Mrs. Little report a significant history of violence and trauma, with at least five family members, including Malcolm's father, being reportedly murdered in racial violence. They also report having their house burned to the ground on two occasions and that Mrs. Little's mother was raped, leading to Mrs. Little's birth. Malcolm also described a positive history of domestic violence between Mr. and Mrs. Little, as well as physical abuse of most of their children, including Malcolm.

Malcolm admits that this pattern of violence has caused significant problems in the family, but reports as much or more concern about how he and his family have been mistreated within the community, especially by his White teachers, neighbors, and social workers. He believes that their actions are often racist, and that they have undermined his family. Both he and Mrs. Little report that she has been increasingly depressed since Mr. Little's murder 8 years ago and with their increasing poverty. He is especially concerned that his siblings have been placed in foster care and about the low expectations that a previously favorite teacher holds for him.

Malcolm has high self-efficacy and an internal locus of control, but an external locus of responsibility; he does not attribute the family's problems to himself or his mother. He sees his current actions as appropriate responses to a racist society that is systematically undermining his family. Malcolm has significant strong leadership skills, is assertive and believes in active responses to stressors, engages adults easily, and responds well to their mentoring when their behavior is racially sensitive.

Given these concerns, barriers to treatment, and individual and familial strengths, the following recommendations are made:

1. The Little family possesses significant strengths and appeared to be functioning very well until Mr. Little's death, which led to a significant loss in family income and social supports. Rather than removing the children to meet their physical and emotional needs, they would probably respond best to referrals to programs that provide financial support and access to food. Foods previously provided have not been sensitive to Mrs. Little's religious beliefs, which should be considered in future referrals.
2. Although Malcolm's current problems may be related to trauma and grief, Malcolm is unlikely to be receptive to traditional forms of psychotherapy. He may accept more active treatments, however, especially treatment that would mentor him and help him identify positive ways of responding to current stressors. He has had very good experiences with Marcus Garvey's church and might be open to efforts to find him a mentor there.
3. As Malcolm has felt that Whites have acted in oppressive and condescending ways, whoever works with him should be responsive to perceptions of racism and oppression in both the stressors that he reports and the services that he receives.
4. Some of the family instability stems from Mrs. Little's current depression and recent hospitalization. Although she is open to treatment currently offered at Kalamazoo State Mental Hospital, many of her symptoms seem to be reactive to the poverty and severe stressors that her family faces. Initial sessions should help her family stabilize, meet their basic physical needs, and develop natural supports in the community.

Respectfully submitted,

Jenevieve J. Swanson, Ph.D.

Licensed Psychologist

MI-5555P

SUMMARY

People exist in a context that influences how they perceive a situation and that directs and limits their responses to it. Failing to assess this context undermines attempts at understanding and empathy.

Four kinds of assessment strategies were discussed in this chapter: (a) psychosocial histories organize diverse information about clients' functioning in a variety of settings in written form; (b) genograms visually organize and present family relationships and family patterns in a way that is easily understood; (c) timelines list major events in clients' lives in a chronological order, which allows easy identification of temporal patterns; and (d) mental status evaluations carefully describe a client's psychological functioning in a number of realms. Each of these assessment strategies gathers information that might otherwise be easily overlooked.

People are three-dimensional beings, although they may come to therapy describing only one part of their lives—usually their symptoms and problems. Broadening the picture of a person by using a range of informants (e.g., client, parents, and teachers) and types of information is often very important to the therapy process. It can both help to generate additional hypotheses to explain why the client is behaving in a particular manner and identify opportunities and potential barriers to change.

How Do These Issues Apply to Your Life and Work?

Choose a problem in your own life and describe your view of factors influencing it. Next, create a psychosocial history, family genogram, and timeline for yourself. How would someone describe your mental status? Identify patterns that emerge from these assessments.

1. What new meanings and understandings emerge as you complete these assessments? How do these strategies change your view of this problem?
2. What psychological resources, social supports, and barriers to the change process do you identify? What factors would you need to consider if you were to decide to make changes?
3. Look at both your initial description of your problem and then the one based on the psychosocial history, family genogram, timeline, and mental status evaluation. How would you feel if someone were to use your initial definition of the problem or to develop the second, more three-dimensional view of you and your presenting problem? Note: Often psychosocial history, family genogram, and timelines are gathered so seamlessly in a session that clients may not even recognize this process.

CHAPTER **7**

Clinical Writing

WHERE ARE WE GOING?

1. Why is clinical writing important?

2. Describe how different types of clinical writing serve different purposes.

3. What characterizes effective clinical writing?

4. How is empathy important to clinical writing?

I'm Just Being a Freak
Claire Fisher, *Six Feet Under*

Claire Fisher (age 17) was referred to her guidance counselor, Mr. Deitman, after having placed a severed human foot in a fellow student's locker (Robin & Garcia, 2001). She is a high school student whose boyfriend's six-year-old brother was killed while playing with his parents' gun. Her boyfriend recently overdosed on a combination of heroin and speed.

Gary Deitman 1: Why didn't you tell me about your relationship with Gabriel Dimas?

Claire Fisher 1: Uh. [laughs] I guess I just wasn't in the mood for a lecture about inappropriate friends.

Mr. Deitman 2: What makes you think I would do this?

Claire 2: Some people don't think he's the greatest influence.

Mr. Deitman 3: What do you think?

Claire 3: I think I'm as much an influence on him as he is on me, so it's not like it only goes just one way.

Mr. Deitman 4: Right. Relating to another person is a way of relating to a part of ourselves.

Claire 4: [pause, looks down and away] He's like an extreme version of me, you know?

Mr. Deitman 5: [nods head] I can see that.

Claire 5: [stares, then quickly shakes head] But what he's going through. It's so much more. I understand, you know, feeling like you've got this shadow over you all the time. [looks up and makes eye contact]

Mr. Deitman 6: What's your shadow?

Claire 6: [frown, nervous laugh] Uhm. Death, I guess. [pause] Death and … silence? [laughs, shaking head] Is that crazy?

Mr. Deitman 7: What's the silence?

Claire 7: [reflective sigh] I don't know. It's like sadness or … [shakes head] fear maybe. [leans forward and speaks more rapidly] It's like, you know, everybody's so scared that they're going to say the wrong thing. Cuz like you know right when you bury someone it's the most sensitive time in a person's life. So, like my family, they're so careful. It's like they almost become invisible. [pause, shakes head, as if to reorient self] That was heavy. [long pause]

Mr. Deitman 8: [leans in] What's going on?

Claire 8: [dismissive] Nothing, I'm just being a freak.

Mr. Deitman 9: You don't have to be afraid that you'll say the wrong thing.

Claire 9: That's just it, I'm not. [laughs, begins gesticulating broadly] I mean, I do say the wrong thing. But, this is going to sound stupid, but I talk so much shit all the time, you know, and that's just another way to not say, whatever … [shakes head]

(continues)

Mr. Deitman 10: To not say what? [pause; CF opens eyes wide while maintaining eye contact, shakes head slowly] I'm not here for the school or for your mom. I'm just here for you.

Claire 10: [slower and quieter] This is confidential, right? [long pause; GD puts his pen down and moves it and his paper pen across the desk towards CF] Gabe didn't OD by accident. [nervous laugh] He did it on purpose, I think.

Mr. Deitman 11: Most ODs aren't really just accidents.

Claire 11: Right, so what can I do as the friend of a person who would do something like that? Like I know, I know all the "I can't save him stuff." I went to the websites. It's all like what you can't do. What <u>can</u> I do? [laughs, looks at him]

Mr. Deitman 12: Try not to make yourself invisible.

Claire 12: [points at herself with both hands] This isn't about me.

Mr. Deitman 13: That's not a very good start, is it? [CF opens her eyes wide, briefly holds her breath, staring] (Robin & Garcia, 2001)

- Identify at least half a dozen things from this scene that you observed about Claire or her guidance counselor.
- What inferences did you draw from these observations?
- How does your worldview influence your perceptions of this scene?
- Write a brief report about Claire using your observations and inferences.

WHY CLINICAL WRITING IS IMPORTANT

I write entirely to find out what I'm thinking, what I'm looking at, what I see and what it means.

—Joan Didion

Writing is a very important part of most clinical jobs—often taking 25% or more of a clinician's work time—and is an overt product reflecting one's clinical skills. Careful clinical writing both develops and reflects contextualized empathy for clients. This chapter describes clinical writing, especially how it differs from other technical or more informal kinds of writing.

Clinical writing is distinct from most other kinds of writing in that it is more formal, objective, and detailed. Its conclusions and recommendations are supported by clinical observations. Because clinical writing systematically organizes information from a number of realms, it offers clinicians an opportunity to develop empathy based in a complex knowledge of the person.

Clinical writing carefully documents and summarizes the clinician's thinking so that other readers can understand his or her conclusions and carry out recommendations. For example, the principal, a psychiatrist, a family therapist, and Claire's mother might each read a report written about Claire and implement some portions of its recommendations. Clinical writing can help the writer and readers develop a shared understanding and work together as a team, even though time and distance may prevent face-to-face contact. Furthermore, because readers and writers may not meet face-to-face, clinicians should be especially careful that their writing is clear and unambiguous.

Clinical writing includes conclusions and recommendations; however, many readers will also want to know the basis for those conclusions and recommendations so that they can evaluate their validity for themselves. As a result, most clinical writing starts out by presenting observations and inferences gathered in response to the particular **referral question**, then draws a clinical assessment of the problem, which is followed by treatment recommendations. This logical organization increases the report's effectiveness and usefulness. As we will discuss further in Chapter 8, referral questions depend on the referral source's concerns. For example, Claire's parents, the school, and her physician might each have different questions underlying their referral. The clinician should specifically address the questions raised by the referring source.

Claire may tell others what she thinks of her guidance counselor, but no one other than the two of them will directly see his clinical work. Instead, other parties' evaluations of his work are based on his clinical writing and his ability to talk clearly, knowledgeably, and empathically about his work. When reports are well-written, well-organized, logical, and complete; when the clinical assessment is contextualized, respectful, and empathic; when the conclusions follow the observations and are consistent with current theory and research—then readers will conclude that the clinician possesses strong clinical skills. One's professional reputation is valuable and should be protected and fostered.

Keeping records is often one of the least favorite aspects of treatment for many clinicians; some choose not to keep records as a result. Moline, Williams, and Austin (1998) explain clinicians' decisions not to keep records in a variety of ways. Some clinicians believe they can maintain confidentiality better without records; some clients ask clinicians not to keep them. Some clinicians fear that clients, attorneys, or insurance companies will disagree with their observations and assessments. Some are confused about what to document and what not to document or are overwhelmed by the time required to do careful documentation. Others, aware that therapeutic records could protect them in court, are convinced they will never go to court, so believe they do not need records.

Moline and her colleagues (1998) fall strongly on the side of thoughtful and accurate recordkeeping. They note that record keeping is a standard set by most professional organizations including American Association for Marriage and Family Therapy (AAMFT), American Counseling Association (ACA), American Psychological Association (APA), and National Association of Social Workers (NASW), as well as by state and federal laws. Records document that treatment occurred and was performed with good judgment, meeting the profession's standards of care. Careful, thoughtful documentation can protect clinicians from malpractice claims, ethics violations, and license reviews. Records can also help clinicians identify progress, remember and track symptoms and issues, and develop assessments.

In sum, clinical writing helps the clinician to build a strong empathic understanding of a client to guide effective treatment, and the clinician shares this clinical assessment with readers so that they can evaluate conclusions and recommendations. As a by-product, it gives readers a glimpse into the quality of the clinician's work. Finally, clinical writing can protect clinicians if faced with legal or ethical charges.

Effective clinical writing takes several different forms; each is related to its specific function in clinical work. Some of these forms are discussed below (i.e., brief report and SOAP note), while others will be discussed in later chapters. Both the form and the content of the writing address the specific purpose of the writing product and respond to the referral question.

BRIEF REPORTS

He doesn't watch, he notices.

—Thomas D'Evelyn

Although your brief "report" for Claire may have been good, it probably was less well-developed than the reports written by most counselors, therapists, social workers, and caseworkers. Most reports are between three and seven single-spaced pages in length, perhaps an amount of detail that initially seems impossible for new clinicians. As described in Table 7.1, they often include unusual behavior during the session, cognitive processes, mood and affect, consistency between verbal and nonverbal behaviors across time, style of relationships and relating, client's goals, willingness to change and more. Each of these aspects contributes to a three-dimensional picture of a person and influences the clinician's understanding of the client, the presenting problem, and resources or obstacles to treatment. A very brief report based on Claire's interview with her guidance counselor can be found in Table 7.2. Note the descriptions of mental status in this report and compare these descriptions to those of Malcolm X in Table 6.5.

TABLE **7.1**
Questions to Consider in a Report.

Referral question:

Why was this person referred for an appointment?

Closing paragraphs should address this question and recommendations should be supported by observations throughout the report.

Background and demographics:

Describe this person in terms of all information that may impact on the referral question or treatment: age, gender, race, language spoken (if not the native language of the community), immigrant status, custody status (for children of divorced/separated parents).

What background conditions may be relevant to the referral? These include a history of violence, family history of alcoholism, and a history of previous treatments.

Physical appearance:

Does the person appear healthy? Are there signs of physical illness or physical limitations?

Is the person well-nourished, undernourished, obese? Tall, short, or average for age?

Is the person well-groomed or, in the case of a dependent child or adult, well-cared for?

What is the person's general manner of dress? Casual? Formal? Appropriate, careless, or inappropriate for the setting?

What are the person's posture and gait like? Unremarkable? Tense? Rigid? Stooped? Slumped?

Symptoms:

What symptoms (e.g., anxiety, depression, inattention, anger, obsessions and compulsions, hallucinations or delusions) are reported? With what frequency and severity?

(continues)

TABLE **7.1**
Questions to Consider in a Report (Continued)

How long has the person had symptoms? Have symptoms remitted in the past? What does this person attribute these changes to?

What treatments (formal or informal) have been used in the past? Which were effective or ineffective?

When does the person *not* have problems? What times of day? What situations? With what people?

What kinds of stressors have been reported? How severe?

What are the person's coping level and normal strategies like? Normal? Resilient? Exhausted? Overwhelmed? Deficient skills? Deficient supports? Growing?

What supports exist? Family? Friends? Church? Co-workers? Social services? Are supports adequate, inadequate, or broad and well developed?

Cognition:

Is the person conscious? Oriented by four (i.e., of person, place, time, purpose of meeting)?

Is the person able to attend? Distractible?

Is the person able to concentrate and persist at tasks?

Were problems/strengths in short-term or long-term memory noted? How? Was information lost, distorted, or never coded? Are defects probably a consequence of dementia, a defense mechanism, problems in encoding or retrieval, or level of intellectual functioning?

What was the person's fund of information like? Was it consistent with the person's level of education? Has this shifted in the past (either by self-report or by history)?

Is reality perceived in a typical manner, consistent with most other perceptions? If not, is this positive and adaptive or otherwise? Is this the result of defensive distortions or psychosis?

Speech:

What is the flow of speech like? Unremarkable? Loud? Quiet? Mute? Blocked? Pressured? Paucity of ideas and content? Flight of ideas? Tangential?

Is the language of the session the client's first or primary language?

How are grammar and word choice? Unremarkable? Other than standard English? Words used or pronounced inappropriately? Fluent, thoughtful, with a well-developed vocabulary?

How coherent were the person's communications? Does A follow B? Are discontinuities evidence of creativity and enthusiasm or a psychotic disorder? How do you know?

What sorts of preoccupations (if any) characterize the person's thought processes? Death and dying? Current stressors? Mental health? Religion? Relationships? Escaping the situation? Sex? Drugs? Physical illness?

Is the person relatively concrete or an abstract thinker? Can he or she follow metaphors? Understand new ideas? Follow the implications of ideas?

Interpersonal presentation and behavior:

What sort of rapport was established? Did it change across the session? In what manner?

Was this person open and honest? If this wasn't consistent throughout the session, when did it shift?

What was eye contact like? Unremarkable? Fleeting? Avoided? Absent? Staring?

How did the person present? As withdrawn? Threatened? Vulnerable? Awkward? Shy? Friendly? Stubborn? Competent? Good?

TABLE **7.1**
Questions to Consider in a Report (Continued)

What is this person's self-esteem like? Are strengths recognized and valued? Self-esteem is rarely all good or all bad. Where is it strongest? Weakest? Physically? Intellectually? Relationally? Socially? Vocationally?

How does this person relate to others? In a warm, trusting manner? Aggressive? Dramatic? Help-seeking? Dependent? Aloof? Self-protective?

Is the person socially mature? Does he or she know and follow social norms?

Does the person have good common sense? Make good decisions? Engage in behaviors that are maladaptive and self-destructive?

What are interpersonal boundaries like? Is this person so reserved that little information is shared or is there an expectation that everything can be asked about or touched?

Mood:

Are emotions responsive to external stimuli? Are moods appropriate to the situation or topic being discussed in form and intensity? How labile are moods? Flat and unresponsive? Restricted? Normal and responsive? Labile and unpredictable?

What are this person's dominant and subdominant moods? Depression? Anxiety? Fear? Anger? Joy? Calm? Surprise? Pride? Guilt? Shame? Relaxation?

When do these moods appear? All the time? When certain topics are discussed? In response to certain triggers? Do these mood states seem (by self-report or report of others) to continue in other situations?

How are these mood states expressed? Pacing? Fidgeting? Body tension? Verbal outburst? Changing the subject?

Is anger or aggression directed inward or outward? With what consequences?

Are self-identified moods (e.g., "I am sad") consistent with interpersonal presentation?

Behavior:

Is he or she on time, late, early?

Does this person do anything that is unusual in the course of your session (or not do something that is usual)? When? How does this relate to your referral question?

What is the person's activity level like? Unremarkable? Slow? Repetitive? Restless? Agitated? Tremor?

Change process:

How motivated is the person to change? Does the person recognize that improvement is possible?

Does the client perceive advantages to changing? What obstacles to change are present? Does the client perceive these obstacles realistically?

What are the person's goals like? Are they clear and realistic? Are they goals that the person feels able to achieve?

Does the person possess insight into his or her behavior and the problems being faced?

Are problems perceived as internally or externally caused? Does the person perceive any ability to control the nature of these problems?

What is the person's level of self-efficacy about these particular problems or problems in general? When has this person changed successfully in the past—both for this problem/issue or others? What made this change possible?

Note: These questions will not always be relevant to your referral question, but they may be things to think about. Certainly, if you were to address each one, your report would be far too long. Based, in part, on Zuckerman (2000).

TABLE **7.2**

Report on Session between Claire and Her Guidance Counselor.

Gary Deitman, MEd

School Counselor

Pasadeno High School

77232 Wood Street

Pasadeno, CA 92401

Interim Report

Claire Fisher (DOB: 7/3/1985) is an attractive 17-year-old Euro American high school junior, referred for counseling by the school after having placed a human foot in her ex-boyfriend's locker. Prior to this incident, she had been being harassed at school after her boyfriend had disclosed that she had fondled and kissed his feet. She was referred for counseling because of the bizarreness of the presenting incident and the suspicion that it might reflect underlying depression or a more serious disease process. Claire has been seen four times as of this report.

Claire is insightful and believed to be of well-above average intelligence, despite spotty grades. She possesses a broad fund of knowledge and observes others well. She thinks abstractly, while also balancing her conclusions with appropriate data. These attributes give her a precocious maturity, which may interfere with her ability to connect with others her age. In addition, her family runs a funeral home, so death is a salient and normal part of her life. This may further distinguish her from others her age.

Claire has strong nonverbal listening skills. She makes good eye contact and her nonverbal behavior is spontaneous and unrestricted. Her affect is broad and responsive to the situation. Her feelings are clearly broadcast on her face and emphasized by broad hand gestures. However, she freely admits that her apparent openness can be a defense against meaningfully connecting with others, relating this to demands imposed by the family business. At the funeral home, her family must be "so careful" of everyone else's feelings that they "almost become invisible." We have a good therapeutic relationship, however, and she is increasingly able to both describe her feelings and be insightful about barriers to expressing them.

Although Claire is emotionally expressive, she still struggles to set reasonable boundaries for herself and meet her own needs in relationships, rather than being primarily other-oriented. In particular, she is struggling to identify how to do this with someone who reportedly recently attempted suicide. Again, this inability to set effective boundaries seems to be related to expectations stemming from the family business, where their clientele are at such a "sensitive time" that her family must put their own needs on hold to take care of the dead person's family. However, Claire is a budding artist and takes an idiosyncratic approach to life. Family and job-related expectations conflict with her own needs and style and she is struggling to find ways to make these more compatible with each other.

Claire's struggles to be real rather than conventional, in combination with the stress of being harassed by her peers, may have led her to place a foot in her ex-boyfriend's locker. As there have been no further problems, what at first appeared to be bizarre acting out, perhaps as the result of some serious psychological problems, now seems to be a way of getting back at her peers with an object close at hand.

In sum, when Claire initially entered therapy she reported being depressed and anxious in a variety of situations. Her family relationships were often formal and superficial. While she continues to experience considerable adolescent angst, her relationships with friends and family are now becoming more meaningful. Although only Claire herself has been seen in treatment, all members of the family are reportedly taking risks to be more "real"—both with others and themselves. This continues to be an ongoing struggle, however, which she is now successfully addressing in counseling.

Respectfully submitted,

Gary Deitman, MEd

School Counselor

Note: This report is loosely based on a scene from the first season of *Six Feet Under*.

The material in the last several chapters provides the foundation for good reports. A clinician's observations should be careful, contextualized, and gathered from a wide variety of sources and settings. Inferences should be based on numerous observations, evaluated relative to multiple **hypotheses**, and drawn only after having considered and challenged factors that could bias conclusions. Clinicians should think about the evidence supporting and challenging their hypotheses.

What Should Be in a Report?

In general, clinicians strive to provide a brief but well-reasoned and complex picture of the client. This picture provides information that is relevant to the **referral question,** but rather than only exploring one side, should examine all hypotheses relevant to the request. For example, is Claire depressed or psychotic? Is her behavior developmentally normal or part of a larger set of problems? If Claire is depressed, we would expect that there would be additional symptoms of depression and that her behavior might be linked to a developmental or environmental stressor. If she is psychotic, there would be other signs of a thought disorder, including a decline in functioning, delusions, and auditory hallucinations.

A strong report is insightful and useful. People enter treatment or are sent for an **evaluation** because of some confusion about what is happening. Claire's putting a foot in a fellow student's locker was bizarre. Her principal needed to know whether Claire was dangerous in order to make sure that she received appropriate treatment to keep herself and her fellow students safe. The report about Claire draws clear and respectful conclusions:

> Claire's struggles to be real rather than conventional, in combination with the stress of being harassed by her peers, may have led her to place a foot in her ex-boyfriend's locker. As there have been no further problems, what at first appeared to be bizarre acting out, perhaps as the result of some serious psychological problems, now seems to be a way of getting back at her peers with an object close at hand.

A strong report is clear and specific, avoiding **Barnum statements**. Note how the following statement appears to be individualized, but in fact is so general that most people would agree that it describes them.

> Although you need others to like and admire you, you tend to be critical of yourself, often fearing that you are failing to meet your goals. Although you have some weaknesses, you are generally able to compensate for them. You have considerable untapped potential that has not yet turned to your advantage. Sometimes you have serious doubts about whether you have made the right decisions or have done the right thing.

Barnum statements are often favorable ("considerable, untapped potential"), vague ("some weaknesses"), and two-headed, including both favorable and unfavorable information ("you need others to like and admire you, you tend to be critical of yourself").

Strong reports are respectful and **strength-based**. In addition to recognizing problems and concerns, they specifically document clients' strengths and successes. They acknowledge the positive intention behind a person's actions (e.g., "Tomas reports yelling at his wife and children frequently. His actions, while counterproductive, seem to be his way of caring for and engaging his family, from whom he often feels disengaged."). No one makes mistakes all of the time, so a strong report notes these exceptions (e.g., "Although Tomas frequently argues with his wife, arguments are worst when one of them is tired or stressed. Furthermore, most fights occur when one member of the family feels that his or her feelings are being dismissed.").

Although at first glance these statements look like Barnum statements, the description of Tomas's behavior is more detailed and takes an explicit stand about his behavior and the cause of his problems. Strong reports are also different in being respectful even while identifying problematic behavior. Favorable and respectful statements are not gratuitous and unnecessary, but useful in building the therapeutic alliance and in identifying treatment strategies that build on these strengths (i.e., that they should find more positive ways of engaging, build in time-outs when one or the other of them is stressed or tired, strengthen coping skills, and improve listening skills).

Food for Thought

• Using the ideas in this section, write a report based on the case material that was presented for Andrea Yates (Chapters 1 and 2).
• How was this report different from your previous report? What did you do better? What could you do that would make the process easier next time?

SOAP NOTES

When you wish to instruct, be brief; that men's minds take in quickly what you say, learn its lesson, and retain it faithfully. Every word that is unnecessary only pours over the side of a brimming mind.

—**Cicero**

Clinicians write many different kinds of reports, depending on the setting and the purpose of your writing. As further described in Table 7.3, an intake report, treatment plan, report to the court, or discharge summary each take a somewhat different form to match its specialized purpose. The report in Table 7.2, for example, might be a letter to the disciplinary board of Claire's school or to her probation officer.

In the course of their work, most clinicians also keep some sort of notes (**progress notes, SOAP notes,** or **DAP notes**). The following discussion will focus on SOAP notes, although many of these ideas also apply to other kinds of notes. SOAP notes are brief notes documenting the content of a single session in a very structured format. While different worksites will structure these somewhat differently, they are often organized in the following manner:

Session objective: Although all agencies do not include this section, it is useful to include the primary objective of the session, both to help other readers track the course of therapy and to keep the clinician on track with the treatment plan.

S: (Subjective) In this section, the most striking and central aspects of a client's subjective experience are recorded. Using the client's own words is often desirable and, when used, should be quoted.

TABLE **7.3**
Common Types of Clinical Writing.

Psychosocial history—An outline of client's status and functioning in a number of realms

Intake report—A report of client's status and functioning in a number of realms, often taking the form of a psychosocial history, but also including other data (e.g., genograms and timelines) and offering clear recommendations about diagnosis, prognosis, and the kind of treatment to be offered (e.g., outpatient therapy, partial hospitalization, residential treatment facility)

Evaluation—A formal administration of a number of assessment tools (e.g., interview, projective and objective personality tests, intelligence and achievement tests), to clearly respond to a referral question

SOAP note—A brief record of a session written in a standard form, focusing on the Subjective experience of the client, Objective observations made in the session, brief clinical Assessment of the client's status and factors contributing to it, and the Plan for the next session(s)

Progress note—A brief record of a session that is often more informal than an SOAP note, focusing on the client's status and treatment administered in session

Treatment plan—A detailed plan for treatment addressing the clinician's and client's short- and long-term treatment goals, planned interventions, and dates that goals will be met

Discharge summary—A brief report summarizing client diagnoses, the course of treatment (e.g., number of sessions and cancellations, interventions used), and factors contributing to the success or failure of treatment

O: (Objective) Objective observations, rather than inferences, are included here. These can include nonverbal behavior, changes in process, recent injuries or changes in symptoms, or summaries of brief assessment tools administered in session.

A: (Assessment) This is where the clinical assessment of the client's current functioning is reported. What can be concluded from direct observations? What might this mean? The clinical assessment should be supported by and follow from the S and O sections. Especially when issues of suicidality, homicidality, and abuse are present, the clinician's decisions and actions should be well documented.

P: (Plan) The plan for the next session is summarized here. What are the objectives for the next session? What homework, if any, was given? When will the next meeting be? This should match the session objective for the next session and should follow from the assessment section for this session. At the end of the note, sign and date it, including professional title.

Table 7.4 contains an example of a SOAP note for a suicidal client.

SOAP notes are brief records of a session for the clinician and other people working at that agency with that client. As you begin writing about sessions, consider the following issues:

Be succinct. Include only the most important aspects of the session. This includes major themes of sessions.

Be objective. Others watching the session should be able to agree with what was described. Observations and conclusions should not be colored by

TABLE **7.4**
A Sample SOAP Note.

Objective for session: Assess suicidality and stabilize client.

S: "I feel like no one cares and that no one really understands me. I'm not suicidal, though." "I'd never kill myself; I know how that only hurts everyone else."

O: Client maintained a closed posture throughout session, with eyes averted. Affect was restricted; she spoke only in response to specific prompts about the no-suicide contract. Nonetheless, she placed ideas for contract in her own words and tailored contract to her situation.

A: Client has become increasingly depressed in the weeks since her mother's suicide. Although she also has a number of risk factors for suicide, most specifically, her mother's recent suicide, she denies serious suicidal ideation or a plan. In addition, she has not attempted suicide since she stopped drinking 4 years ago, is aware that her suicide would "kill" her best friend and does not want to hurt her, is not using any substances, is not impulsive, and agreed to a no-suicide contract (see chart). Our strong therapeutic alliance and her supportive relationship with her best friend are additional protective factors.

P: Continue to monitor suicidal ideation and adherence to medication and no-suicide contract. Identify additional ways of stabilizing her. Homework: Monitor mood on scale of 1–10 throughout day, increasing support and asking for help when suicidality is above 6. Next: Tuesday, 2/19, 3 pm. 2/26/10 Carmen D. Gabriel-Rodriguez, Ph.D., Licensed Psychologist.

the clinician's biases. Inferences should be supported and reflect an awareness of and rejection of competing conclusions.

Be strength-based. Clients have the right to read what was written about them; therefore, clinicians should write as they would like others to write about them. In addition, writing in a strength-based manner is a good habit to foster and increases the clinician's ability to be hopeful during clinical work. This does not mean that they should lie, play Pollyanna, or be obscure; instead, they should be clear, honest, and respectful.

CYA.[1] Clinicians should document a client's suicidality, homicidality, and anything done to keep the client and significant others safe. Careful documentation of decisions and the decision making process can reduce clinical risk of ethical complaint or legal proceedings (Bennett et al., 2006; Youngren & Gottlieb, 2008). Dr. Gabriel-Rodriguez's reasonable and competent interventions documented in Table 7.4 would protect her from legal suit and ethical complaint if this client had completed suicide after attending their appointment.

CYCA.[2] Not every piece of information needs to be in the note. This is especially true for irrelevant information that might embarrass clients if it were to end up in court. As clinicians consider whether to include potentially embarrassing information, they should think about whether that information is relevant to their work with the client.

---

[1] Cover your ***.

[2] Cover your client's ***.

Food for Thought

Return to Eminem's interview (Chapter 5) or the transcript of Claire's therapy session. Write an SOAP note for one of these. How does this segment of clinical writing differ from what you might have written for another purpose?

OTHER CONSIDERATIONS

Practice, practice, practice writing. Writing is a craft that requires both talent and acquired skills. You learn by doing, by making mistakes and then seeing where you went wrong.

—Jeffrey A. Carver

Making observations and writing reports about others should be done carefully, as the recorded observations and conclusions often have significant consequences for clients. These are things that clinicians should keep in mind while writing about clients and clinical interviews.

Be tentative about those things that are unknown. Clients will say many things, some of which are the truth, others that they may believe to be true. They will tell white lies and outright deceptions. When they say something that has not been confirmed elsewhere, especially if this appears to be a place where there may be some question about what they say, clinicians should make appropriately tentative statements, prefacing their statement with verbs like "reported," "stated," or "said." For example, *Ms. Durrant reported that her husband became very suspicious and angry when she prepared a fancy dinner for the two of them.* Her clinician does not know whether he became suspicious and angry or whether she just believed he did.

In addition to misrepresenting others' behaviors and intentions, clients may also intentionally or unintentionally inaccurately report their own thoughts, emotions, and behaviors. If Ms. Durrant says that she is very committed to treatment, unless there are other observations supporting this conclusion, the strongest statement one can make is, *Ms. Durrant stated that she was very committed to addressing her use of alcohol at the present time.* If her clinician believed she was very committed, he should give the evidence for his conclusion,

> Ms. Durrant appears to be very committed to addressing her use of alcohol at the present time. She reports wanting to do "whatever it takes" to stay clean, has attended every scheduled session, and has completed all homework assignments. Her husband and children are very supportive of her sobriety without either nagging her or making the changes for her.

When no additional observations directly support this conclusion, smart clinicians keep in mind that most people in substance abuse treatment programs are ambivalent about change. She has many reasons to deceive herself and her clinician.

Remember that there are multiple explanations for any single observation. Smart clinicians make sure that they have considered all reasonable hypotheses for observations and that their conclusions are justified. They consider both evidence supporting their conclusions and that countering it, while being fair.

> Although Ms. Durrant appears very committed to change and has been working hard in treatment, she has been in a very supportive setting and has not been exposed to any of the triggers that have put her at risk in the past. Furthermore, she has many reasons to claim to be committed to change even if she is not, chief of which is her fear that her husband will leave her if he believes that she is using again.

Don't be afraid to draw reasonable conclusions. Despite the warnings in the previous points, clinicians are (or will be) paid to draw conclusions. They should draw reasonable and supported conclusions that are responsive to the referral question and give their readers the evidence for their conclusions.

> Although Ms. Durrant continues to have occasional slips, she has worked hard in treatment, attending sessions regularly and going well beyond requirements for homework assignments. Because she has done well in treatment and has no history of neglecting her children, even when drinking, her children should be returned to her as soon as possible. However, as her drinking has the potential for negatively impacting her children, she should continue to be involved with treatment and her treatment compliance should be considered in future custody decisions.

Be respectful. Empathic clinicians treat clients with respect, as people rather than objects. This does not mean that clinicians whitewash what they say; however, they should not demonize clients for having symptoms or making mistakes. They recognize and write about both their clients' weaknesses and strengths, using strengths to guide treatment. They observe exceptions to the problem, as exceptions may provide opportunities for treatment. They use **person first language** in their descriptions (see Table 7.5).

> In the last 90 days, Ms. Durrant reports having "slipped" three times, drinking between one drink and a bottle of vodka on each occasion. Nonetheless, she has called her sponsor each time and has increased her attendance at AA meetings. She has noted which situations put her at risk and has been either avoiding or changing these situations so that they are less problematic. She has identified a series of coping mechanisms that she is increasingly consistently using in order to prevent relapses. She also reports catching her slips earlier in the cycle. Last week she called the Center when contemplating taking a drink but before she had actually taken one.

Address referral questions. Reports should clearly answer the referral question. Irrelevant information should not be included even though it may be interesting. For example, it may be interesting and noteworthy that Ms. Durrant has a history of being sexually abused, but in discussing her ability to work well within a Twelve-Step Program (Alcoholics Anonymous, 2009), anything beyond a quick mention of her history is probably gratuitous and could be damaging, depending on the audience. On the other hand, when clinicians believe that their ability to work effectively in treatment will be compromised by Ms. Durrant's flashbacks and difficulties with trust, they would be remiss in not discussing her history.

TABLE **7.5**
Principles to Guide Respectful Writing and Speech.

Principle One: Use Person First language.

Place the focus on the person rather than the problem. The person has a problem, but is not defined by the problem. This distinction is especially important when helping people change. People who see symptoms as internal and unchangeable are less able to change than those who see symptoms as external and temporary.

Avoid: Schizophrenics, autistics, the mentally retarded.

Use: People with schizophrenia, autism.

The woman who is depressed.

Principle Two: Avoid describing things as "handicaps."

The word "handicap" suggests an inability or an obstacle. Blindness, deafness, and other disabilities may be handicapping, but primarily in response to societal oppression and environmental barriers. This word suggests that there is a right way to approach life and overlooks other strengths and compensations.

Avoid: He is physically handicapped.

Use: She is paralyzed.

He uses a wheelchair.

Principle Three: Everyone is normal in many ways.

Avoid describing people as either normal or abnormal; even people with problems are typical in many ways. Furthermore, people with autism challenge limited views of normality, suggesting that those of us without autism are not normal or better, just neurologically typical.

Avoid: He is a normal 5-year-old.

Use: She is a 10-year-old with no reported intellectual or behavioral deficits.

His development is within normal limits.

Principle Four: Avoid terms with unnecessary negative connotations.

The words we use can have important meanings for how people see themselves and how we see them. Avoid language that projects pain, suffering, or struggle when it is absent. Obviously, if someone is in pain, it is OK to note this.

Avoid: Victim, cripple, defective, deformed, restricted to a wheelchair, afflicted with, stricken with.

Use: She is paralyzed.

He has a cleft lip.

She sees herself as a victim of child abuse. (This acknowledges that it is a perception rather than a necessary aspect of the person.)

He has a history of physical abuse.

Note: Modified from Folkins (1992).

Consider the audience. What Ms. Durrant's therapist will need to know is significantly different from what her children's teachers need to know. Just because Ms. Durrant is in treatment does not mean that she should lose her right to privacy. In fact, disclosing protected health information without permission is both illegal and unethical and could leave a clinician liable to lawsuit.

Choose tense thoughtfully. Use past tense to describe things that have already happened (things that occurred in the session or before it). For example, *She appeared anxious during the session and frequently fiddled with her pearls. Despite this, she was open in disclosing problems*. Use present tense to describe things that are currently happening (i.e., their current age, where they are employed). That is, *Ms. Durrant is a 46-year-old African-American mother of two, currently employed as a nurse practitioner at a local hospital*.

Proofread your writing carefully. Counseling and therapy are often done behind closed doors. Because of this, people's conclusions about the quality of clinical work are often based on clinicians' records and reports. When writing and the thinking in it are sloppy, readers generally assume that the work is also sloppy and unprofessional. Learning to write quickly and well is worth it!

WHY EMPATHY?

In Chapter 1, we described May's (1967) view of effective clinical work as combining both objectivity and subjectivity (i.e., empathy). Many assessment reports, however, err on the side of objectivity. We suspect that overzealous objectivity is an attempt to be careful, cautious, and professional. However, one can be careful, cautious, professional, *and* empathic.

An empathic approach to developing a clinical assessment has consequences for the clinician's work, the client, and the reader. Empathy strengthens the therapeutic relationship, leading to better and more helpful disclosures from clients. Although clinical writing must be based in observations and facts, it should also help readers understand clients—who may feel crazy to themselves and others (e.g., the story from Raymond Corsini, that started off Chapter 6). When reports express a truly empathic understanding, readers are more likely to understand clients, engage with them, and respond empathically themselves.

SUMMARY

Effective writing about clients takes several different forms; each is related to its specific purpose (e.g., a progress note, a report, treatment plan, discharge summary, and so on). Some of these forms have been discussed here (e.g., SOAP note, brief report), and others will be discussed in later chapters. Both the form and the content of the writing address the specific purpose of the writing product and answer the referral question.

Clinical writing should be succinct, objective, and strength-based. SOAP notes and progress notes, for example, are especially succinct and objective styles of writing used to document interviews and therapy sessions. Clinical writing should balance the needs of both the client and the clinician. They should include enough information to document that the helper assessed and intervened competently, without including material that unnecessarily embarrasses clients or puts them at risk if another party were to read the note or report. In addition, clinical writing should recognize multiple explanations for observations and should be appropriately tentative. Nonetheless, clinicians should draw reasonable conclusions, even while acknowledging the limitations of conclusions.

Readers draw conclusions about clinical abilities based on a clinician's writing style and inferences. Therefore, effective clinicians write carefully, accurately, and respectfully, addressing both referral questions and the needs and understanding of their audience. A clinician's reputation depends on the quality of his or her clinical writing and is worth protecting.

How Do These Issues Apply to Your Life and Work?

1. Observe how you hear others described over the next week. How do these descriptions differ from the kinds of descriptions that mental health professionals would include in a report? What descriptions from either professional or nonprofessional sources make you uncomfortable? Why?

2. As you begin working on your writing, pay attention to the things you do well. What would you like to improve? How can you further strengthen your writing? Develop a plan for improving your observational and writing skills.

CHAPTER 8

Addressing Referral Questions and Identifying Goals

WHERE ARE WE GOING?

1. What factors often make changing difficult?
2. How does clients' readiness for change affect the change process?
3. How do relapses and lapses differ and what are their implications for treatment?
4. How do referral questions guide treatment and treatment goal development?
5. What are the characteristics of good treatment goals?
6. What happens when clinicians' goals are incompatible with their clients'?
7. How can you identify goals towards which clients will work?
8. How do developing shared goals build empathy?

Jail was My Saving Grace
Reymundo Sanchez

In Chapter 3, Lil Loco (b. 1963) talked about his involvement with gangs in Chicago. When he was 21, he was sent to prison on drug charges. He described this period as "my saving grace," a "blessing in disguise." His nightmares stopped and he began to think differently. Thinking about the bad things in his life, paradoxically, now made him aware of the ways that he had been lucky, rather than only cursed.

> Because all my life I had felt I was cursed, I never knew what a blessing was. Being at peace allowed me to begin to understand. I remembered guns pointed at me at point-blank range that never fired. I recalled bullets shot at me that did less damage than a bad fall or the beatings at the hands of my own gang. I compared them with the events that had taken the lives of so many others but had somehow spared mine. Then I thought about the huge amounts of drugs I had poured into my body, yet I was still alive. It was these thoughts that made me realize the meaning of a blessing. It was then that I started to consider my conviction [on drug charges] as a blessing. It was actually the first blessing I counted. (Sanchez, 2003, p. 73)

Two older men served as mentors to Reymundo—one when he was in jail, another when he was on work release. They helped him think about the directions in which he might go, although in very different ways. King Leo, a member of the Latin Kings, serving a life sentence at Shawnee Correctional Center, took Rey (as he was now called), under his wing. Rey had begun writing poetry, an outlet for his frequent pain and anger. Leo supported his writing and encouraged him to connect his writing and drawing with his newly emerging sense of inner peace. Leo said,

> "Look at those brothers over there,"… looking in the direction of the weight pile. "All of them short-timers, a couple of years and they're back on the street. *Son pendejos, mi pana* (They are idiots, my partner). *En ves de enfuenzar sus mentes, enfuerzan sus cuerpeos* (Instead of strengthening their minds, they strengthen their bodies). They leave just as stupid as they came in, only stronger." Leo turned to face me. Most of them will come back, some of them lifers like me. *No seas haci de pendejo* (Don't be an idiot like that)," he concluded. I understood, and I stayed on the course I had chosen to reinvent myself. (Sanchez, 2003, p. 84)

His other mentor, Kalil, was Jamaican-born and Muslim. He was a member of another gang, the El Rukn. Rey met him while they were on work release. Kalil said,

> "Can you deny that the time you spent in jail was the salvation for your life? Not many brothers can say that, nor can they even begin to think it. Allah works his miracles for those who seek them faithfully."
> "But I don't believe in or even recognize Allah," I responded.
> "Call him what you will," Kalil answered. "It's faith that will lead us all to the promised land. As I sit here talking to you, all my questions regarding the

(continues)

(continued)

> path my life suddenly took are being answered. Your journey has just begun, young brother. Just be faithful, even when faith seems not to exist." Of all the conversations I had with people who tried to give me advice on where and how my life should go, Kalil's words were the ones that stuck with me the most. (Sanchez, 2003, p. 113)

He now believed that his life had a future. He wrote:

> I didn't want to do anything that would risk my losing the new freedoms I had gained. I could smell total freedom just ahead in my life, and I lived every day with the intention of gaining it and keeping it. (Sanchez, 2003, p. 112)

- How would you describe Rey's readiness to change at this point? How is this different (or similar) to his readiness for change during the period described in Chapter 3? How do you know?
- What did Kalil and Leo do that were so powerful for Rey? Would they have had the same impact if Rey had been mandated into treatment and his suburban-born counselor had said these same things? Why or why not?
- If you were working with Rey, how might you tailor your interventions for him in a way that was genuine for you and effective in helping Rey change?

CHANGE

Most people readily identify what others can do to change, although they may see their own problems as difficult to change. Sue Monk Kidd (2006)—who very much wanted to change—talked about the process in this way:

> My husband, Sandy, was as exasperated as he was bewildered. He wanted things to go back to the comfortable way they were before. He wanted me to "snap out of it." I did too, of course. I had ordered myself to do just that numerous times. But it was sort of like looking at an encroaching wave and telling it to recede. Demanding didn't make it happen. (p. 5)

Failures in empathy, such as this, can make changing even more difficult.

Often the change process is emotion-laden. Some people may feel overwhelmed and stuck, unable to change. Others may believe that the problem is unchangeable or that they cannot control that change (Bandura, 1997). They may be ambivalent about change, recognizing both its benefits and also the losses they will incur (Prochaska, 1999; Prochaska & DiClemente, 1982). They may see numerous barriers to change, including financial and transportation barriers (Reust, Thomlinson, & Lattie, 1999). Such views can determine the outcomes of treatment. For example, in a study of cancer patients, perceived barriers to changing differentiated those people who profited from a pain intervention from those who did not (Ward et al., 2008). In addition, previous negative experiences in the mental health system can prevent people from returning, as can difficulties with setting an appointment or accessing insurance (Reust et al., 1999).

Despite the real and imagined costs of change, many people *are* able to change. Reust and her colleagues (1999) reported that people who identified a problem, had social support for changing, perceived mental health professionals positively, and believed that they would get something positive from changing were more likely to set and keep their appointments.

STAGES OF CHANGE

Just do it!

—Nike

"Just do it!" is a good advertising campaign, but as Sue Monk Kidd (2006) observed, it is not an effective way to help people change. To change, people must recognize that they have a problem and be committed to change. Like Reymundo Sanchez (2000, 2003), clients vary markedly on these two dimensions. Clinicians must tailor interventions to match their clients' readiness for change (Prochaska, 1999; Prochaska & DiClemente, 1982).

Change is often a gradual process rather than a one-time decision (see Table 8.1). Clients' location in this process can be assessed by carefully listening to their discussions of the problem and change (e.g., "I can't see doing that," "I just don't have the energy right now," or "I'm going to start now!"). Amrhein and his colleagues (2003) observed that the way substance abusers speak indicates readiness to change and predicts treatment outcomes.

Recognizing clients' readiness for change is important for developing a strong empathic understanding of them. Clinicians who fail to recognize their clients' ambivalence about change may leave their clients feeling frustrated and hopeless about meeting their goals. Furthermore, clinicians are likely to feel frustrated or angry when they believe their clients are more ready to change than they actually are. They may justify their frustration and anger by attributing their clients' lack of change to **resistance** or noncompliance (Bohart, 2001).

Precontemplation

At some point most people have had what other people would identify as a "problem," but have been unaware of its negative consequences. Prochaska (1999; Prochaska & DiClemente, 1982) calls this stage **Precontemplation**. People in the substance-abuse field often call this lack of insight "denial." Clients in this stage may appear uninterested, unaware, or unwilling to change, even though friends and relatives are often very aware of the problem. When they end up in treatment, it is often because a third party (e.g., parents, an unhappy spouse, or a judge) has forced them. Clients at this stage may say things like, "I don't know why I should change. They're the ones with the problem!"

Clients must first recognize that they have a problem. Questions like, "How would you know that this is a problem?" can be useful at this stage (Zimmerman, Olsen, & Bosworth, 2000). Supportive and empathic responses are often helpful, while confrontational and conflict-laden responses increase resistance and interfere with treatment (Beutler et al., 2001; Moos, 2003; Serran, Fernandez, Marshall, & Mann, 2003).

TABLE **8.1**

Stages of Change and Their Impact on the Selection of Treatment Goals.

Stage of change	Characteristics of stage	Focus of treatment
Precontemplation	No intention to change in the foreseeable future. Often there is little or no awareness of the problem. May enter treatment because of another party (e.g., a family member or the court).	Increase awareness of problem and its consequences.
Contemplation	Aware of the problem, seriously considering change, but has not yet made a commitment to do so. Evaluating options; significantly ambivalent about changing.	Address ambivalence and identify barriers to change.
Preparation	Committed to change and intends to take action in near future.	Develop behavioral skills and alternatives to negative behaviors, elicit support from others to change, information, resources to overcome obstacles. Address barriers to change and identify small changes that prepare clients for change.
Action	Actively changing behaviors, beliefs, experiences, or situations to overcome problem	Identify strategies for making change and support making it.
Maintenance	Recognizes need to maintain changes and is willing to do so.	Discuss change process, especially that change is not permanent without work to maintain it. Distinguish between lapses and relapses. Identify situations that put clients at risk of relapse and ways to avoid, change or handle these.

Note: From Prochaska, 1999; Prochaska & DiClemente, 1982.

Contemplation

Even when clients have identified a problem, they may not necessarily be willing to change. Many people acknowledge that they are having difficulty, but also recognize the significant costs associated with change and experience ambivalence about accepting those costs (Prochaska, 1999; Prochaska & DiClemente, 1982). For example, a woman in a violent and abusive relationship may know that her relationship is unhealthy, but also worry that if she leaves her husband she will be unable to pay her bills, will receive disapproval from her family, friends, and church, and will lose a father for her children along with the financial and emotional support that he offers. She may be afraid that she cannot parent their difficult children on her own, will not find a job that will support the family, does not have the skills to keep their bills paid and their car and house running smoothly, and will not find another man who will love her as much. She may also feel guilty that she has not done enough to make their relationship work better.

Clients in **Contemplation** recognize a problem, but are not yet ready to change. They need to assess barriers to change as well as identify the potential benefits of changing. Questions like, "What are the benefits of changing at this point in time?" and "What might keep you from changing at this point?" are helpful for clients in this stage (Zimmerman et al., 2000). The goal of treatment is to heighten motivation and tip the balance towards committing to change.

Preparation

Once clients have identified obstacles as well as motivators for making change and have worked through their ambivalence about change, they often need to prepare to change. During **Preparation** the water is tested, often by making small changes first (Prochaska, 1999; Prochaska & DiClemente, 1982). This stage is characterized by planning, getting information, getting support, problem-solving, and making sure they have the skills they need.

Action

Prochaska (1999; Prochaska & DiClemente, 1982) defines **Action** as the stage when the target behavior (e.g., leaving one's husband or quitting smoking) has occurred for at least one day. Although the focus in Precontemplation and Contemplation is on motivating clients, in Action, clinicians need to help clients identify behavioral strategies that will help them change more effectively.

Even though clients in Action are committed to change and are actively changing, the change process can still be difficult. Clinicians need to be generous and genuine with positive feedback. For example, in working with a client who is quitting smoking, a clinician might remark, "Wow! It's been a week since you last smoked! What are you doing that is making this happen?" Some clients may attribute their change to luck or chance. Clinicians need to empathize with their client's *feeling* that the change was outside their control, but help to search for the client's contribution to the change (Walter & Peller, 1992). For example,

> I know it feels like *someone or something else* made the change happen, but I want you to think about what *you* did, so you can do it again. What changes did *you* make—no matter how little—that caused this week to be such a good one?

Notice the active, first person focus of the question. Also note that this clinician ended with an **open question** (i.e., questions beginning with what, how, when, and why). If it had been a **closed question** (i.e., questions beginning with is, are, could, and do), the client might have accepted that an extreme and dichotomous response was acceptable: "Nothing!"

Maintenance

It is easier to initially stop drinking/lose weight/become more assertive than to maintain that change. Mistakes and lapses are normal parts of life, but how clients perceive them makes an important difference in treatment. They can be seen as indicators that long-lasting change will never happen (a **relapse**, a full-blown return to the problem behavior) or as opportunities to fine-tune the change process (a **lapse**, temporary slips that can be learned from). Transferring skills to other situations, maintaining them across time, and preventing relapses are other important tasks in **Maintenance** (Prochaska, 1999; Prochaska & DiClemente, 1982).

About 75% of people who stop using and abusing substances use them again within one year's time, at least briefly (McLellan et al., 1994). There are two essential aspects to preventing and reducing the frequency and impact of slips: (a) reducing **triggers** to the problem behavior and (b) challenging negative cognitive and emotional responses to slips. Slips do not occur at random, but in predictable situations. These include periods of boredom, loneliness, interpersonal stress, and exposure to other triggers (Laudet, Magura, Vogel, & Knight, 2004; Sharkansky, Brief, Peirce, Meehan, & Mannix, 1999). Some triggers can be avoided (e.g., bars, for people who are trying to quit smoking or drinking); others can be minimized or prevented (e.g., stress and fatigue).

People with high self-efficacy and positive self-attributions following a lapse are less likely to have a second one (Shiffman et al., 1996). It can be useful to pay attention to clients' successes in order to modify their attributions and build their self-efficacy, as illustrated in the following excerpt:

Shane 1: It sounds like Friday was a really hard day for you. What happened?

Trish 1: I don't know. I had had a hard day at work and was bored and antsy. My friends were hanging out and planning on going to the bar and I just thought, "I've been too good, too long!"

Shane 2: You said, "I don't know," but you did a really nice job describing what happened. [pause] In addition to being bored and at loose ends, you were with friends who were encouraging you to have fun. [Uh huh.] I'm also curious about your statement about having been "too good." It sounds like you're seeing staying sober as being in conflict with having fun.

Trish 2: Yeah, it feels like all I do anymore is work, go to meetings, and sleep. I'm still a kid—at least I feel like one—and I want to have fun too!

Shane 3: It sounds like you're saying that one of the things you need to do, along with continuing to address your triggers, is look at some ways to have fun without drinking.

REFERRAL QUESTIONS AND TREATMENT GOALS

God grant me the serenity to accept the things I cannot change; courage to change the things I can; and wisdom to know the difference.
—Reinhold Niebuhr

Imagine that Andrea Yates was referred to you shortly after drowning her children. This referral could have come from numerous sources—her attorney, the court, her psychiatrist, her family, the prison system, or even from herself. Each of these individuals or groups might have different referral questions that they would want you to address. For example,

- The court might want to know whether she was **competent** to assist in her defense. Does she understand the legal system and the decisions that she will have to make in the course of her trial? Can she identify facts that are relevant to the case? Can she think rationally about her situation?

- Both the prosecuting and defense attorneys would want to know whether she was sane at the time of the murders according to the definition used in Texas. Legal definitions of **sanity** are substantially different from psychiatric ones and generally focus on whether the person recognized at the time of the crime that the act was wrong and whether they believed they could prevent it.
- Her psychiatrist might want to know whether her psychotic symptoms are associated with schizophrenia, major depressive disorder, bipolar disorder, or some other cause, and may also ask for treatment recommendations.
- The prison might want to know whether she can be maintained effectively in their system or whether she needs a more secure setting.

Each of these questions guides the assessment process in a different direction, determining the questions asked during interviews as well the assessment strategies administered. The reports written in response to each of these referral questions would differ in important ways, as illustrated in Table 8.2.

TABLE **8.2**
Hypothetical Summary Statements in Response to Three Possible Referral Questions with Regard to Andrea Yates.

With regard to her competency to stand trial:

Ms. Yates is a 37-year-old female who was referred for an evaluation of her competency to stand trial following drowning her five children. She is a bright woman who is college educated and, despite her current severe depression and past psychosis, understands the legal system and the implications of abstract court actions. Her significant guilt about how she was raising her children, however, may lead her to make decisions that could hamper her case.

With regard to her sanity at the time of the murders:

Ms. Yates is a 37-year-old female who was referred for an evaluation of her sanity following drowning her five children because she believed that "they were doomed to perish in the fires of hell" as a result of her poor parenting. She admits to having hallucinations both at the time of the murders and on several occasions in the past and reports feeling compelled to drown her children in order to "save" them. Nonetheless, she recognized that her actions were wrong by the larger society's laws and values, thus calling the police after drowning her children.

With regard to whether she can be maintained in the prison system:

Ms. Yates is a 37-year-old female who was referred to determine whether the current prison wing is appropriate given her mental health needs. In particular, it was unclear whether she was an ongoing danger to herself or others. Ms. Yates is a highly moral person—in terms of her own belief system—so is unlikely to harm anyone else unless she was to believe that she was saving them, as she reports believing she was doing in her acknowledged murders of her children. However, she is currently mostly mute, very passive, reports feeling extreme guilt about her "poor parenting," and committed an act that many of her fellow prisoners will likely find heinous and reprehensible. As a result, it is highly probable that she would be an easy victim within the prison system and would not act to keep herself safe.

Food for Thought

What problems would you want to address in the course of treatment with Ms. Yates? What do you think she would see as important problems to address? Your goals should derive from the problems you identify as most important. These might include:

- Decreasing the severity of her depressive symptoms;
- Decreasing the frequency and intensity of her psychotic symptoms;
- Increasing her compliance with her medicines and therapy;
- Identifying positive strategies for coping with her feelings of depression and guilt;
- Building a positive support network in prison;
- Identifying a sense of direction and purpose for the future.

Which of these goals would you want to work on first? Would your decision be influenced by whether you expected that she would be released from prison? Would her wishes influence your decisions? Would it be enough that she stopped some behavior (e.g., having hallucinations)? Would you also want her to make a positive change of some sort? Why?

WHAT ARE GOOD GOALS?

If one does not know to which port one is sailing, no wind is favorable.

—Lucius Annaeus Seneca

Effective goal setting requires listening to the client's values and preferences to identify treatment goals together. Notice how Leo and Kalil did this with Reymundo Sanchez in the case material at the beginning of this chapter. In particular, treatment goals should be culturally relevant, individualized, and collaboratively set with clients. They should be client-centered, concrete, and measurable. When these criteria are met, clients can give truly informed consent and work harder towards meeting treatment goals.

Well-defined goals take a specific form (Walter & Peller, 1992). Goals should be under the client's control and expressed in the form of behaviors, in the positive, specific, and present-focused (see Table 8.3). In addition, they should use the client's own words and metaphors. When this occurs, clients can see where they are going and work toward meeting their goals.

Goals under Clients' Control

Clients often think about ways that their lives would be better if *others* were to change. Although this may be true, clinicians cannot directly change clients' families and friends. They can, however, help change the person in the consulting room. That person's change, in turn, may cause others to behave differently. Clinicians cannot make a client's husband stop his abusive tirades. They can help her change how she reacts to them. She can examine her behavior and

TABLE **8.3**
Criteria for Good Treatment Goals.

Criteria	Key words	Sample questions or responses
Under the client's control	"You"	"What can you do to make that happen?"
Behavioral	"How," "ing"	"How will you be doing this?"
In the positive	"Instead"	"What will you be doing instead of yelling?"
As specific as possible	"Specifically"	"Describe, as specifically as possible, what you're going to do differently."
In the present	"Now," "on track"	"As you leave here today, and you are on track, what will you be doing differently?"

Note: Modified from Walter & Peller, 1992.

identify the grain of truth in his accusations. She can respond assertively, rather than aggressively, to his requests. She can hear the pain behind his tirades.

Behavioral Goals

Strong goals are behavioral in nature. They are actions rather than end results and usually can be phrased as a verb (e.g., studying more, running daily). Grades and weight loss are often at least somewhat outside clients' control, but they can change their study habits, exercise patterns, and diet. In their assessments, clinicians might ask questions like, "What will you be doing differently when you're on track?" or "How will you be thinking differently?"

Positively Phrased Goals

Rather than focusing on what *not* to do, good goals have clients focus on the changes they want to occur. What will they be doing instead of yelling? What will they be doing instead of being anxious? Phrasing goals in terms of positive actions facilitates the change process by clarifying the direction of treatment.

Specific Goals

The change process is often difficult to see. Because clients may not see what they should do, they often provide vague goals that are poor guides for treatment (e.g., "I want us to be happier."). What, specifically, will clients do differently? To the extent possible, the desired change should be framed in terms of concrete, observable behaviors (e.g., "I'm going to start asking her about her day when she comes in the door. I want her to see how important she is to me."). Specific goals are objective and quantifiable, which helps people to monitor the extent to which they are on track.

Present-Oriented Goals

Rather than waiting for change to happen magically at some distant point in the future, effective clinicians encourage clients to think about how they can begin to change right now. Clinicians might ask, "As you leave here today, and you are on track, what will you be doing differently?" This focus encourages clients to commit to changing now rather than at some indeterminate point in the future.

Goals Phrased in Client's Own Words

Rather than communicating using psychological jargon, effective clinicians use clients' metaphors and key words as much as possible. Clients' words reflect their worldview and describe their familiar ways of looking at the problem. As seen in the following example, using their words communicates the clinician's understanding of them and their problems. Sharing this understanding strengthens the therapeutic relationship.

Miguel 1:   There's a wall between the two of us, like we will never get close again. She just doesn't talk to me any more.

Javier 1:   You feel like there's a wall between the two of you, and you don't know what you can do to climb over it or to tear it down. (Yeah.) What can *you* do *now* to make a door through what often feels like an impenetrable barrier?

Miguel 2:   Maybe we could try to understand each other...

Javier 2:   What could you do *today* to begin to tear down that wall?

Miguel 3:   I could tell her how much I've missed having her in my life.

Note, although Javier accepted Miguel's metaphor (J1), he didn't accept that the wall was permanent or impenetrable. He expanded Miguel's way of thinking about his problem in J2 by using a standard aspect of walls (e.g., that they have doors, can be climbed over, or can be torn down). His questions also helped Miguel develop a concrete picture of what he wanted to change and what he needed to do to get there.

Food for Thought

- Look at your description of your treatment goals for Ms. Yates from earlier in this chapter. How well do these goals match Walter and Peller's (1992) recommendations?
- How might you negotiate any differences between your goals and Ms. Yates' goals for herself?

CONFLICT IN GOALS

Conflicts may be the sources of defeat, lost life and a limitation of our potentiality but they may also lead to greater depth of living and the birth of more far-reaching unities, which flourish in the tensions that engender them.

—Karl Jaspers

Perhaps it is surprising that it can be difficult to identify who the client is. Court-referred clients may not be the "real" client; instead, the court and probation or parole office may have mandated the client into treatment and set the treatment goals, which may be different than the client's own goals. For example, Latino immigrant parents are more collective in their approach to school situations than their children's Euro American teachers, disagreeing on the importance of individual achievement, the use of praise rather than criticism, the relative importance of academic rather than social skills, and individual expression rather than respect for authority (Greenfield et al., 2006). Hmong immigrants and their U.S. physicians often differ both in goals for treatment and in acceptable strategies for approaching it (Fadiman, 1997). Children and their parents may have different, even conflicting, treatment goals, and clinicians must find a way of contracting for treatment with each (Hawley & Weisz, 2003; Reyes, Kokotovic, & Cosden, 1996). Similar issues arise in the course of marital therapy, where one partner may be more committed to change than the other, and work with suicidal or psychotic clients, who may actively reject their clinician's efforts to keep them alive or reduce their psychosis.

Even willing clients may have goals for themselves that are different from those aimed for by their clinicians. Lent (2004) describes one such case:

> I am reminded of a supervisee whose client admonished her for moving too quickly toward prescribing actions to help the client feel better. After a figurative tug-of-war in one session, the client announced, "I know how to get myself to feel better. And I know how to make decisions. What I could use your help with is figuring out how I get myself into messes like this to begin with."
> (p. 489)

Clinicians and clients must make decisions about what to talk about during treatment, how to talk about it, and what approach to take. They may also have different and contradictory values. Liszcz and Yarhouse (2005), for example, have highlighted the role of clinician values in the treatment goal-identification process for work with clients questioning their sexuality. Religious clinicians and those specializing in work with gay and lesbian clients each tended to choose treatment goals consistent with their own values and attitudes about sexual orientation. Even when there was a conflict in goals, clinicians tended to choose goals consistent with their own values over their clients' goals.

These difficulties in collaboration can affect goal setting, treatment plan development, and clients' feelings of being understood. The following case material illustrates how differences between clients and clinicians' worldviews may lead to difficulties in empathy as well as problems in collaborating and setting mutually acceptable treatment goals.

Conflicts between Hmong Immigrants and U.S. Physicians

In discussing the Lee family's story, Fadiman (1997) described the numerous ways that the worldviews of Hmong American families and Western medicine can conflict. Although this conflict is sometimes due to misinterpretations of one another's intentions or language problems in communication or translation, it is also due to differing beliefs about the causes of disease and appropriate responses to symptoms. A Hmong American's refusal to go to the doctor or follow the prescribed treatment may be due to concerns about the medical treatment used, but, equally likely, may be about diverging views of health and appropriate treatment of bodies and problems with authority that have their roots in conflicts stemming back thousands of years. As Fadiman notes, the Hmong tend to see everything as connected (see Table 8.4).

(continues)

TABLE **8.4**

Comparison of Hmong American and Euro American Cultural Values.

Hmong Americans	Euro Americans
Time	
• Time is relatively elastic	• Time is precise, prompt
• Take a day at a time or as it comes	• Plan for tomorrow; future-oriented
• Are more past-oriented	
Relationships	
• Tend to focus on extended family	• Tend to focus on nuclear family
• Are more interdependent	• Are more individualistic
• "Correct" social relationships	
Group	
• Are more adult-oriented and respect old age and authority	• Are relatively youth-oriented
• Are more interdependent and group-oriented	• Are more independent and autonomous
• Are more shame conscious	• Are more guilt conscious
Approach to world	
• Worldview is more holistic, emphasizing harmony with others and nature	• Worldview is more reductionistic, valuing analysis and the scientific method
	• Emphasize competition and survival of the fittest; humans control nature
Therapeutic change and process	
• Are more status quo-oriented; weigh and internalize community needs, problems, and frustration in deciding whether to change	• Moral code and values are relativistic and situational
	• Are more change-oriented; are more willing to express needs and problems publicly

Note: From Faderman, 1998; Fadiman, 1997; Lao Family Community of Minnesota, Inc., 1997.

The Hmong view of "symptoms" can be very different from that of U.S. physicians. The Lee family saw their daughter's epilepsy as indicating that she would be a healer, a *txiv neeb* (Fadiman, 1997). Faderman (1998) described how the parents of a child with clubfoot were sued for failing to get him "appropriate" medical treatment. The parents, on the other hand, had seen his clubfoot as saving them from other curses. Hmong Americans perceive the U.S. schools and health system as "conflating parental discipline with child abuse" and undermining their authority (Faderman, 1998, p. 13).

U.S.-educated physicians expect to be listened to and respected. Although they believe listening to *symptoms* is part of their job, listening to proposed *treatments* is not. One Hmong American ruefully commented, "Doctor is like earth and sky. He think, you are refugee, you know nothing" (Fadiman, 1997, p. 62). When recommendations made by U.S. physicians are ignored, the physicians feel disrespected—just as their Hmong Americans patients often feel when their views are not taken seriously or understood.

Unlike U.S. physicians, a Hmong shaman does not request payment for services; the family is expected to know this and remunerate him appropriately. He was "a model for the rest of the community who, ideally, cared much more about the undoubted powers of the unseen world than the remote possibilities of riches in this world" (Faderman, 1998, p. 27). Faderman described the relative valuing of spirituality and money in these two cultures with two stories: a Hmong who gave up treasure discovered in the mountains, because obtaining it would have disturbed a spirit's resting place, and the U.S. decision to build an airport in a sacred place—"at the time the god was still living there"—causing their soldiers to get sick and have nosebleeds (p. 30).

Relations between U.S. physicians and Hmong Americans may also be complicated by unusual patterns of communication (by U.S. standards). For example, asking questions to clarify meaning is often seen as disrespectful; thus U.S. workers and physicians need to make sure that their Hmong Americans patients understand their meaning clearly (Lao Family Community of Minnesota, Inc., 1997). Furthermore, "Yes" does not always mean "Yes," but may simply indicate that the listener has heard the speaker. Because "No" is perceived as disrespectful, a Hmong American might counterintuitively indicate "No" by saying "Yes." Some Hmong Americans smile when criticized or reprimanded, which could be misunderstood as ridicule or a failure to take a person seriously, although their smiling instead might indicate embarrassment, sadness, or insecurity.

- Compare the worldviews of Hmong Americans and their physicians, as described in these Hmong statements, earlier discussions, and Table 8.4. How does the clash between the two worldviews lead to problems in their work together?

(continues)

(continued)

- Compare your worldview with the Hmong worldview. Where would you run into problems working with the Lee family (Chapters 5 and 10)? How could your worldview and personal style be successful in your work with them?
- How do cultural or social values give meaning to how clinicians see a disease and how they intervene? Can you identify other examples of how cultural and social values influence the conceptualization and approach of illness or health?
- What would need to change so the Lee family and other Hmong Americans can hear their physicians and vice versa? What could Lia Lee's doctors do to work more effectively with this family?

IDENTIFYING A COMMON GOAL

*Let us never nego-
tiate out of fear.
But let us never fear
to negotiate.*

—John F. Kennedy

Although clinicians and clients may be unwilling partners in treatment and have difficulty negotiating mutually agreeable goals, clinicians need to look for ways to engage clients in treatment. The following strategies can help clients and clinicians find common ground and work effectively together.

Work from Where the Client Is

Clients must feel understood and safe enough to change. Clinicians can create this sense of safety by listening carefully to their clients and accepting their perceptions of the world. Only when clients feel understood can clinicians begin to intervene to help them perceive their situation or problem differently (Ivey & Ivey, 1999). Notice how Liam's drug and alcohol counselor handles this.

Ryan 1: What is your goal for being here?

Liam 1: The judge and social worker think I should be here.

Ryan 2: I hear you saying this was their idea. I wonder why they think you need to be here.

Liam 2: They took my kids because they said I was neglecting them. [pause, clenching jaw] The judge says that if I want to get my kids back, I have to see you.

Ryan 3: [Gently] This is hard.

Liam 3: Yes, real hard. All I have is my children. I think about them all the time—whether they are safe, what they're doing. I just want them back.

Ryan 4: You want them back. [pause] They're saying you need to parent differently? Is this your goal too?

Liam 4: I suppose. Yes, I think so. [pause] I need to stop drinking, too. When I'm drinking, I'm not such a good parent.

Notice how Ryan listens to Liam and shares his understanding (in R2)—and Liam recognizes this (in L3). Once Liam recognizes and accepts Ryan's understanding, Ryan can begin to get Liam to identify and set goals (in R4).

Build Clients' Commitment to Change

Clients in Precontemplation do not perceive the problem that the court or their parents, spouse, or employer sees (Prochaska, 1999; Prochaska & DiClemente, 1982). Clients in Contemplation are ambivalent about change, seeing both the pros and cons about changing. Clients in any stage may have different goals than their clinician or referral source.

In the exchange between Ryan and Liam, Ryan accepted Liam's feelings and listened seriously to him. He respected Liam's choices while holding him responsible for the consequences of his decisions. If he had been forced to enter a parenting class, Liam might have dug in his heels and refused. When it was his choice, he was willing to commit to make changes. Ryan also helped build Liam's commitment by noting and highlighting Liam's motivation to change (in R3 and R4), "This is hard.... You want them back." Still, Ryan let Liam set his own goals.

Address Obstacles to Change

From the outside, change looks straightforward and easy. From the inside, it's often hard. Liam may want to change, but in becoming a better parent, he has to develop new skills, which takes time and comes with no guarantee of success. He also has to admit that he has made mistakes as a parent and that some other approach may be better than his current one. Liam might have to tell others that his drinking has been a problem and that he has made mistakes. He needs to identify triggers to his drinking and find ways of changing his behavior during those situations. He needs to find better ways of handling stress and other strong emotions that he muted with alcohol. He might have to make new friends and find new pastimes in place of drinking.

Assuming that Liam is in Contemplation about stopping drinking, Ryan needs to recognize and address both sides of Liam's ambivalence, both his desire to change and the barriers to doing so. Many clinicians are hesitant about raising and addressing problems, believing that doing so might undermine a client's self-efficacy. Talking about ambivalence can be done without undermining hope.

Ryan 5: It sounds like you want to stop drinking and that getting your children back would be a real incentive for doing so. I'm wondering, though, what things we should be prepared for. What might make stopping difficult for you at this time?

Liam 5: [putting face in hands] I hate thinking about this...

Ryan 6: Thinking about this *is* difficult, but it can help prepare you to cope with problems. [pause] You've tried quitting before? What happened?

Liam 6: Uh, ok. [pause] The hardest thing last time was my friends. They all drink and I could either go out with them or sit home alone. I hate being alone.

Ryan 7: Those are important things that we should address in treatment. Anything else?

Respect Clients' Strengths and Contributions to Treatment

Recognizing and using client strengths is often essential to treatment. These activities build hope, self-confidence, and self-efficacy; strengthen the therapeutic relationship; and increase the probability of recovery (Asay & Lambert, 1999; Lambert, 1992; Dunn & Dougherty, 2004; Lopez & Snyder, 2003).

As seen in the last exchange, there are many places where clinicians can acknowledge and use client strengths. Liam is committing to changing both his drinking behaviors and parenting and is willing to work on each goal, even though doing so is difficult for him. He is socially oriented and insightful, readily describing some situations that have previously put him at risk of relapsing. Ryan recognized these strengths, normalizing the difficulty of discussing these issues in therapy (R6), but also acknowledging the importance of the patterns Liam had already observed and described (R7). Liam is open and honest with Ryan and they appear to be developing a good relationship.

Build Self-efficacy and Mastery, Starting with Goals with a High Probability of Rapid Success

Clients often enter treatment with a number of "failures" under their belt, sometimes believing they will never be able to change. Assignments with a high probability of success can increase clients' perceptions that therapy can be successful and that they can change. Ryan's request that Liam consider where he has run into problems abstaining from alcohol in the past could be framed as a homework assignment that will be successful whether Liam is abstinent, craves alcohol, or drinks. This allows Ryan to normalize Liam's cravings and reframe them as useful observations rather than as a problem in motivation.

Ryan 8: Liam, I'm impressed with your ability to observe when and where you've run into problems abstaining from alcohol. [pause] Could you expand this and think about when and where you crave alcohol this coming week? Record your observations throughout the week. Including as much detail as you can will be helpful. [OK.] I also want you to observe the times when you *don't* have cravings. You're probably doing something special there that we want you to develop and expand.

Focus on the "Forest," While Respecting Clients' "Trees"

Many clients bring in the "crisis of the week" to discuss. It is important to see the big picture, but clinicians must also take their clients' crises seriously. Paying attention to the big picture addresses treatment goals; discussing the current crisis clarifies the context that might otherwise be missed and can strengthen the therapeutic relationship. Such discussions can help clients recognize their clinician's commitment to empathy and understanding.

Ryan 9: Liam, it sounds like you lost it when you couldn't find a sitter when you'd planned to go to a meeting, but that you eventually pulled things together, smoothed things out with your kids, and made it to a later meeting. Right? ([Uh-huh]) Have you thought about how this relates to the issues we've been talking about for the last several weeks?

Liam 9: Yeah. Things don't go as I plan and I lose it. I didn't drink this time, I didn't hit my kids, but I thought about it.

Ryan 10: But you didn't do it. That's a big change from a month ago.

Notice how Ryan first paid attention to Liam's crisis [beginning of R9], making sure that he and Liam were on the same page, but then related this to the larger treatment goal [end of R9]. In doing so, Ryan developed a shared understanding with Liam, which allowed him to intervene and successfully reframe Liam's behavior.

SUMMARY

Change is often difficult, as people may have mixed emotions about change and identify a number of obstacles to change. Helping people change requires a strong understanding of the change process. People enter treatment at different places and with different motivations to change (Prochaska, 1999; Prochaska & DiClemente, 1982). Recognizing these different levels of commitment to change helps identify appropriate styles of intervention for individual clients. These stages are:

- **Precontemplation**—Clients entering in this stage are unaware that they have a problem. Clinicians must first increase their clients' awareness that their behavior has negative consequences and is under their own control.
- **Contemplation**—Many clients enter therapy ambivalent about change; they may want change, but be afraid of its consequences, see major obstacles to change, or feel safe and comfortable where they are. Clinicians working with these clients must address these obstacles, help them weigh the costs and benefits of changing, and work through this ambivalence.
- **Preparation**—During Preparation, clients begin to make small changes that prepare them to make larger changes: planning, getting information, getting social support, problem-solving, and making sure they have the needed skills.
- **Action**—Clients are ready to change and actively begin changing. Their clinicians help them identify behavior change strategies to guide their change process. They may start slowly first, which when reinforced can become more substantial change.
- **Maintenance**—Most change requires more than making the initial change: a continuing commitment to change or to maintain that change. Clinicians help clients acknowledge that change is an ongoing process and that they must prevent or handle slips, helping them become lapses rather than lapses.

Not all goals are useful, nor are they necessarily goals that clients will willingly work towards. Good goals are (a) under the client's control and described (b) in the form of behaviors, (c) in the positive, (d) as specifically as possible, (e) in the present, and (f) in the client's own language (Walter & Peller, 1992).

However, clients and clinicians may identify different goals that may reflect differences in values or a clinicians' poor assessment of the client's stage of change. Wise clinicians work from where their clients are, strengthen their clients' commitment for change, address obstacles for change, respect their clients' strengths and contributions to treatment, and build their clients' self-efficacy and sense of mastery. While they pay attention to their clients' individual concerns, they also are able to see how weekly crises relate to the larger issues that brought clients to treatment.

How Do These Issues Apply to Your Life and Work?

Consider your own experiences with change:

1. Identify your stage of change for a change you made or attempted to make. How difficult was it to change? How was this level of difficulty influenced by your readiness to change?
2. Are there changes that others think you should make that you don't see as important? How have you handled these potential conflicts?
3. For a current "problem" in your life: What are your goals for handling it? How can your strengths be useful in approaching or resolving it? What do exceptions to the problem tell you about how you can handle it?

CHAPTER 9

Developing Case Conceptualizations and Treatment Plans

WHERE ARE WE GOING?

1. What factors contribute to strong case conceptualizations?

2. How can case conceptualizations become biased? How can clinicians reduce this bias?

3. Why is recognizing strengths important to treatment?

4. Why should clinicians write and use treatment plans?

5. How do clinicians write treatment plans?

6. How do clinicians assess treatment?

Yates Verdict Can Serve as Warning to Prevent Future Tragedies

The National Organization for Women is troubled by the March 12 guilty verdict in the Andrea Yates trial and its implications for the one in 1,000 new mothers who will suffer from postpartum psychosis. Our society cannot wash its hands of this tragedy by locking up Yates for life, or putting her to death.

Who shares in the responsibility for these five deaths and possibly another? What about the hospital that sent a dangerously psychotic woman home? What about the doctor who inexplicably stopped Yates' anti-psychotic medication 13 days before this tragedy? What about the weak support system that left Andrea Yates, delusional and suicidal, alone with five young children? The health care system and the medical establishment failed all of them.

Will we take action before this story repeats itself?

This case is not an isolated situation. We desperately need research into the cause and treatment of postpartum psychosis and we need a health care system that doesn't cut corners when it comes to the mentally ill. These women and their families need full medical attention, complete information on the condition and its risks, assistance at home, and widespread public education. The warning signs were there with Andrea Yates and they will be there again for another woman—increased treatment and support could prevent a mental health crisis from turning deadly.

Prosecutors conceded that Yates was mentally ill at the time she drowned her children, yet the jury convicted her of capital murder, which could carry the death penalty. Unfortunately, the jury had to make their decision within the narrow framework of Texas law and as members of a society that has little understanding of mental illness in general and postpartum psychosis in particular.

In the sentencing phase of the trial, the jury must choose the death penalty or life in prison for Andrea Yates. In Harris County, Texas, where Yates was tried, more people are executed than in any other county in the U.S. NOW hopes that the jury will reject this barbaric trend by refusing to add another death to this tragedy. (Gandy, 2002)

1. Who or what caused the murders from Ms. Gandy's point of view? What recommendations does she make about how Andrea Yates should be treated?
2. Does Ms. Gandy's perspective differ from yours? If so, how? If you were writing two treatment plans from these different case conceptualizations—yours and Ms. Gandy's—how would they differ in terms of identification of problems, goals and interventions?
3. Did Ms. Gandy's argument change your view of Ms. Yates? If so, how? What, if anything, does this suggest about the case conceptualization process?

CASE CONCEPTUALIZATIONS

If we are facing in the right direction, all we have to do is keep on walking.

—Buddhist Proverb

Gandy's (2002) description of Andrea Yates provides a radically different viewpoint than that generally drawn. It clarifies the nature of **case conceptualizations**. Gandy's statement, like other case conceptualizations, is an integrated and developed set of hypotheses about the forces driving the person and the causes and treatment of the presenting problem. Like Gandy's statement, case conceptualizations lead to some sort of an action plan; hers specifically to political action. In clinical work, case conceptualizations naturally lead to a plan for treating the individual or family.

Strong case conceptualizations are based on the assessments of, interviews with, and observations of the client. Strong conceptualizations lead to the identification of some problems, goals, and interventions. As Gandy's statement highlighted, not everyone will draw the same conclusions about the nature of the problems to be addressed and appropriate goals for treatment. Different theoretical viewpoints lead to different useful pictures of the person and symptoms (c.f., Allen, 2005; Chasin, Grunebaum, & Herzig, 1990; Saltzman & Norcross, 1990). For example, rational-emotive behavior therapists emphasize the role of irrational beliefs; cognitive-behavior therapists emphasize thought patterns and skill deficits. Structural family therapists emphasize the hierarchies and boundaries in the family system, while feminist therapists emphasize issues of power and oppression and the social and political contexts in which they occur (see Table 9.1). Case conceptualizations are also influenced by the available research and client and clinician preferences. Clients and clinicians may also choose among possible interventions on the basis of time, costs, and possible side effects.

As seen in Table 9.1, there is no single "correct" way of conceptualizing a person's problems; most people can be well-understood from the viewpoint of a number of theories. This can be frustrating for many beginning clinical students, who often are more comfortable with knowing the "right" answer. Developing multiple conceptualizations of clients, however, strengthens clinicians' understanding of the role of research and theory, as well as increasing their ability to intervene flexibly.

Organizing interview and historical data into a psychosocial history can identify hypotheses that have been overlooked and make the case conceptualization process more productive and thorough. Gathering a broadly conceptualized psychosocial history can challenge biases and prevent clinicians from missing information that does not readily fit their case conceptualizations. Kottler (2004) describes the importance of careful assessments:

> It's not that you are procrastinating when you hesitate to answer her query about how you will help her; it is just that you would be foolish to attempt any intervention without fully understanding what you are attempting to accomplish. It would be as if you went to see a doctor complaining of a stomachache and she immediately scheduled you for surgery without running appropriate tests to determine what might be wrong. (p. 198)

In the following case material, imagine how Ruthie Schlimgen's doctors, therapist and social workers might have decided to intervene when she was diagnosed with rheumatoid arthritis. How could this information guide their case conceptualization and treatment?

TABLE **9.1**

Examples of Theoretical Explanations for Andrea Yates' Depressive Symptoms and Corresponding Treatment Approaches.

Biological model. Ms. Yates had a biological vulnerability to depression, especially following the hormonal changes accompanying childbirth. These changes can be countered through a variety of medical treatments, including antidepressant and antipsychotic medications and electroconvulsive therapy.

Psychoanalytic model. Ms. Yates' childhood encouraged her development of a strict, overly rigid superego and led her to ignore her own needs. Her marriage reinforced this pattern. Her ego was relatively weak and unable to negotiate between her demanding superego and her often-ignored and "unacceptable" impulses. She often handled these conflicts by using projection. Treatment should focus on setting more reasonable expectations and strengthen her ability to negotiate between id impulses and her rigid and demanding superego.

Cognitive model. Ms. Yates held rigid and unreasonable expectations and beliefs about herself and her children. These were often dichotomous (good vs. evil) and unrealistic. Treatment should teach her to recognize her beliefs and how they influence her interpretations of situations, especially during periods of extreme, negative emotions. Then she can learn to challenge her irrational beliefs and identify healthier ways of observing and thinking about herself and her world.

Person-centered model. Ms. Yates was raised in a demanding environment that failed to accept her for who she was. As a result, she learned that she had to appear to be someone other than who she truly was in order to be accepted by others. Listening to her empathically and genuinely, accepting her for who she is—someone who is imperfect, a woman who murdered her children—will allow her to begin to accept herself as she is and, paradoxically, to begin to make changes to actualize her self-concept.

Multicultural model. Ms. Yates can be understood in terms of her race, gender, class, religion, and other cultural influences that, in sum, caused her to set high, unrealistic standards for herself; repress anger and avoid discussions of concerns and problems; take care of others while making her own needs a low priority; and, ultimately, to murder her children. Treatment should simultaneously help her to recognize these influences and identify more flexible ways of responding to these pressures.

It's Not So Simple

Ruthie Schlimgen

Ruthie Schlimgen (43) was recently diagnosed with rheumatoid arthritis. When she was first diagnosed, she believed she had a benign and nonprogressive form of the disease. Given that belief, she took her medicine only when it was absolutely necessary—when she could no longer do her job or tolerate the pain. This decision made sense in terms of earlier events in her life.

Although she was a powerful and outspoken woman who was often very assertive about individual and social injustices, Ruthie was ambivalent about her body and its treatment.

(continues)

She had been physically, emotionally, and sexually abused as a young girl. She learned to mistrust others and not ask for help. At some level, she also learned that her needs were unimportant.

This message was consistent with other family and cultural messages. Her mother took care of everybody else before taking care of herself. Like her mother, Ruthie put herself "last on her list" and became, as she described herself, a "German, stoic idiot." She believed she could offer people only one thing: her ability to take care of them. She wondered whether she deserved to be cared for. Would anyone step in to take care of her if she needed it?

Ruthie also had a heart condition that was undiagnosed until she was 13. Until it was diagnosed—and even afterwards—she was encouraged to ignore her body and what it was telling her. Although she received tens of thousands of dollars' worth of tests for HIV, heart conditions, brain cancer, breast cancer, bone cancer, leukemia, lupus, multiple sclerosis, Lyme disease, and other autoimmune diseases, her vague physical symptoms went undiagnosed until she was 43. At each flare-up of her symptoms she was told that there was no problem. She felt that her body was not her own and that others did not respect her opinions about it. She was "catastrophizing." She was a "hypochondriac."

As Ruthie had a long history of psychiatric problems, her physicians also wondered whether her cardiac arrhythmias were due to panic disorder and whether her pain was psychogenic in origin or secondary to depression. Nonetheless, she had been moderating her moods and relationships well—on a very stressful job—and had been getting by well without psychiatric medicines for three years. Still, the very thing that she did to keep herself healthy—take care of her psychological self—put herself at risk physically:

> I was focusing on psychological things. I was focusing on not getting depressed, because that was always a pretty big thing for me. I did a pretty good job of ignoring that crap, but then ignored physical cues that were screaming at me, that I overlooked to keep working and to take care of other people. So in that way I got out of balance.

Ruthie is the mother of two adult children who were living on their own and is a lesbian in a committed relationship of 15 years. She had considerable support from her family and friends, but also frequently faced discrimination and prejudice. The conservative congregation of her church told her that she was going to hell when she came out to them. Her daughter's inner-city high school had refused to allow her partner to attend parent-teacher conferences. Her partner had domestic partner benefits on her health insurance, but the insurance company challenged these benefits when Ruthie's health care costs escalated. Their apartment door and windows were occasionally vandalized. Ruthie learned to stand up for her rights and, simultaneously, to bite her tongue.

(continues)

(continued)

At the time of her diagnosis, Ruthie and her partner were applying to buy a house. It was difficult for her to admit that she was having significant health problems while continuing to pursue buying a house with her partner. Her ambivalence about sharing her concerns with her partner, with whom she had previously shared everything, was further complicated by the fact that her partner had been seriously depressed and suicidal in the past year.

Ruthie's ability to hear her diagnosis and to pursue treatment options was also influenced by work and financial issues. Ruthie managed the human resources department of a small corporation that paid just enough to put her above the poverty level. She could not afford to quit her job because she needed her health care benefits. Their other bills accounted for a large percentage of her salary each month and, to pay them, they often robbed Peter to pay Paul. She could not afford to take a day off work just because she was in pain, so often had to work through the pain.

Ruthie also had a significant history of narcotic abuse that began in her teens and continued into her 30s. She now worried about becoming an addict again. She often preferred to stay in pain and, rather than worrying her family and friends, kept her mouth shut.

With some chronic pain disorders, medication is a choice. Treatment may include learning how to tolerate or transform pain, or to distract oneself from it. Rheumatoid arthritis is different, however. The pain associated with rheumatoid arthritis generally indicates a flare-up of the disease process, especially joint inflammation. Much of this inflammation is chronic and progressive. Therefore, when someone with rheumatoid arthritis experiences pain, the disease process is attacked immediately and aggressively. A flare-up that lasted weeks, like hers, meant considerable additional damage. Her doctor was angry that she failed to follow his directions and compromised her health. On the other hand, she hadn't "heard" him tell her these things. "[I was] doing self-care on many levels, but still not doing what I needed to do about what was obviously a pretty serious disease. I didn't understand how serious it was."

So, how do you report symptoms when you haven't been believed in the past? How can you be a patient when it will put a greater burden on your family? How do you ask for help when you have not been encouraged to express your needs or to expect that your needs will be met? (Case material and quotations used with permission)

1. Develop a timeline and psychosocial history for Ruthie. What other information would you want? Why? How might the factors identified in the timeline and psychosocial history impact her preference for treatment strategies?
2. What is your conceptualization of the problems Ruthie is having in handling her health? How did your case conceptualization consider and

(continues)

reflect the context of her life? Develop at least one other case conceptualization from another theoretical viewpoint.

3. If you were her health psychologist, what would be your goals for working with her? Why? Do you think she would she be willing to work with you on these goals? Why or why not?

4. Her physician wanted to aggressively treat her rheumatoid arthritis at any cost, which she was unwilling to do. If you were a social worker working in this doctor's office, how would you address this conflict between the two of them?

5. How did Ruthie's readiness to change shift during the diagnosis process? What helped her make that shift? What would you do to help her commit to change?

RESEARCH INFORMS TREATMENT

You certainly usually find something, if you look, but it is not always quite the something you were after.

—J. R. R. Tolkien

When developing a case conceptualization, clinicians frequently draw on the research on an issue, problem, or group. This research helps clinicians develop their understanding and case conceptualization. What **comorbid** disorders can be expected? What kinds of typical obstacles can be anticipated in the course of treatment? What treatment strategies are most effective? What ancillary treatments increase the effectiveness of treatment? What makes treatment less effective? What risk factors should be considered? What role, if any, does medicine have in treatment?

Clinicians should also consider the client's culture(s). What challenges or stressors do people of the client's cultural backgrounds typically face? What values are commonly shared? What messages do people of this culture generally receive about self, family, sex, parenting, and their bodies? What resources and supports are commonly available? What are unavailable? As discussed in Figure 4.2, many people identify with multiple groups. For example, Ruthie Schlimgen identified as a woman, a lesbian, a German American, a mother, a recovering addict, and a person with rheumatoid arthritis. Andrea Yates identified as a Christian, a wife, a mother, a daughter, and a woman.

In most practices, a number of clients present with similar problems or issues (e.g., depression, anxiety, substance abuse, or cognitive impairments). The knowledge that clinicians gain through researching these problems develops an expertise helpful to many clients. Even when working with a relatively homogeneous population, clinicians will pick up clients with new presenting issues. For example, at an in-home family therapy program, many children and teens may be depressed or oppositional, and have school or legal problems; however, occasional clients may be enuretic or diagnosed with obsessive-compulsive disorder. A clinician may generally work with an African-American population, but sometimes work with Latinos. As new issues and populations present, wise clinicians do additional research.

Food for Thought

- Depression often accompanies rheumatoid arthritis (see Table 9.2). Given this brief summary, how would you approach treating Ruthie Schlimgen's depression? How does the research summarized here fit with your case conceptualization?
- What does the research on postpartum depression generally conclude? How would this research inform your treatment of Andrea Yates? How would this knowledge interact with and complement your understanding of her personal style, cultures and context?
- Look at the research on post-traumatic stress disorder. How might this research impact your understanding of Reymundo Sanchez's behavior? How might his background as a Puerto Rican male, raised in Chicago, and active in a gang influence how you conceptualized his behavior?

TABLE **9.2**

Summary of Research Findings on Psychosocial Consequences of and Interventions for People with Rheumatoid Arthritis (RA).

RA is associated with mild to moderate levels of depression, although not necessarily more so than for other chronic diseases.

Even RA patients with low levels of depression have unusually high use of medical services, decreased functional activities, fatigue, and diminished quality of life.

Both RA-related and RA-unrelated negative attributions are related to depression.

Social-stress levels are closely related to whether a person with RA is depressed.

Optimism both reduces the risk of additional health problems for people with RA and seems to be related to better outcomes.

Dissatisfaction with current ability to perform previously valued physical tasks, rather than disability *per se*, is the most important predictor of depression in people with RA.

People with RA who use active coping and religious coping have less pain and depression and better psychological well-being than those who tend to rely on passive coping strategies.

Involving family members in treatment seems to be somewhat helpful for the person with RA and may also be helpful for the rest of the family as well.

Note: From Abraído-Lanza, Vásquez, & Echeverría, 2004; Chaney et al., 2004; Murphy, Dickens, Creed, & Bernstein, 1999; Neugebauer, Katz, & Pasch, 2003.

EVERYONE HAS STRENGTHS

Success is achieved by developing our strengths, not by eliminating our weaknesses.

—Marilyn vos Savant

When clients present for therapy, they are generally not at their best. In crisis, their attention may be focused on the things that are not working. They may rely on maladaptive coping strategies. They may describe only the parts of their life that are problematic, either because they believe that is what their clinician is interested in, or because they want to make sure that their clinician recognizes the significant help they need. Sometimes clinicians fail to look for or ask about strengths.

Although the field of **positive psychology** is still in its infancy, Lopez and Snyder (2003) assume that everyone has strengths. They note that the early evidence suggests that using and developing client strengths increases school achievement; leads to meaningful, productive work; and improves mental health. Clinicians need to pay attention both to people's strengths and to their weaknesses, each equally valid aspects of the person (Evans, 1993; Lopez & Snyder, 2003; Lopez, Snyder, & Rasmussen, 2003).

Look at the glass of water in Figure 9.1. Is it half empty or half full? The nature of this question illustrates the dichotomizing tendencies of humans. The glass is no more one than the other. Each aspect—its emptiness and its fullness—are valid ways of looking at the glass of water. Similarly, our strengths and weaknesses, problems and exceptions to problems, successes and failures, are equally valid aspects of who we are.

The importance of identifying strengths can be seen in an example. Jayne (age 14) was molested by a neighbor when she was 13. Because she felt guilty about putting herself at risk, because she felt dirty and ashamed, because she felt unsafe in most situations, Jayne closed down, refused to talk to the people around her, and began fighting with her parents. Her father, with whom she had had a long and healthy relationship, was surprised when, relatively late in treatment, Jayne's therapist noted that it was nice that he and Jayne were beginning to develop a better relationship. Her father observed that

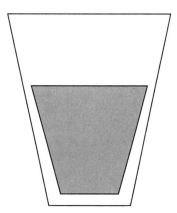

FIGURE **9.1** Is this glass of water half-empty or half-full?

they had had a positive, supportive relationship until Jayne was molested and had begun to withdraw.

Her therapist's failure to recognize that Jayne and he had had a strong relationship was hurtful to her father, but, more importantly, it meant that her therapist formed a weak case conceptualization that undermined her empathy for Jayne's parents. As a result, she failed to tap an important resource for treatment. Jayne's therapist might have asked herself these questions:

- Although Jayne and her father frequently fight, do they always? Have they always?
- What distinguishes between the bad and better times?
- What do Jayne and her parents do well? How can their strengths be used as resources in treatment?

As this example illustrates, looking for strengths and exceptions to problems has multiple benefits. In particular, it can lead to the development of a stronger case conceptualization, identify resources for treatment, build empathy, and strengthen the therapeutic alliance.

Food for Thought

What strengths does Ruthie Schlimgen have? How could these be used in the course of treatment? What about Reymundo Sanchez? Andrea Yates?

WHY WRITE TREATMENT PLANS?

Without goals, and plans to reach them, you are like a ship that has set sail with no destination.

—Fitzhugh Dodson

Treatment plans are a standard part of treatment, often required by agencies and insurance companies. Why should clinicians write them? Treatment plans help client and clinician develop collaborative goals that help them recognize that they are both working well together. Developing short-term goals and **interventions** provides client and clinician with a "map" that helps them identify where they are in treatment and when goals have been met. Treatment plans can increase client hopefulness and self-efficacy. They can make change easier to recognize.

Without a treatment plan, treatment can be rudderless, going hither and yon with the weekly concerns of a client: for example, fighting with husband, children who are disrespectful, being bypassed for a promotion at work. Treatment plans remind clinicians to step back and see the forest, rather than only individual trees. In our example, each of these symptoms (i.e., the fighting, disrespectful children, and work problems) might be seen as problems with effective and assertive communication. Focusing on the big picture can help clinicians develop a consistent course in treatment and ensure that the client's full range of concerns is addressed (L. Seligman, 2006). Collaboratively developing treatment plans with clients can build the clinician's understanding of the problem and empathy for the client, ultimately strengthening the therapeutic alliance.

DEVELOPING A TREATMENT PLAN

Reduce your plan to writing.... The moment you complete this, you will have definitely given concrete form to the intangible desire.

—Napoleon Hill

A treatment plan is a very useful therapeutic tool for both clients and clinicians. Generally, treatment starts with a client identifying a problem and preferred long-term goals. Often, **problem statements** are phrased in the client's own words (e.g., "Our marriage is in trouble because he never talks to me. He treats me like I'm a maid and nothing more."). Phrasing the problem in the client's own words helps clinicians see the problem from the client's own viewpoint. Notice how different the conceptualization might be if this client had instead said, "We fight like cats and dogs, each wanting to be King of the Hill—but then we have wonderful makeup sex and seem to have a common vision of where we want to go. If only we could get there without killing each other first!"

Asking people to imagine their preferred future can sometimes be useful, as with the **miracle question**, which asks clients to imagine that a miracle happened and how they would first know that the miracle had occurred (Berg, 1994; de Shazer, 1988).

> Imagine that you go home tonight, do the dishes, go about your daily life, go to sleep, and a miracle happens. The problem that brought you here has disappeared! What would be the first thing that you would notice that would let you know that this miracle happened to you?

This exercise allows clients to imagine change, recognize where the miracle is already happening, and visualize the steps that need to be taken to make it happen more frequently. Asking clients what they were doing differently after "the miracle" can help them more concretely identify what they can do to change. Clinicians can follow the miracle question with a **scaling question** in subsequent weeks to assess where the client is relative to the desired change, "On a scale from one to ten, with 0 being the day that you called to make your appointment and 10 being how it will be the day after the miracle, where are you today?" When a client's response is different from the previous one, ask, "What is different?" This series of questions gets people thinking about change and what they can do to place it under their control and make it happen.

Goal Statements

Two different problem statements have been described, from which **goal statements** can be inferred.

> **Problem for Person 1:** He never talks to me. He treats me like I'm a maid and nothing more.
> **Long-term Goal 1:** I want him to talk to me and treat me as his partner, someone who he loves.

and

> **Problem for Person 2:** We fight like cats and dogs, each wanting to be King of the Hill.

> **Long-term Goal 2:** I want us to work together well and have a common vision of where we want to go.

Of course, these statements are inferences and would need to be checked out, before going further (e.g., "What I hear you saying you want is... Am I on track?").

There are stated goals for each of these problem statements, but do these **long-term goals** match Walter and Peller's (1992) criteria (i.e., a behavioral goal that is under the client's control, stated as a specific behavior to be added rather than only one to be removed, in the present, and in the client's own language)? (see Table 8.3). Goal 1, for example, is specific, positive, in the present and in the client's own language, but it is not under the client's control. Goal 2 is positive, in the present and in the client's own language, but is not specific. The second half of this goal statement (i.e., a common vision) is not a behavioral outcome and needs to be described in more specific behavioral terms. Furthermore, it's not clear whether the client has control over the outcomes. This might be a good goal for couples' therapy, but should be more clearly under the client's control if this is a goal for individual counseling. Goal 1 could be better phrased as:

> **Long-term Goal 1:** I am going to begin taking myself more seriously and ask that others do so too.

Goal and problem must match. Finally, the problem and long-term goal must fit each other. Sometimes clients and clinicians choose goals that do not address the issue identified in the problem statement. A student with poor grades may say that she needs to study more (although she cannot concentrate when she *does* study). A man who is overweight may believe that he needs to eat less (although he eats a normal number of calories, but rarely exercises and consumes more than 1200 calories per day in beer). A father may conclude that he needs to be stricter with his daughter (in fact, he is strict enough, but fails to tell her that he loves her).

Note how the last version of Long-term Goal 1 only partially matches the problem. Perhaps a more complete description of Problem 1 would be

> **Problem for Person 1:** He never talks to me and treats me like I'm a maid. I think about myself in this way, too, and allow others to treat me that way.

This new version of Problem 1 helps the client to recognize her role in the problem and identify what she can do to change.

Food for Thought

- Are you satisfied with Long-term Goal 1? What could be done to make it clearer and more specific (i.e., How would she know that she had been treated seriously?).
- Rework Goal 2 to meet Walter and Peller's (1992) recommendations.

Good goal statements depend on a strong and accurate assessment of the problem. Timelines, genograms, psychosocial histories, and behavioral observations can broaden clinicians' and clients' perspectives, so they can look past symptoms and problems to the larger concerns (i.e., past individual trees to the larger forest).

Short-Term Goals

Although goal statements are useful, they do not provide a detailed plan for treatment. They are like trying to travel the country without a map. Most clinicians expand client goal statements by identifying **short-term goals** that move the client closer to meeting long-term goals (e.g., "Client will learn and practice cognitive therapy techniques to challenge irrational beliefs."). Even short-term goals are often broken into smaller steps—the interventions that will be used to meet these goals. These goals and interventions should, if the treatment plan is well-designed and carried out, help clients meet their goals.

As discussed earlier, goals are generally written using concrete action verbs ("ing" words), reflecting the idea that treatment is a process, rather than a place or state of mind (Walter & Peller, 1992). Furthermore, not all action verbs are equivalent. Many clinicians organize their goals with Bloom's (1984) taxonomy in mind (see Table 9.3). Rather than only knowing or understanding a concept (lower order cognitive tasks), clinicians generally want clients to *apply* their knowledge and understanding (Application) and *think critically* about their life and problems (Analysis, Synthesis, Evaluation).

TABLE **9.3**

Bloom's (1984) Taxonomy of Learning and Goal Statements Associated with Each Level of Cognitive Processing.

Level of processing	Action verbs	Possible goal
Knowledge	Define, name, list, tell	"Identify three approaches to parenting."
Comprehension	Explain, discuss, identify, recognize	"Discuss the role of self-talk in emotion."
Application	Apply, practice, illustrate, use, demonstrate	"Practice assertiveness skills in settings outside the office, starting with easier situations first."
Analysis	Distinguish, analyze, criticize, relate	"Distinguish between the emotional responses elicited by validating and invalidating responses."
Synthesis	Design, plan, propose, organize	"Design an approach to responding to your child's anger that uses the skills discussed today."
Evaluation	Judge, evaluate, choose, measure	"Determine whether your approach to parenting meets your description of 'effective parenting.'"

Food for Thought

What short-term goals would follow from Goals 1 and 2?

Clinicians want to help clients extend their understanding outside the office and increase their ability to independently use the skills they learn there.

Treatment Planning: An Example

Although there are different formats for presenting a treatment plan, one common way of doing so is presented in Table 9.4. Problem and goal statements are generally described above a row of cells, which include the short-term goals and interventions. Dates to meet goals and outcome measures may be included in additional cells.

When Jayne (age 14) entered treatment, she was neither willing to work directly on trauma or abuse issues nor willing to work on family issues or her frequent absences from school. She *was* willing to change her depressive style of thinking, improve her coping skills, and address the relationship problems she was having, especially with her boyfriend. How she and her clinician agreed to approach these problems is described in Table 9.4.

TABLE **9.4**
Treatment Plan for Jayne, Who Is Depressed, Coping Poorly, and Having Significant Relationship Problems.

Problem 1: I am sad much of the time and have difficulty getting out of bed in the morning. I'm not enjoying the things I used to.

Long-Term Goal 1: I want to be able to be happy and enjoy life again.

Short-Term Goals	Interventions	
1a. Client will challenge irrational beliefs contributing to depression.	1a(i).	Discuss relationship between beliefs and emotional and behavioral consequences.
	1a(ii).	Monitor and analyze connection between beliefs and emotional and behavioral consequences, especially during periods of strong emotion.
	1a(iii).	Recognize irrational beliefs and their impact on emotions.
	1a(iv).	Challenge irrational beliefs, first in the supportive environment of the therapy room, then in balance of life.

TABLE **9.4**
Treatment Plan for Jayne, Who Is Depressed, Coping Poorly, and Having Significant
Relationship Problems (Continued)

1b. Client will engage in regular self-care.	1b(i). Discuss the importance of regular self-care in maintaining mental health.
	1b(ii). Identify self-care behaviors that are personally relevant.
	1b(iii). Engage in at least one self-care behavior per day, noting both consequences of using them and obstacles to doing so.

Problem 2: When I get stressed or upset, I react in negative ways. I see drama all about me—and I cause it. I yell and scream. I push people away from me. I cut or burn myself.

Long-Term Goal 2: I want to be able to cope with my feelings in a less impulsive, healthier manner. I want to be able to cope without ending up in the hospital again.

2a. Client will accept and validate his or her feelings, even when others invalidate them.	2a(i). Discuss adaptive aspects of both positive and negative feelings, distinguishing between emotions and how we act on them.
	2a(ii). Discuss ways that feelings can be invalidated, observing ways that self or others do so, and the consequences of being invalidated.
	2a(iii). Challenge invalidating responses from self and others, substituting more validating responses, noting consequences of doing so.
2b. Client will cope more effectively with stressors.	2b(i). Discuss coping mechanisms, evaluating their impact on self and valued outcomes, including but not limited to relationships.
	2b(ii). Increase use of adaptive coping strategies, evaluating their success, identifying better ways of coping as necessary.
	2b(iii). Discuss and practice meditation and mindfulness techniques.

Problem 3: I have difficulty identifying anything good about myself, so doubt that anyone else could love me. My boyfriend and I often end up in fights, because I twist everything to mean that he's leaving me.

Long-Term Goal 3: I want to be able to feel good about myself and to have a close, rewarding relationship with my boyfriend and others.

3a. Client will see herself accurately and value who she is.	3a(i). Identify positive aspects of self and behavior, validating positive intentions of less negative aspects.
	3a(ii). Challenge dichotomous thinking when discussing problems.
	3a(iii). Identify and use believable daily affirmations to focus on strengths and goals.
3b. Client will identify and use more positive ways of relating to others.	3b(i). Identify self-talk leading to more negative interactions, first challenging self-talk in session, then practicing self-talk under less controlled settings.
	3b(ii). Discuss assertiveness, distinguishing it from passive, aggressive, and manipulative behaviors. Practice assertiveness in controlled settings first, then move up hierarchy.
	3b(iii). Identify qualities present in client's ideal relationship, evaluating whether current relationships reasonably approach these ideals.
	3b(iv). Discuss and practice ways of developing more satisfying relationships.

It is rarely advisable to work on goals that a client finds unacceptable. Many clinicians discuss trauma issues directly. Clients may become more willing to discuss this trauma, however, as the therapeutic alliance becomes stronger and they become more confident about their ability to change (Walter & Peller, 1992). Furthermore, treatment of abuse and trauma is generally approached multidimensionally; school, work, family, and grief issues often each have to be addressed (Faust & Katchen, 2004).

GETTING THE BIG PICTURE

Details create the big picture.

—**Sanford I. Weill**

Initial assessments help develop a broad, contextualized picture of what is happening. This assessment process should include identifying expectations for treatment, previous therapy relationships, current and past substance use and abuse, current and past suicidal ideation and behaviors, strengths and weaknesses, exceptions and exacerbations to the problem, and the nature and strength of the social support network (Park & Slattery, 2009; Slattery, 2004).

While developing this case conceptualization and treatment plan, clinicians should also consider the meaning of symptoms and problems to the client in order to further build empathy (Kottler, 2004). Why is the client asking for help now rather than at some other point? What were things like before the problem began (or got to this level)? How is this problem affecting the client's work, school, relationships, or functioning in the community? What are the costs and benefits of symptoms or problems? What would happen if the problem were resolved? Who else is invested in the client changing (or staying as is)?

Most problems and symptoms can be addressed in several ways. Treatment plans should consider the nature and level of services appropriate for a particular client (Kottler, 2004; L. Seligman, 2006):

- What intensity of services is necessary to stabilize the client (i.e., outpatient, partial hospitalization, inpatient, or residential)? What option would be least restrictive *and* most helpful?
- Is counseling appropriate? If so, what kind (i.e., individual, family, or group)? In what setting should it be offered?
- What community services are available to help stabilize the client (e.g., housing, transportation, medical assistance, parenting classes)?
- What natural supports can be engaged to help stabilize the client (e.g., grandparents, babysitters, softball coaches, and ministers)?
- Might medication be appropriate? Should a psychiatric consult be requested?
- Are adjunct drug and alcohol services necessary? Could drug and alcohol issues be solely addressed in the primary treatment relationship?
- Has the client had a recent physical? Could some unidentified medical syndrome cause or complicate the client's symptoms?
- How might already identified medical syndromes influence—or cause—the client's symptoms? Could symptoms be caused by prescription (or recreational) medications?

Food for Thought

For the people discussed in Chapters 8 and 9 (i.e., Ruthie Schlimgen, Reymundo Sanchez, Lia Lee, and Andrea Yates):

1. What do they want? What would they be willing to work towards?
2. How do their goals differ from their society's goals for them? How might their goals differ from your goals for them?
3. Write a treatment plan for one of these individuals (a) using goals that he or she would find acceptable; (b) recognizing current strengths and exceptions to the problem(s) faced, as well as current symptoms; (c) breaking the goal into concrete, recognizable steps that build on each other; and (d) considering natural supports, substance use, and health issues.

- Does the client express strong preferences for the gender, race, or religious background of the clinician? If not, is there a reason to consider these issues when assigning a clinician?

Some issues are especially complicated and may require multiple types of interventions. Because trauma and abuse affect many dimensions of a person's life, treatment should focus on multiple aspects, including safety planning, grief work, and family functioning (Faust & Katchen, 2004). Treatment should both address patterns that put clients at risk and symptoms that arose in response to the trauma. Often, therapy should challenge problematic thoughts while also building skills. Because trauma can affect work and school performance, treatment should also consider functioning in these realms.

Although adjunct services can be very helpful, more is not necessarily better. To be most helpful, there must be a shared, consistent picture among the treatment team and other professionals involved. This can be accomplished through phone contacts or by sharing written reports. Furthermore, many clients can be overwhelmed when too many workers and services are offered at the same time. Therefore, it is best to approach treatment using a sort of triage model: identifying and working first with those issues or services that will most rapidly stabilize the client or create movement.

ASSESSING PROGRESS

Know what's weird? Day by day, nothing seems to change, but pretty soon ... everything's different.
—**Calvin from "Calvin and Hobbes"**

Weltner (1998) argues that a good assessment of the problem leads to a treatment plan that is easy, efficient, and effective. Plans are not necessarily useful and efficacious, however, no matter how carefully they have been developed. Plans might not be effective because the problem was poorly or incompletely assessed, the treatment plan does not really address the problem, the client and clinician do not identify the same problem, the proposed plan was unacceptable to the client, or the plan was poorly implemented. As a result, after developing and implementing a treatment plan, it is important to evaluate on a regular and ongoing basis whether the plan helps clients meet their **treatment goals**.

There are a variety of ways to determine whether treatment has been effective. The easiest way to assess whether treatment is effective is to ask a client. There are also short satisfaction questionnaires that are aimed at either an adult or child (e.g., Client Satisfaction Questionnaire [CSQ]: Larsen, Atkisson, Hargreaves, & Nguyen, 1979; Youth Satisfaction Questionnaire [YSQ]: Stuentzner-Gibson, Koren, & DeChillo, 1995).

Unfortunately, satisfaction questionnaires like the CSQ and the YSQ are only weakly related to either therapist perceptions of outcomes or client behaviors. The poor validity of these measures has been attributed to several factors. Clients, family members, and therapists might each focus on different aspects of a client's behavior (e.g., subjective depression, energy levels, or sick days taken). Clients can focus on the connectedness in the relationship, rating therapy well, even though little change was made. Clients might also give unduly rosy feedback to protect a therapist's feelings. Despite these problems, most clinicians believe that monitoring client satisfaction is one important aspect of assessing the effectiveness of treatment, even though it might not mean what it appears to mean.

Change can also be assessed with paper and pencil measures at intake and some later point in treatment. For example, if a client's treatment is effective, one might expect that his or her score on a depression assessment (e.g., Beck Depression Inventory [BDI]: Beck, Steer, & Garbin, 1988) would decrease. Self-reports like the BDI are short and easy to respond to and score, although because their intent is fairly transparent, they are easily biased by the desire to look good or bad or by client denial and lack of insight about the problem.

One can also monitor change using behavioral measures. Again, assuming the outcome measure is a good assessment of this change, there should be a visible change in the frequency or rating of the behavior across time.

Clinicians may also assess change in treatment using more than one measure and at more than one point. Borckardt and his colleagues (Borckardt et al., 2008), for example, recommend a daily or weekly measure of distress, as well as standardized outcome measures like the BDI or the Outcome Questionnaire-45 (OQ-45: Lambert, Gregersen, & Burlingame, 2004). A family therapy program might use measures of both child and family functioning (e.g., Child and Adolescent Functional Assessment Scale [CAFAS]: Hodges, Doucette-Gates, & Liao, 1999; Family Assessment Device [FAD]: Kabacoff, Miller, Bishop, Epstein, & Keitner, 1990). Using multidimensional scales such as the FAD or CAFAS and multiple outcome measures is useful because they can identify both growth and strengths, while also identifying relative weaknesses. Behavior in the home, as assessed by the CAFAS, might not be a problem, although functioning in school could continue to be problematic. Furthermore, a child might have made considerable progress in the home, school, and community, as assessed by the CAFAS, but the family might still be struggling to set healthy rules and roles, as assessed by the FAD.

For example, Sommer, Jayne's therapist, wondered whether treatment was effective and moving toward treatment goals. She hypothesized that if it was, monthly ratings of depression as assessed by the BDI should decrease, as should incidents of self-injurious behaviors, the number of school absences, and hospital admissions. As shown in Figure 9.2, some of these measures changed while others did not change as much, which may indicate that the treatment plan needs to be fine-tuned to further target these behaviors.

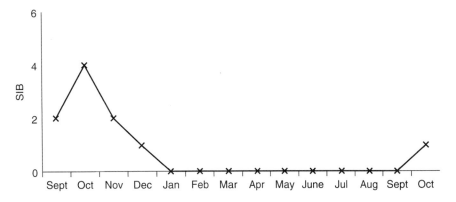

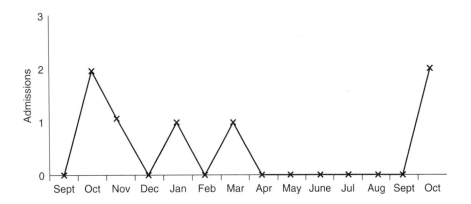

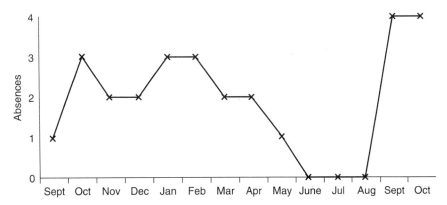

FIGURE **9.2** Effects of treatment on four of Jayne's target behaviors: incidents of self-injurious behavior (SIB), hospital admissions, school absences (excluding hospital days), and monthly assessment of depression on the BDI.

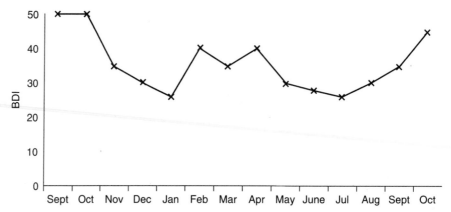

FIGURE **9.2** Effects of treatment on four of Jayne's target behaviors: incidents of self-injurious behavior (SIB), hospital admissions, school absences (excluding hospital days), and monthly assessment of depression on the BDI (Continued)

Furthermore, these measures can also be additional assessments of the problem. As seen in Figure 9.2, Jayne seems to have an easier time in the summer, when no target behaviors occurred, although reported levels of depression were still somewhat elevated. Of course, these measures cannot distinguish from among several possible causes of the continuing problems: elevations during the fall could be related to the transition into the school year, interpersonal problems when around more people, a social phobia, or anxiety about school performance. Nonetheless, it does suggest that some school-related factors are involved. Furthermore, they suggest that the problem does not completely decrease over the summer and that the current use of anti-depressants and therapy interventions have not completely addressed depression. These graphs might also be used to discuss treatment goals. Although Jayne had previously refused to contract for school issues, seeing and discussing these graphs might cause her to reconsider her decision.

SUMMARY

Treatment plans prevent client and clinician from getting lost among the daily crises and guide treatment towards meeting treatment goals. The content of treatment plans should be mutually decided by the client and clinician and be a function of the clinician's theoretical viewpoint, research on the problem, and the client's strengths and resources—as well as those of the clinician. While balancing these competing factors, clinicians should gather as broad an assessment as possible and address sources of bias. Often this means that clinicians should gather information from multiple sources.

Treatment plans, like other pieces of information about clients, should be written as a way of documenting that careful, thoughtful treatment planning occurred. When possible, plans should be written collaboratively with clients in order to help client and clinician develop collaborative goals, identify that both client and clinician are working towards the same goals, and develop a map for treatment.

Most treatment plans have the following parts:

- **Problem statements**, generally expressed in the client's own words (e.g., "He hit me again and I'm so afraid.").
- **Goal Statements**, the long-term goals. These should both match the problem and the client's unique situation and preferences (e.g., "I just want to get away from him," "I want to be able to be assertive with him," or "I want to understand him.").
- **Short-term goals**, the immediate subgoals that help the client move toward accomplishing long-term goals (e.g., for the first goal statement, "I want to strengthen my support system," "I want to develop skills to take care of myself and my children financially," and "I want to develop more confidence in my opinions and actions).
- **Interventions**, the specific strategies that client and clinician will use to meet their goals.

In effective treatment plans, problem and goal statements match, while the interventions help the team meet short-term goals. When all short-term goals are satisfied, long-term goals will also be met and problems will be resolved.

Treatment progress and outcomes should be regularly assessed, preferably from the beginning of treatment and along several outcome dimensions. Satisfaction questionnaires are useful, but can be biased. Multidimensional scales and multiple measures (self-reports, paper and pencil measures, and behavioral outcomes) can identify strengths, weaknesses, ongoing issues, and alternative interpretations of problems.

How Do These Issues Apply to Your Life and Work?

1. Consider a time when you worked with someone who did not share a clear "treatment plan" with you (e.g., a course without a syllabus, a vacation without destinations or plans, medical interventions that were not clearly described). How did this experience feel? If this lack of planning felt good under some circumstances and was uncomfortable at other times, why? What was different across situations?

2. Do some research on a problem that you would like to change. What do you learn? How does this influence how you might think about changing it.

3. For a "problem" that is important to you, write a brief treatment plan. As you do so, pay attention to the research on the problem, exceptions to the problem, and strengths that may be useful in resolving the problem. Pay attention to your conceptualization of the problem. Develop concrete, recognizable steps toward meeting your goals. Your treatment plan should consider contextual issues including natural supports, substance use, and health.

4. How would you assess progress towards your goal? How have you identified change on a goal you have previously addressed?

PART IV

Clinical Skills for Expressing Empathy and Facilitating Positive Change

Part 4 of this book focuses on the skills that clinicians need to effectively communicate their understanding to those with whom they are working and to help bring about positive change. We begin this section by outlining the relational and structuring skills that clinicians use to engage clients (Chapter 10). The therapeutic alliance is built by the clinician's careful and empathic listening to clients and by creating a clear and safe structure for treatment. Clinicians create a clear and safe structure by setting effective boundaries for treatment, using a thoughtful informed consent process, and working collaboratively with clients.

Empathy must be conveyed in order to be effective. Chapter 11 describes the verbal skills that clinicians use to obtain and communicate empathic understanding. Chapter 12 describes the common issues that cut across different therapeutic approaches and common strategies used to help clients change. This chapter also describes how clinicians handle client strengths, exceptions to problems, and barriers to treatment. Chapter 13 reviews strategies for ending treatment well, including preventing relapse and helping clients own their treatment progress, and identifies ways of responding to difficult terminations.

CHAPTER 10

Building the Therapeutic Alliance: Listening Nonverbally and Structuring Treatment

WHERE ARE WE GOING?

1. What strategies do clinicians use to develop their ability to be empathic?

2. Why is the therapeutic alliance important?

3. How do effective listeners express empathy nonverbally?

4. In what ways do clinicians create an effective structure for treatment and thus build the therapeutic alliance?

Everyone Needs to Feel Understood and Supported
Anna J. Michener

As an adult, Anna Michener (see also Chapter 11) says that she feels "very glad to have reached a point in my life where I feel fairly secure and comfortable with my beliefs about myself and no one who disagrees with me can seriously impact my life or my sense of self anymore" (A. J. Michener, personal communication, January 17, 2005). Nonetheless, she remains angry at the events that led to her hospitalization for more than a year while a teenager:

> … I can't help also considering it very important to point out the inescapable differences between dealing with two adults with such conflicting viewpoints and dealing with an adult and a child. What child has more personal capabilities, more external resources, more options with which to deal with such conflicts than an adult? Everyone needs to feel understood, validated, and supported, but children most of all. Children are in the process of developing their personal identity. This is such a difficult process for everyone, but exponentially more so for a child who lacks positive assistance and support and/or is struggling to deal with excessive negative input. Of course caretakers deserve empathy for and support with their monumental task of raising children, but can't this be done in a way that also helps, rather than harms, an inherently less powerful and more needy child?
>
> I believe the first step to such an achievement would be to actively seek and consider, in all cases, other views of a child in question than that of the primary caregivers—especially the view of the child. Anyone who reads [this] has more information about my viewpoint and has considered it more carefully than almost everyone involved in my case as a child. If only they had at least consulted my teachers or other adults who knew me they would have received an entirely different picture of me than that provided by my family. And now I have the starkly contrasting experience of seeking psychological counseling for myself as an adult and seeing exactly how listening to me and considering my viewpoint valid results in strikingly different, and actually helpful, diagnosis and treatment than that which I was given in my childhood. (A. J. Michener, personal communication, January 17, 2005)

• Ms. Michener felt misunderstood and objectified by her family and clinicians. How might this have affected her treatment? How might she have shown whether she felt understood and accepted (or not)?

LEARNING EMPATHY

Your neighbor's vision is as true for him as your own vision is true for you.
—**Miguel de Unamuno**

Strupp (1996) observed that clinicians' attitudes about their clients profoundly influence clinicians' diagnoses, estimates of prognosis, nature of the treatment plans, and empathic quality of their statements. He further noted that clients perceive these attitudes and react in kind, for example, reacting negatively towards clinicians who hold negative attitudes about them. How do helpful initial attitudes develop? By listening carefully, contextually, and from the client's point of view.

Some people believe that one either *is* empathic or one is not. We disagree. Although people vary in their *initial* propensity to behave empathically, everyone can learn to become more empathic.

However, expressing empathy well is a skill requiring more than just book learning and memorization (Pedersen et al., 2008). Sometimes, empathy develops as a result of similar experiences. This can be a useful approach for developing empathy, but there are two problems limiting its usefulness. First, having empathy that is drawn purely from one's own experience severely limits the types of clients with whom one can work. From this viewpoint, clinicians and clients would need to share both backgrounds and concerns. Second, even if a clinician's experience of an event matches that of a client's, each might perceive that situation very differently. In fact, while sometimes helpful, assuming understanding based on similar experiences or shared group membership can actually interfere with clinicians' abilities to see the world from their clients' point of view.

Life experience is *one* way of developing empathy, but experience must be balanced by other skills and practices. One of the most basic of these is an attitude of curiosity about others (Blatner, 2002). Effective clinicians are curious about what values, beliefs, and goals inform and motivate their clients' behavior.

Clinicians' understanding can be further developed through book learning and research, reading memoirs and novels, traveling, and listening to friends. Perhaps more importantly, empathy can be increased through sensitively observing clients' words and behavior. People reveal their views of themselves and their world in many ways—what they discuss and fail to discuss; their juxtaposition of topics and their manner of discussing them; changes in facial, postural, breathing, and spatial cues; and what and how they do within a session as well as patterns of change within and across sessions (Mozdrzierz et al., 2009; A. G. Rogers, 2001; A. G. Rogers et al., 1999).

Finally, empathy can be increased by sensitively observing one's own emotional and cognitive reactions in a situation (Rothschild, 2004; Strupp, 1996). Changes in the *clinician's* breathing, mood, fantasies, thoughts, and activity might be important cues about a *client*. These physical, cognitive, and emotional cues can be difficult to interpret, however, without well-developed insight into one's own thoughts, feelings, dynamics, and motivations. This self-awareness increases one's ability to use internal cues effectively and to distinguish between reactions that are primarily due to the clinician's own "stuff," either historical or current, and the client's. Being self-aware can help clinicians identify what is in the client's best interests and what instead serves the clinician's needs and purposes (Strupp, 1996).

THE THERAPEUTIC ALLIANCE

Let us watch well our beginnings and results will manage themselves.
—Alexander Clark

It takes two, however, to create empathy. Empathic understanding depends on both the clinician's understanding and the client's willingness and ability to be emotionally expressive. People who are empathic can accurately understand people who are emotionally expressive and can read them better than can people with low levels of empathy (Zaki, Bolger, & Ochsner, 2008). However, most people, even those with higher levels of empathy, have difficulty understanding people who are less emotionally expressive. This suggests that to be effective in developing empathic understanding of clients who are not very emotionally expressive, clinicians need to look for ways to help those clients to be more honest and open in expressing their emotions and concerns. In general, developing an empathic understanding depends on a strong therapeutic alliance.

Clients entering treatment are often ambivalent about treatment and unsure whether their new clinicians will be able to understand and help them. In addition to other initial treatment goals—assessing the problem, developing mutually acceptable goals, and formulating a plan to meet these goals—clinicians must join with their clients in order to work together effectively as a team. **Joining** fosters the therapeutic alliance. Although this relationship can be assessed from either the client's or clinician's viewpoint, a *client's* assessment of the quality and strength of the therapeutic alliance appears to be a somewhat better predictor of therapeutic outcome than the clinician's perceptions (D. Y. Lee et al., 1985). Fraser and Solovey (2007) concluded that between 21 and 26% of the variance in therapeutic outcomes is related to clients' perceptions of this alliance. In fact, in their **meta-analysis** of the literature, Martin, Garske, and Davis (2000) concluded that therapeutic outcomes were moderately strongly related to the quality of the therapeutic alliance, regardless of who is rating the alliance.

Joining with new clients can be difficult, because both clients and clinicians enter the treatment process with their own diverging agendas, goals, and values. As Ms. Michener described, this divergence is especially true for children and teens, who are often mandated into treatment by parents, Child Protective Services, or Juvenile Justice agencies. Criticism, confrontation, and judgment undermine the therapeutic alliance (Beutler et al., 2001; Serran et al., 2003; Strupp, 1996). Clients respond to such approaches by discrediting their clinician, devaluing the issues raised, or superficially agreeing to change while failing to make changes (Serran et al., 2003). By listening to and working with clients, clinicians powerfully and directly communicate that they are on the same side and want the same goals (Fraser & Solovey, 2007).

Effective therapeutic alliances are built on mutual trust, liking, respect, caring, and perceptions that the clinician can be helpful. Clients view clinicians who have difficulty forming therapeutic alliances as rigid, self-focused, blaming, belittling, aloof, distracted, bored, exploitive, critical, moralistic, or defensive (Ackerman & Hilsenroth, 2001). When clinicians focus on the therapeutic alliance, they acknowledge that clients need to feel safe and trust them before they can risk changing. Martin and his colleagues (2000) suggest that initial sessions are an especially important time to focus on the therapeutic alliance, but that this relationship must also be fostered throughout treatment.

Although a strong therapeutic alliance is almost certainly an important and even necessary precondition to change during counseling and psychotherapy (C. R. Rogers, 1957/1992), there are significant individual and cultural differences in what people want in a clinician—compare the Lee family (next case), Reymundo Sanchez (Chapters 3 and 8), and Annie Rogers (Chapter 11), for example. Some clients prefer more authoritative relationships, while others prefer more egalitarian ones. Some prefer a business-like consultation, while others want warmer and more empathic relationships (Lazarus, 1993). Otherwise skilled and strong clinicians can be ineffective when they fail to match their style to individual clients.

Joining can be accomplished in many different ways. The listening and structuring aspects of this process (i.e., setting safe boundaries, getting informed consent and collaborating on treatment goals and methods) are described later in this chapter. However, clinicians often take small yet visible steps to help their clients recognize that they are being heard and understood and that their contributions to treatment are valued. Some ways of joining are described in Table 10.1.

TABLE **10.1**
Joining Strategies.

Listening carefully
Example: "It sounds like you've had a very stressful week and have had some difficult times, but also that you've had some positive periods and handled the week better than usual."
Example: "OK, let me see if I can hear you better. It was a challenging week, but you experienced what you see as a surprising amount of success."
Example: "When you were talking about your mother, you dropped your eyes and your voice got quieter. Can you tell me what was happening for you?"

Inquiring about client strengths
Example: "You said that you had three fights this week. What about the rest of the week? What made it better?"
Example: "You're very quick to tell me about the problems you're having. Tell me what you do well."

Offering choices
Example: "What things are you wanting to work on here?"
Example: "Do you want to use the red crayon or the blue one?"

Checking in with clients to see how they are doing
Example: "We've been talking about some difficult issues today. How are you doing? Can we continue or should we take a break and work on something else?"
Example: "We talked about a lot of things last week. What was most important to you?"
Example: "I know that you've been doing well the last couple of weeks. How is your level of depression this week?"

Respecting clients and their cultural values
Example: "I know that next week is Yom Kippur. Do you still want to meet at this time or is there a better one for you?"
Example: "It sounds like your *abuela* [grandmother] is very important to you and a frequent source of support."
Example: Including artwork and décor that are inclusive of the genders, ages, and cultural groups served by the agency.
Example: Learning about your client's culture.

Paying attention to the nonsymptomatic and nonproblematic parts of clients' lives
Example: While shaking hands and making good eye contact, "Nice to see you again, Mr. Johnson, Mrs. Johnson. Wow! I really like your new haircut, DeMar!"
Example: "I see you had a good time at the beach this past week!"
Example: "What a nice picture of your children! They look like they really love each other!"

Specific Issues in Joining

In general, joining with clients depends on clinicians' genuineness and empathy for their clients, along with their abilities to create a safe physical and emotional space to change and to formulate a plausible explanation for symptoms and treatment (Fraser & Solovey, 2007). These are overlapping issues, but all point to the clinician's ability to understand a client and create an individualized setting that facilitates change to meet the client's needs.

Clinicians must do two apparently contradictory things in treatment. On the one hand, in order to foster the therapeutic alliance, they must validate the client's concerns and rationale for choosing a particular approach to solving a problem, yet on the other hand they must also help clients find a different approach to the problem (Fraser & Solovey, 2007; Ivey & Ivey, 2003). In general, people tend to become more firmly entrenched in problems and preferred solutions rather than trying a different approach (Fraser & Solovey, 2007; Watzlawick, Weakland, & Fisch, 1974). The difficulty is in how clients see the problem or stressor—not in the problem itself. Helping clients change depends on clinicians providing clients with explanations of the "problem" and treatment that are consistent with clients' worldviews, that clients find plausible and believable, and that motivate clients to try a different approach (Fraser & Solovey, 2007).

Clients who have weak alliances with their clinicians and do not share their clinicians' treatment goals or believe in the treatment approach are less attentive to and involved in treatment, more likely to drop out, and less likely to generalize skills outside of the therapy setting (Garcia & Weisz, 2002; Weisz & Hawley, 2002). As discussed previously, clinicians generally help their clients change their thoughts, feelings, and behavior by first listening to and understanding them. Listening to and responding within clients' values and goals helps clinicians join well and intervene effectively.

NONVERBAL LISTENING SKILLS

Only when the clamor of the outside world is silenced will you be able to hear the deeper vibration. Listen carefully.

—**Sarah Ban Breathnach**

Change is an inherent and necessary part of life: Seasons change, the calendar moves relentlessly forward, and people grow older. Nonetheless, many people find change difficult and inherently risky. Many people find it difficult to step into the unknown, have difficulty believing that they can change, and believe that change involves real risks as well as possible benefits. Often, staying in a bad situation can seem easier than trying something new.

As Ms. Michener described in the opening case material, failing to listen carefully damages the therapeutic alliance. Therapeutic empathy predicts successful treatment outcomes, perhaps by helping clients feel safe enough to risk changing (Friedlander, Escudero, & Heatherington, 2006; L. S. Greenberg et al., 2001). In fact, hearing clients well and communicating one's understanding is a clinician's first step to implementing any effective intervention (Ivey & Ivey, 2003).

An important part of listening is nonverbal. Nonverbal listening strategies serve three functions in treatment situations: They (a) help clinicians focus and listen well, (b) communicate interest, respect, and empathy, and (c) build and strengthen the therapeutic alliance.

What do effective listeners do? In Western cultures, effective listeners have several qualities in common. Their posture is relaxed and open, their arms and legs uncrossed. See Figure 10.1. They maintain a slight forward lean. Warm facial expressions and smiling help clients feel comfortable enough to do the work of treatment (Young, 2005). Smiling, head nods, an interested facial expression, eye contact, and relaxed and open posture are related to client perceptions of clinician trustworthiness, expertise, and attractiveness (D. Y. Lee et al., 1985). Although effective listeners are not rigid or tense, they are relatively still and avoid fidgeting and other nervous habits. The physical space between clinician and client is relatively small, reflecting the intimacy of the relationship.

As seen in the following example drawn from the Internet, poor listening skills can have a very negative impact on the therapeutic process. Notice how, despite treatment being very good in other ways, this clinician's behavior influenced the client's feelings about her clinician, what and how she discloses, and whether she will return to treatment.

> I have a question regarding a therapist I have seen three times. He's definitely good at what he does and in a short time has displayed good insight. He has

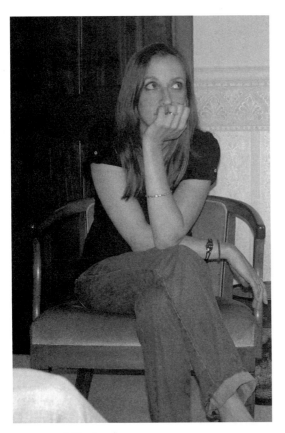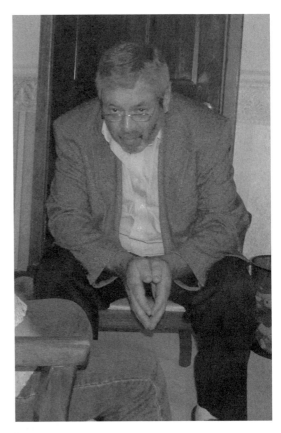

FIGURE **10.1** Closed (left) and open postures (right).

managed to get me to think about certain things [which have] led to some important revelations. Basically, I am very happy with him. The only problem, and it's leading to an apprehension on returning for another session, is I feel that he is displaying signs that he either doesn't like me or is offended in some way. I make sure not to use foul language and I have not discussed anything of a sexual nature. Yet, I have noticed that he sits with his legs crossed at the knee, pointed away, and will at times cross his arms over his chest. I tend to have an open posture as I want him to know I am open to his thoughts and/ or suggestions. I don't know if I'm reading too much into this or not. It's not that I'm looking for a therapist who totally likes me, but I really don't want to see one who has a strong dislike either. It's kind of uncomfortable and not really conducive to revealing innermost thoughts and feelings. (Anonymous, 2008)

Strong listening skills can help clinicians listen to clients more effectively. One particularly effective way of listening nonverbally is **mirroring** clients' posture, movements, breathing, language use, and paralanguage (May, 1967). Many people do this naturally—speeding up their speech when talking to someone excited, for example, and speaking more slowly and quietly when talking to someone who is depressed and silent. Although mirroring too closely can make some people uncomfortable, observing breathing and other nonverbal behaviors can be an important route to both gaining and communicating empathy (Lakin & Chartrand, 2003; van Baaren, Holland, Kawakami, & van Knippenberg, 2004).

Difficulties in Understanding Nonverbal Behaviors

One difficulty in displaying or interpreting nonverbal listening cues effectively is that different cues can be at odds with one other. A person who has an otherwise relaxed and inviting posture may have dry skin that causes fidgeting. Another may listen well but look away while thinking.

Even when nonverbal behavior is clear and consistent, communications may be misinterpreted. For example, people diagnosed with borderline personality disorder or paranoid disorders may have difficulty trusting others, regardless of the effectiveness of the other person's listening style. People with worldviews that undermine interpersonal relationships may be much more aware of and reactive to signals of problems in relationships (e.g., fidgeting, poor eye contact) than to signals of effective listening.

Some clinicians believe that they listen better using other styles of listening; however, many clients find it difficult to believe that people who are fidgeting, doodling, looking away, sitting in a closed posture or who fail to mirror them are listening and taking them seriously. Their rate or level of disclosure can be affected by their perception that they are not being heard. As counseling and psychotherapy are about the client rather than the clinician, clinicians need to find ways to communicate their understanding genuinely and in ways in which their clients will understand, even when those ways initially feel awkward to the clinician.

Culture influences how nonverbal behaviors are interpreted. Euro Americans generally see eye contact as respectful and its absence as a failure to listen, but people from other cultures, especially Asians, Native Americans, and older African Americans, may see eye contact as disrespectful under some circumstances (Paniagua, 1998). Touch can be comforting or anxiety-provoking, depending on a client's history of abuse and violence. Some clients are comfortable with long silences, while others, especially adolescents, find them uncomfortable. Effective clinicians monitor their behavior and observe its impact on their clients, modifying their listening style so that it is effective with that particular client.

Responding to Both Content and Process

The most basic of all human needs is the need to understand and be understood. The best way to understand people is to listen to them.

—Ralph Nichols

One of the difficulties of using nonverbal behavior to understand another person or to communicate one's own understanding is that nonverbal behavior is ambiguous and can mean many different things. Is a client's failure to make eye contact due to feelings of shame or discouragement about ever being understood, to poor social skills, or to low self-esteem? Is his silence due to embarrassment, a failure to find words to respond, or respectfully giving the other person space to speak? Collecting other kinds of information can help answer these questions.

People generally focus on words and vocal tone to understand others' thoughts and visual nonverbal behavior to recognize feelings (Hall & Schmid Mast, 2007). Paying attention to the client's **content**, the overtly expressed thoughts and feelings, is one important path for developing an empathic understanding. Robbie might paraphrase Anna Michener's verbally expressed concerns in this way:

Robbie: It sounds like you wish that they had asked people other than just your mother, in order to get a fuller, more valid picture of you. If they had really *listened* to you, they would have developed a more helpful diagnosis and you would have received more helpful treatment than you had ever had been given.

Robbie's paraphrase both communicates his understanding and builds his relationship with her. It facilitates further disclosures by indicating that she can be understood without being judged or rejected.

Although the client's overt content is important, clients embed indirect messages in their statements. Ms. Michener used few feeling words; however, her statement had a very passionate and emotional tone. When she said, "Everyone needs to feel understood, validated, and supported, but children most of all," she suggested that she had not felt understood, validated, or supported. When she asked, "Can't [supporting parents and caretakers] be done in a way that also helps, rather than harms, an inherently less powerful and more needy child?" she suggests that she felt harmed by the support that her mother and grandmother received. Perhaps Robbie would respond like this:

Robbie: It sounds like you felt alone, misunderstood, and unsupported during that period. Their support of your mother and grandmother might have been helpful to *them*, but you were *hurt* by it.

If this reflection of feeling was effective, Ms. Michener might have listened, relaxed, nodded, and expanded on what she had been saying, perhaps, "Yes, I felt like no one cared." If it had been off-track, she might have stopped, held her breath, broken eye contact, and responded by correcting her clinician,

"Well, I really felt more *guilty* asking for any help," changing the subject, or making a relatively superficial response. As seen in this example, the client's **process**—changes in nonverbal behaviors across time and juxtapositions of content, emotional and behavioral reactions, etc.—can be very helpful in identifying and clarifying a client's meaning.

Ms. Michener's ability to label the harm that she experienced and her contrast between her past and present experiences suggest that not only was it "strikingly different," but also more positive and that she is feeling less harmed. Robbie might continue by saying,

Robbie: Although you felt very alone then, being heard and understood *now* seems to be both helpful and also *healing.*

Robbie's responses rely not only on Ms. Michener's words, but also on the unverbalized emotions that are below the surface. His **challenge** attends to the discrepancies between one aspect of what she said and another, thus allowing him to communicate a fuller, more complete and more accurate picture of her experience.

What clients say is modulated and modified by process variables, including changes in nonverbal behaviors and discrepancies between words and nonverbal behavior. How was Ms. Michener sitting as she talked? Did she use an open posture with a forward lean, or was she turned away with a tense, closed posture? What was her tone like? Flat? Expressive? Tentative? If her tone or posture changed during a session, when did it change? What was she talking about at that point? Perhaps if Ms. Michener had had a tense but open posture and had spoken tentatively but without obscuring her ideas, Robbie would have instead responded somewhat differently:

Robbie: Although you felt very alone then, it sounds like you're feeling heard and understood now. It is still scary to believe that you'll be understood, yet you're willing to take some small risks.

Finally, earlier client statements and nonverbal behaviors can contextualize and illuminate later ones; these change interpretations about clients' intentions and meaning (Gesn & Ickes, 1999). For example, imagine if Ms. Michener had said, "*Of course* caretakers deserve empathy for and support with their monumental task of raising children," Is she saying this is obvious or is she criticizing the mental health system? Her meaning can be deciphered by considering her typical use of **verbal underlining,** her previous use of sarcasm, and earlier discussions of this topic. However, while knowing someone well can help one make more sophisticated and useful inferences, it also increases the tendency to fit new observations into preexisting hypotheses. Clinicians who recognize the natural tendency to engage in an expectancy confirmation process can take steps to avoid getting stuck in old and unhelpful patterns of thinking about clients (Trope & Thompson, 1997).

This section has discussed the multiple modes that clients use to communicate. Additional verbal and nonverbal behaviors that can build understanding are outlined in Table 10.2. When clinicians listen carefully to their clients, recognizing the layers of messages inherent in clients' speech, clients are more likely to feel understood in a manner that builds the therapeutic alliance.

TABLE **10.2**
Verbal and Nonverbal Behaviors That Can Help Clinicians Develop Empathic Understanding.

- **Content.** The overt message communicated by the client's words alone. When contradicted by other indicators, may indicate what they believe or would like you to believe.
- **Word choice.** The client's words provides overt clues to emotional tone and the client's meaning (e.g., "I feel so alone").
- **Verbal underlining.** Words in the same sentence can be emphasized differently (e.g., "*He* is important to me," "He is *important* to me"), changing the meaning.
- **Paralanguage.** Speed, volume, and changes in intonation (e.g., speaking rapidly and dropping the volume at the end of the sentence) provide clues about communication style, personality variables, and more acute emotional states, including depression, anxiety, power, and assertiveness.
- **Discrepancies.** Discrepancies can occur between words, among nonverbal behaviors, or between words and nonverbal behaviors. Discrepancies "fatten" the client's meaning by hinting at two poles of a client's beliefs or feelings (e.g., "Well, it's time to go now," while hesitating and not moving, or "I like you," while leaning back and looking away).
- **Rate and volume of breathing.** Breathing reflects autonomic nervous system activity and associated levels of stress or anxiety. Slow and deep breathing indicates relaxation; more rapid and shallow breathing indicates stress or anxiety. Changes in breathing within a session may point to particular topics that are associated with increased or decreased anxiety.
- **Eye contact.** Eye contact is an important nonverbal behavior, but can indicate many different emotions, including interest, challenge, respect, disrespect, or anger. Breaks in eye contact can mean shame, poor self-esteem, respect, guilt, boredom, disinterest, or needing to gather one's thoughts. The meaning of eye contact can be identified through contextual cues and knowledge about the person's behavior across time.
- **Facial expressions.** Raised eyebrows, smiles, wrinkled foreheads, and other facial expressions influence the meaning of other verbal and nonverbal behaviors. These are ambiguous behaviors, though, with multiple meanings. Tension around the jaw, eyes, and mouth influence the specific interpretation.
- **Posture.** Open posture is characterized by less body tension, uncrossed limbs, and often a slight forward lean. Closed posture is characterized by greater body tension and crossed limbs (see Figure 10.1).
- **Personal space.** In general, larger personal space suggests a more formal or less intimate relationship or difficulties with trust. Smaller personal space suggests greater trust and intimacy or a less formal setting.
- **Touch.** Can express intimacy or reassurance; be soothing; send sexual messages; or demonstrate power or aggression depending on speed, pressure, size and speed of gesture, and its relationship to other verbal and nonverbal communication.

Clients' Contributions to Treatment

I know that you believe you understand what you think I said, but I'm not sure you realize that what you heard is not what I meant.

—Robert McCloskey

Clinicians make an important contribution to the therapeutic change process, but change is not done *to* clients, but *with* clients. Earlier parts of this book described clinicians' assessment process. Although this process is important, *clients'* assessments of their clinicians and the change process is perhaps more important (Fraser & Solovey, 2007; D. Y. Lee et al., 1985).

> [The client] is determining whether he can trust the clinician with his assumptive world. He operates with a set of criteria that are based on his unique experiences with others and previous helpers. Before he will allow the therapist to be admitted into his inner sanctum, the part of him that is within his self-protective system, he needs to have a sense of the therapist's personhood. Is the therapist a person who is capable of understanding his problem? Does the therapist genuinely care about him and respect him despite his problems? Is the therapist

genuine and congruent, or is there the hint of a hidden agenda? Does the clinician seem competent? Does the therapist know what [to] do about the client's problem? (Fraser & Solovey, 2007, p. 89)

Clients must be hopeful and believe that they can change, as opposed to only wanting to change (Frank & Frank, 1993; Goldfried, 2004). Although clinicians can act in ways that provoke hope, clients must have their *own belief* that they can change. Clinicians can care about their clients, but clients must *feel* cared for (Goldfried, 2004). Clinicians must accept their clients, but clients must *feel* accepted. Clinicians can listen carefully to their clients, but clients must be willing and able to express their emotions so they can be heard (Zaki et al., 2008). Moreover, while clinicians' personality style and listening behaviors predict the strength of the alliance, clients' motivation to change and their ability to be open and cooperative rather than resistant and defensive are better predictors of positive therapeutic outcomes (Taft, Murphy, Musser, & Remington, 2004).

Problems in joining do occur. When treatment gets off-track and clients are not compliant with clinicians' treatment plans, many clinicians attribute problems to clients (Bohart, 2001). Labeling clients as treatment resistant will, in and of itself, interfere with treatment, as will other critical and judging interventions (Beutler et al., 2001; Serran et al., 2003; Strupp, 1996). Bohart argues that joining should be more than just obtaining compliance with the clinician's treatment plan; it must involve developing a true collaboration between client and clinician. When clinicians recognize that they are having a difficult time hearing and empathizing with their clients or seeing strengths as well as symptoms and problems, they should step back and focus on the therapeutic alliance.

Joining should be a continuous and ongoing process, with clinicians frequently checking in on and assessing the quality of the therapeutic alliance. Joining takes place within each session: at the beginning, when clinicians ask about the weather or the drive; in the middle, as clinicians listen sensitively to their clients' point of view; and at the end, when clinicians set homework that is consistent with their clients' skills, needs, and individual treatment goals. Joining occurs in the first session, but clinicians must also assess and foster the therapeutic alliance in later sessions. In reading about the Lee family (see also Chapters 5 and 8), note how some people focused more on their own treatment goals than on understanding the Lees and recognizing and addressing barriers to treatment. How did this affect the treatment process? Pay attention to styles of relating that helped clinicians join well with the Lees.

Joining with a Hmong American Family
The Lee family

The ways that U.S. workers were able to be effective with the Lee family and other Hmong American families is instructive, in that some workers were clearly able to be effective with this population—despite not being

(continues)

Hmong—while some of the Hmong translators or cultural liaisons were strikingly ineffective (Fadiman, 1997). Anne Fadiman chose May Ying as interpreter and cultural broker.

> [B]y virtue of our gender and ages, [we] constituted a decidedly low-status team. That turned out to be an advantage. I didn't need more status in the Lee home. If anything, I needed *less* status. Ever since they had arrived in the United States, the Lees had been meeting Americans who, whether because of their education, their knowledge of English, or their positions of relative authority, had made them feel as if their family didn't count for much. Being belittled is the one thing no Hmong can bear.... With May Ying at my side, I was not an official, not a threat, not a critic, not a person who was trying to persuade the Lees to do anything they did not want to do, not even someone to be taken very seriously. My insignificance was my saving grace. (pp. 96–97)

Sukey Waller, a psychologist, attributed her own success with the Hmong American community to the match between her worldview and personal style and that of many Hmong:

> The Hmong and I have a lot in common. I have an anarchist sub-personality. I don't like coercion. I also believe that the long way around is often the shortest way from point A to point B. And I'm not very interested in what is generally called the truth. In my opinion, consensual reality is better than facts. (Fadiman, 1997, p. 95)

One would expect that the Lee family would dislike Jeanine Hilt, the Child Protective Services worker who removed Lia from their home. Nonetheless, the Lees liked her for numerous reasons, treating her

> ... not as Lia's abductor but as her patron, "the person who gave Lia her disability money."... [She was one of two Americans who] I talked to who didn't describe the Lees as closemouthed and dim; not coincidentally, she was also the only American I ever heard Foua or Nao Kao refer to by name.... She responded by learning the names of all eight of Lia's siblings.... [She] seemed warm and unpretentious. Even her size—five feet one and comfortably rounded—was closer to the Hmong scale. (Fadiman, 1997, pp. 112–113)

Ms. Hilt had the further advantage of being able to make house visits. There she was able to use May, the Lee's daughter, as interpreter. Further, May was able to repeat and explain what had been said even after Ms. Hilt left.

1. Anne Fadiman, Sukey Waller, and Jeanine Hilt each adopted different tactics for working successfully with the Lee family and the Hmong American community. What were these tactics? Did they have any commonalities?
2. Your size and age might not help you join effectively with the Lees. How could you use your unique qualities to join well with the Lee family?

STRUCTURING TREATMENT

Even if you're impro-
vising, the fact that
beforehand you know
certain things will
work helps you make
those improvisations
successful.

—John Cale

For many people, developing a safe structure also strengthens the therapeutic alliance (Fraser & Solovey, 2007). Three aspects of this structuring are discussed here: creating a safe environment with effective boundaries, informed consent, and treatment plan development. Others are described in Table 10.3. In each case, when these processes are performed well, the increased clarity they provide helps clients feel respected and more able to take the risks of treatment.

Creating a Safe Setting for Treatment

Change is a risky venture and clinicians must help clients feel safe enough to take the necessary steps to change (Friedlander et al., 2006). When clinicians are genuine and sincere and believe in the efficacy of the interventions they offer, when they make a serious effort to understand their clients—and their clients feel that their clinicians are trying to understand them from their own point of view—clients believe that clinicians can help them change (Fraser & Solovey, 2007). Safety is further developed by creating a physical environment promoting safety, fostering client perceptions of clinician competence, and making the counseling environment comfortable and free of judgment and criticism.

Clinicians create a safe physical setting by using noise screens, having client entrances that protect client confidentiality, creating client-flow patterns within an office that reduce the probability that clients will run into each other, and lighting parking areas well (Friedlander et al., 2006). Starting and ending sessions on time and avoiding multiple relationships with clients sets safe emotional boundaries for treatment. Furthermore, making self-disclosures, accepting gifts, and hugging clients only with the client's needs and best interests at heart reinforces effective boundaries (Knapp & Vandecreek, 2006).

Clients draw conclusions about a practice from the way that the office is set up and decorated. See Figure 10.2. Some of these conclusions concern the

TABLE **10.3**
Strategies for Structuring Sessions Well.

- Carefully inform clients both orally and in writing to gain their consent to treatment. Continue this process across treatment, as necessary.
- Create a safe setting (e.g., closed doors, curtains on windows, noise screens, private entrances, locked file cabinets, and lighted parking lots).
- Respect clients' personal space, moving chairs neither too close nor too far apart for an individual client.
- Keep track of treatment and session goals, making them salient for both clinician and client. Work steadily towards these goals.
- Stay within the allotted session time, whatever that is, starting on time and ending on time whenever possible.
- Demonstrate that confidentiality is important and respected, both by getting signed permissions to release information and protecting clients' confidentiality (e.g., talking about clients only in places and ways that maintain confidentiality; putting charts and appointment books in places where client names cannot be identified).
- Collect bills and co-pays in a timely and predictable fashion.
- End treatment in a careful and safe way, generally by discussing termination in the weeks prior to doing so.

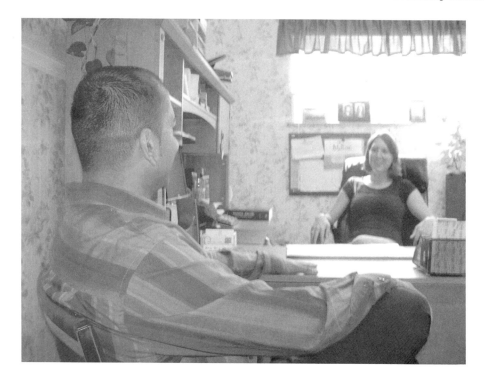

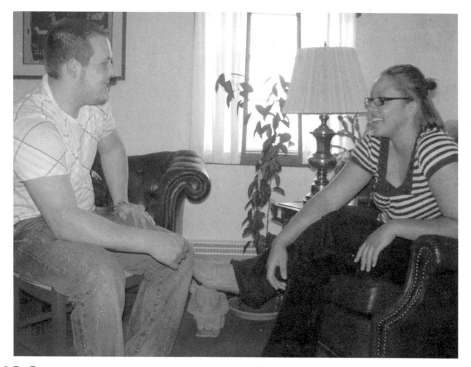

FIGURE **10.2** Office settings may impact perceptions of safety, competence, and comfort, as well as the nature of the relationship.

clinician's competence. Obtaining informed consent for treatment, displaying licenses and diplomas (as required by U.S. law), having books that are relevant to the nature of the practice, using appropriate assessment measures, and following accepted clinical practices communicate that the clinician is competent and that clients will be safe receiving treatment.

Although concrete objects and practices can signal safety, safety must be reinforced at the level of client disclosures. Consider the following short scene from the *Clumsy Counsellor*, paying attention to your reactions as you read (Walker, Jacobs, & Crisp, 1992).

Client: There is something that has really been troubling me. I've been under such pressure recently. I'm just afraid that something is going to snap and that I'm going to harm the children.

Counselor: I can understand that you're under such pressure, but you know as well as I do that you mustn't do anything like that. (Scene 5)

This client might have felt judged and believed that her counselor saw her as incompetent and stupid. As a result, she would probably have a difficult time disclosing other potentially embarrassing or shameful thoughts or emotions. Note that she did not indicate that she was planning to hurt her children, only that she was afraid she might. People have many thoughts and emotions that they would never act on, but that they worry about nonetheless.

Engaging Clients through the Informed Consent Process

In an episode of the TV show *House*, an agoraphobic man with an intestinal blockage refused to leave his home (Blake & Yaitanes, 2008). To save his life, the medical team finally decided to anesthetize him for surgery, then, *without his consent*, take him to the hospital. This intervention ultimately saved his life, but imagine how he might feel awakening in an unexpected place after explicitly refusing the move.

In general, in counseling and psychotherapy, failing to obtain informed consent prior to treatment is unethical. Clients have the right to know what treatment they will receive as well as the benefits and risks they can reasonably expect. They have the right to know what other treatments are available and to receive a referral to those alternative treatments when appropriate. Other issues that might be addressed—such as the clinician's fees, training, cancellation policy, and decision-making process about medications—are described in Table 10.4. Acting without a client's consent is acceptable only under extreme situations, such as involuntarily hospitalizing homicidal or suicidal clients. In fact, a similar situation occurred in the previously described *House* episode, where without intervention, the man with the intestinal blockage would have died. Even under such extreme circumstances, clinicians should attempt to get consent and intervene in the least coercive manner possible (Knapp & Vandecreek, 2007).

The informed consent process assists clients in becoming a true partner in treatment, encourages collaboration, enhances client autonomy, and can lead to more trusting relationships between clinicians and clients (Getzinger, 1993). Informed consent helps clients make thoughtful and knowledgeable choices about their mental health care and forestalls lawsuits. Provision of informed consent should not be thought of as occurring at a single point in time; instead, multiple informing and consenting cycles might occur over the course of treatment, as decisions about alternative treatments, medication, or psychiatric hospitalizations arise (Raphaely, 1991). As Pipes, Blevins, and Kluck (2008) observed, however, some of these decisions are true choices (e.g., "Do you want this treatment or that one?"), while others simply allow clients to acknowledge that they have been informed about the clinical process (e.g., "If you report child abuse, I am mandated to report this to Child Protective Services."). Their choices in the latter situation are few: either accept these rules or refuse treatment. Nonetheless, although a client might not *choose* to initiate a mandated report, being informed beforehand that this is a possibility can reduce feelings of betrayal in the event that a report is made.

By informing clients about the treatment process, sharing expectations, and addressing common concerns from the very beginning, the informed consent process can also forestall another serious problem for many clinical practices, that of cancellations and premature termination (Barrett, Chua, Crits-Cristoph, Gibbons, & Thompson, 2008). Almost 40% of people who schedule a therapy appointment fail to attend their first session (Hampton-Robb, Qualls, & Compton, 2003). In addition, as many as 57% of people who attend an initial session fail to attend a second (LaTorre, 1977). This problem has been attributed to a number of factors, including confusion about the process, poorly developed intentions about treatment, and the stigma surrounding mental health diagnoses and treatment (Barrett et al., 2008; Hampton-Robb et al., 2003). Educating people about the process of psychotherapy—what they can expect and what is expected of them—can strengthen the therapeutic alliance and reduce cancellations and premature terminations, as well as increase motivation and decrease perceived barriers to treatment (Barrett et al., 2008; Hampton-Robb et al., 2003). In reviewing the literature, Barrett and her colleagues concluded that unattractive and crowded waiting rooms; inaccessible offices; and culturally-insensitive assessment, joining, and treatment reduced return rates.

Premature terminations from therapy may be an overt indicator of an even bigger problem. As many as 50% of people who report intending to perform a behavior fail to do so (Sheeran, Aubrey, & Kellett, 2007). Follow-through is highest when people know specifically what they are going to do and when and how they will do it. Furthermore, one study found that when clients expected positive outcomes from what they did, they were more likely to follow through with treatment recommendations (Sheeran et al., 2007).

One reason that people fail to attend treatment sessions is a fear of being perceived as stupid or crazy (Sheeran et al., 2007). A letter sent to clients with their initial psychotherapy appointment and intake materials can speak to these problems, as follows:

> Many people feel anxious or concerned when preparing to attend their first appointment. Some may feel that their concerns aren't important enough to justify taking up an appointment or, conversely, that they will be seen as crazy. These feelings are perfectly normal and understandable and are shared by many people

TABLE **10.4**
Information that Might Be Covered in an Initial Informed Consent Form
or in an Ongoing Informed Consent Processes.

Therapy

- What type of therapy is used? How was it learned? Where? How does it compare with other kinds of treatment? How does it work? What are the possible risks?
- What percentage of clients improves with this treatment? What percentage gets worse? What percentage of clients improves without therapy?
- How long does therapy generally take? What should be done if therapy does not seem to be working?
- Will tests be used? What kind? Why?
- Is a therapy manual with predetermined steps used? Why or why not?
- Is therapy done over the phone or Internet?

Alternatives to therapy

- What other types of treatment are available? What are the risks and benefits of these other approaches? What are the risks and benefits of *no* therapy?
- How is this type of therapy different from other options?
- Is medication prescribed? Do you work with people who do prescribe? If clients are already taking medication, do you work with the prescribing doctor? Are you knowledgeable about medications?

Appointments

- How are appointments scheduled? How long are they? Are fees higher for longer sessions?
- How can you be reached in an emergency? If you are not available, who should be called?
- What happens in the case of bad weather or illness? What happens when an appointment is forgotten or intentionally missed?

Confidentiality

- What kinds of records are kept? Who has access to them? How is confidentiality maintained?
- Under what conditions can confidential information be disclosed? Do family members have access to information about treatment?

Money

- What are your fees? How are they paid for? Must missed sessions be paid for? What about telephone calls, letters, and e-mails?
- What are your policies about raising fees? Can fees be lowered if a job or insurance coverage is lost? What happens if fees are not paid as agreed?
- How much and what kind of information about sessions are shared with insurance companies? How much influence do insurance companies have on therapy? How are disagreements about treatment with insurance companies resolved?
- How would therapy be different if paid for directly rather than by the insurance company?

General

- What is your training and experience? Are you licensed? Are you supervised? Board certified?
- What is your professional background? What are the advantages and disadvantages of your credentials?
- Who should clients talk to if they have a complaint that cannot be resolved?

Note: Modified from Pomerantz & Handelsman, 2004.

entering a new situation for the first time. Remind yourself that this is normal although, if you're comfortable doing so, tell me about these feelings at your first appointment.

This sort of intervention was found in one study to decrease cancellations and no-shows by 12%–26% (Sheeran et al., 2007).

Collaborating on Goals and Methods

Setting goals and collaborating on treatment plans can be another strategy for building the therapeutic alliance. Many clients find the process of being listened to and collaboratively developing treatment goals that are consistent with their own values and goals is different from their experience in other parts of their lives. Notice how the clinicians who collaborated well with the Lee family were more effective than those who were less collaborative. Sukey Waller, like the Lees, believed "that the long way around is often the shortest way from point A to point B," and was willing to set treatment goals that were consistent with the Lees' worldview (Fadiman, 1997, p. 95). Jeanine Hilt, the Child Protective Services worker who removed Lia from their home, helped them get disability money, learned their names, and expected that they would collaborate on treatment. Effective clinicians were not "softer," but were more collaborative in their goal-setting and overall approach.

Setting goals and collaborating on treatment plans is not just something to be done at the beginning of treatment but also something to be done in the middle of treatment and at its end. It occurs both at the beginning of a session in response to a client's entering crisis and also later in a session as a clinician redirects the focus to the treatment goals. For example, Lia Lee's doctors' primary treatment goal was to reduce the number and severity of her seizures; however, if the Lees brought Lia to an appointment with a fever and her doctors failed to first attend to that, her doctors would not be able to engage the family and identify ways to reduce the seizure activity.

In addition, in some places the client's crisis is a particular example of the problem being addressed by the treatment plan. For example, the Lees had difficulty giving Lia's medicine consistently and as prescribed. One treatment goal might have been to identify obstacles to taking medicine consistently and develop more effective strategies. If Lia had been taken to the emergency room during a grand mal seizure, stabilizing her would have been her physician's immediate goal. Ms. Hilt, however, might have used this incident as an opportunity to identify obstacles to treatment and to collaborate with Lia's physician to develop a more effective medication and dosing regimen.

SUMMARY

Essential to effective treatment, empathy is not an unchangeable trait, but a style of listening and responding that can be learned. Empathy is developed through one's experiences, book learning, careful listening, and introspective processes. It is fostered by an attitude of curiosity as well as by the recognition that people may react differently to superficially similar situations and similarly in superficially different ones.

Clients often enter treatment with some feelings of ambivalence about the process and about change. Listening and validating clients' concerns, although not necessarily agreeing with their perceptions and conclusions, strengthens the therapeutic alliance, while criticism, confrontation, and judging undermine it. Clients tend to respond to the latter approaches by discrediting their clinicians, devaluing the issues raised, or by only superficially agreeing to change. In addition to being genuine and empathic with their clients, clinicians strengthen the therapeutic alliance by creating a safe physical and emotional space to change and providing explanations for the problem that are plausible from the client's worldview.

Nonverbal listening strategies help clinicians to (a) focus and listen well; (b) communicate interest, respect, and empathy; and (c) build and strengthen the therapeutic alliance. In Western cultures, effective listeners maintain a relaxed and open posture, with a slight forward lean and few nervous habits. They maintain good eye contact and a warm and responsive expression. To build understanding, effective clinicians pay attention to the overt content in clients' statements, but they also observe the process reflected in the clients' word use, juxtaposition of topics, and nonverbal behaviors, as well as changes in affect, mood, and relational style.

Informed consent contributes to the joining process by helping clients make thoughtful and knowledgeable choices. It encourages collaboration, enhances client autonomy, and can forestall lawsuits. Informed consent should not be thought of as occurring at a single time; instead, multiple informing and consenting cycles often occur over the course of treatment. By informing clients about the treatment process, sharing expectations, and addressing common concerns from the very beginning, the informed consent process can also decrease cancellations and premature termination.

Finally, developing a treatment plan together and implementing it in a way that is responsive to a client's needs strengthens the therapeutic alliance. Fine-tuning the treatment plan to reflect the client's goals can strengthen the alliance. Keeping the treatment goals in mind can help clinicians maintain a consistent and more effective course in treatment even when responding to individual crises.

How Do These Issues Apply to Your Life and Work?

1. Describe a change you have made in your own life. How did it feel to make that change? What made it easier or more difficult to change? Compare your experience with that of your friends or fellow students. What do you conclude in comparing your story with theirs?

(continues)

2. If someone—a parent, friend, minister, teacher, or therapist—helped you change, what did he or she do that seemed helpful? What characteristics and behaviors seemed particularly helpful? Compare your experience with that of your friends or fellow students. Which of these characteristics would you like to further develop in order to become a better helper? What steps could you take to make these changes (B. C. Murphy & Dillon, 2003)?

3. How do you recognize that you are being treated respectfully? Would being treated respectfully be different in therapy than in other parts of your life? If so, how? If you would like to be more respectful of others, especially in the counseling and psychotherapy process, what changes would you need to make? What steps could you take to make these changes?

4. Observe people talking to each other. What do you notice? Can you identify good listeners and poor listeners based on their nonverbal listening skills? How do others react to them?

5. Videotape yourself while talking to someone else. Turn off the sound and only watch your nonverbal behavior. What do you observe? Watch your partner's responses to your nonverbal behaviors. What do you observe?

6. Practice your mirroring skills by paying attention to other people's breathing patterns and making postural shifts that match theirs. What do you learn about them? How do they respond? Make your changes both subtle and respectful.

7. Speak quickly and loudly with someone who is speaking quietly and slowly. Sit up straight with someone who slouches. How connected do you feel? How does the other person react? Make sure to debrief them afterwards.

CHAPTER 11

Techniques for Communicating Empathy

WHERE ARE WE GOING?

1. What types of barriers can interfere with successfully communicating empathy?

2. How do clinicians express empathy verbally?

3. How can clinicians recognize when their understanding is on track?

4. How can clinicians develop their empathic understanding even when clients have a difficult time expressing their thoughts and feelings verbally?

5. How do positivity and validation contribute to empathy?

You Must Have Had a Very Good Reason
Annie G. Rogers

Annie Rogers is a gifted therapist in her own right but was hospitalized after a psychotic break. When releasing her from the hospital, her doctor made her promise to stay on her medication and away from psychotherapy: "What's wrong with you can be changed only with medication and time" (A. G. Rogers, 1995, p. 121). In less than a week, she broke her promise—"the need to understand what is happening to me overrode my promise" (A. G. Rogers, 1995, p. 122)—and made an appointment to see Dr. Blumenfeld, who would become her new therapist.

... Dr. Blumenfeld lean[s] in a little to listen, as if he is hearing what I have not said, what are not, in all honesty, even my thoughts. I don't look directly at him. On the periphery of my horizon of awareness, I pick up every gesture and every shift of breath. I have learned that this way I know far better what someone is thinking and feeling.

"I took a gun and a knife to my therapist and I threatened to kill her." These words come out of me into the room, the first words I have spoken. They startle me even as I speak them.

"You must have had a very good reason for wanting to do that," Dr. Blumenfeld says calmly, as if this is true.

"I didn't want to. There were voices that told me to do that, and I, I felt compelled to follow them."

Even my straightforward explanation frightens me.

He laughs, a light laugh. "Ah, they must have had a very good reason."

"No!" I say. Yet in the silence that follows, I find that I believe this myself. He sounds as if he is on their side, which is also my side.

I look up. His eyes are blue-gray, almost the lilac color of the sky before it snows. The silence wraps itself around us.

"I can hear you in whole sentences!" I exclaim. "My hearing has been messed up. Sometimes I can't hear people in whole sentences. In my journal, there are a few lines like that, whole sentences. But they are surrounded by— words that make no sense to me— gibberish!" I spit out the word, hating the sound of it. "And no one in the hospital could understand me when I spoke."

"No one there knew that gibberish is a language too?"

His questions come, like little animals, up into my lap. Tears abruptly fall down my face, and I want to stop them. I have the sense that it is not me who is crying, but I look for a Kleenex.

"I don't have any," he says. "I don't want you to wipe them away. Let the tears be."

I sit and let them drip off into my hands.

After a long time, I begin my story again, from another angle. "The woman who was my therapist, she won't see me, not ever again."

"She has abandoned you," he says simply.

"No, she loved me," I argue, swallowing hard.

"Love? What is love then?" he asks.

(continues)

(continued)

The room tilts, as if a huge wave hit us. "I don't know. I don't know what love is, or what is real anymore."

"How could you possibly know?" he asks.

His words come to me like my own unspoken thoughts. I am dizzy, then flooded with relief. (A. G. Rogers, 1995, pp. 123–124)

- What do you think about Dr. Blumenfeld's work? What do you like or not like about it? Why?
- If you had to briefly summarize the message that he was giving Dr. Rogers at this, their first meeting, what would it be? Does she accept it or reject it? How do you know? Do his responses seem to fit with her worldview?
- What did you think about his interpretations (e.g., "No one there knew that gibberish is a language too?" or "[The voices] must have had a good reason.")? What information informed his interpretations? Did they seem to be effective? How do you know?

BARRIERS TO COMMUNICATING EMPATHY

Giving connects two people, the giver and the receiver, and this connection gives birth to a new sense of belonging.
—**Deepak Chopra**

Understanding someone, while helpful, is not enough. For empathic responses to be useful, they must be shared. Regardless of how accurate Dr. Blumenfeld's insights were, if he had sat on his hands, maintained a poker face, and kept his ideas to himself, Annie would not have recognized that he understood her.

Clinicians face a number of barriers to listening empathically and sharing that understanding. Hearing someone well requires being willing to set aside one's biases and life stressors to listen carefully and recognize that another person's perspective may be different from one's own (Mordecai, 1991; Pedersen et al., 2008). Listening empathically can be disconcerting, because becoming open enough to hear someone carefully and sensitively can leave the listener feeling more visible and vulnerable. Listening empathically can make one feel intimate, thus frightening for some clinicians; in addition, some men may see this intimate sharing of emotions as inconsistent with the male gender role. For some people, intimacy can also create feelings that can be misinterpreted as sexual (Celenza, 1995; Sherby, 2009).

Cultural norms in the United States often discourage openly acknowledging problems; people avoid talking about difficult emotions in order to protect relationships: "Nice people" do not see bad things and do not talk about them. Seeing and discussing problems can feel intrusive and like an invasion of another person's "emotional space." Discussing problems can feel like confrontation, with which many people also have difficulty. Some clinicians retreat behind the therapeutic role in response to these norms and perceived barriers and simply nod their heads and respond woodenly.

These barriers and misperceptions indicate the difficulties that people have in really feeling heard by someone else in the rest of their lives, especially during periods of crisis. In summarizing his career's work, Strupp

(1996) noted the profound influence the quality of this connection has on diagnoses, estimates of prognosis, the nature of the treatment plan, and the empathic quality of the clinician's statements. Genuinely listening to and hearing someone can create connections between two people, foster feelings of belonging and understanding, and may itself be healing. This chapter describes not only basic skills for communicating empathy but also more advanced skills, including recognizing and responding to client ambivalence and unrecognized feelings.

VERBAL STRATEGIES FOR SHARING UNDERSTANDING

You only listen and say back the other person's thing, step by step, just as that person seems to have it at that moment. You never mix into it any of your own things or ideas, never lay on the other person anything that person didn't express.

(Gendlin & Hendricks, n.d., quoted in C. Rogers, 1980)

There is a variety of verbal strategies that we use to communicate our understanding of someone else's experience. The most important of these verbal listening **microskills** are encouragers and minimal encouragers, paraphrases, reflections of feeling, open and closed questions, and summarizations (see Table 11.1).

TABLE **11.1**
Verbal Listening Skills.

- **Paraphrase.** Promotes discussion by summarizing the essence of what a client has said over a short period of time, both to demonstrate the clinician's understanding and to check out that understanding. *"You said that you began the semester smoking only three cigarettes a day, but smoked more and more as the semester went along, especially when you were stressed."*
- **Reflection of feeling.** Promotes focus on and discussion of emotions. Communicates understanding but does so by selectively focusing on the client's feelings. *"You sound very confused and frightened as you talk about this." "You sound pretty overwhelmed."*
- **Minimal encouragers.** These simple sounds help people feel heard or understood without or with few words. These include "uh-huh," "awww," "oooh," "yes," and "ah."
- **Encouragers.** Very quickly encourages elaboration of ideas and emotions by repeating one or a few of the client's main words. *"Suddenly?"*
- **Questions.** Techniques used to draw out specific information rapidly.
  - **Open questions.** Used to bring out major data and facilitate discussion. Generally begins with "what," "how," "why," or "could." *"How did you come to choose psychology as a major?"* Generally, try to avoid Why questions, which may make them feel blamed.
  - **Closed questions.** Quickly obtains specific data, stops lengthy discussion, often answered in a few words. Often begins with "do," "does," "is," "could," and "are." *"Are you almost finished?"*
- **Summarization.** Repeating the client's facts and feelings from a relatively longer part of a session or treatment in such a way to organize it and check out understanding. Very useful at the beginning and end of a session, as well as at periodic intervals in between. *"What you described last time is your concern about your daughter's ability to concentrate and focus. It seems that she is always moving from one thing to another and, as a result, you are feeling pretty hopeless about having the kind of family you would like to have."*

Paraphrases

Paraphrases are brief summaries of the content of what a person says. They promote discussion by sharing the clinician's understanding of the client's experience. They are often followed by a **check-out**, which further clarifies the clinician's understanding of the content the client discussed. Paraphrases often take the form of (a) a sentence stem where the clinician takes ownership for what he or she heard ("It sounds like …" or "It seems like …"); (b) the essence of the content of the client's communication; followed by (c) a check-out, which clarifies the clinician's understanding ("Is that right?" "Am I following you?" "Am I on track?"). Generally paraphrases are in the clinician's own words; however, occasionally using clients' words and metaphors strengthens the paraphrase and increases the probability that it will be useful.

Because clients' discussions are often long and include several ideas, paraphrases can go in different directions, including focusing on different aspects of the client's message or the client's underlying meaning. Choosing from among these directions should be determined by what goals are most important to the client and what will best further treatment goals.

Sherman:	We just found out that we can never have a child. They've done all the hormones and in vitro fertilizations that they can do. That's it. [silence] How do you go on after your whole world has been centered around making a baby for four years?
Clinician A:	You've been doing fertility treatments and focused on that, but now you've learned that you cannot have a child. Is this right? (paraphrase, check out)
Clinician B:	It sounds like having a child has been the center of your world for the last four years and now that you can't have a child, you're looking for purpose and meaning. Am I hearing you OK? (paraphrase, check out)

Clinician A's response could be very helpful in getting the facts out clearly so that he can develop a strong, shared understanding of Sherman's story. Clinician B's focus on the underlying meaning would be especially helpful once she had developed a good understanding of the facts. This response would focus the ongoing discussion on purpose and meaning.

The sentence stem and check-out frame the paraphrase and communicate understanding. Once comfortable using paraphrases, clinicians can begin dropping the sentence stem and check-out, like this: "Your world has been centered around making a baby and you're wondering what you can do to go on."

Reflections of Feeling

Reflections of feeling also further discussion and communicate understanding, but do this by selectively focusing on feelings. Like paraphrases, they often begin with a sentence stem (e.g., "It sounds like …" or "It feels like …") and are often followed by a check-out (e.g., "Am I understanding you?"). In between them is a phrase reflecting the emotion or emotions that the client is talking about, implying, or expressing nonverbally, often followed by a statement of what caused the feelings ("You're feeling pretty angry" + "since losing your job"). The basic form of a reflection of feeling is, "It sounds like" + "you're feeling _____" + "since _____." + "Is that right?"

Sherman:		It's just been so crazy. [pause] We focused so much of our time and energy on making a baby for so long and it's like I don't know what to feel or do now. Sometimes I'm angry at what we've lost. Sometimes I'm depressed. Sometimes I'm almost relieved—then I feel guilty because I feel relieved.
Clinician A:		It seems like you've been feeling a lot of different things—anger, frustration, depression, relief and guilt—since you found out that the two of you can't have a baby. Am I understanding you OK? (reflection of feeling, check out)
Clinician B:		It feels like you're really confused about what you feel now. Sometimes you feel numb, but other times you feel angry, depressed, relieved, or even guilty. Am I on track? (reflection of feeling, check out)

The feeling is the essential aspect of a reflection of feeling; the other three parts can be dropped after clinicians have developed greater therapeutic skill, especially when there is a strong therapeutic alliance between the clinician and the client. For example, a clinician might occasionally say, "You're feeling really blue today," but he should also observe the client to see whether he is on track.

Clients signal that a therapeutic response is on track by nodding and smiling, leaning forward, saying "Yes," or expanding on the discussion (Thomas, 2005). They signal that a response is off track by saying "No," then correcting the misunderstanding, leaning back, hesitating or stuttering, changing the subject, engaging in nervous laughter, or briefly breaking eye contact. Other clients respond to off-track responses by beginning to talk about more superficial or meaningless topics (see Table 11.2).

After a reflection of feeling, clients are likely to explore and feel their emotions more intensely. Following paraphrases, clients tend to discuss content rather than feelings. Therefore, reflections of feeling are more appropriate

TABLE **11.2**
Strategies for Deciphering Mixed Messages.

	Expression	Meaning
Strong positive feedback	Strong, clear, congruent positive message (e.g., smiling broadly and maintaining eye contact while saying, "Yes, I agree.").	Agreement with interpretation or suggestion.
Mixed positive feedback	Increased emotional or physical energy; speech quickens; eye contact increases (e.g., quick outburst, staring at clinician, "That's the craziest thing I ever heard!").	Agreement with interpretation or suggestion, although agreement is muted by ambivalence or anxiety.
Mixed negative feedback	Affect is flat; speech is flat, hesitant or slowed; movement slows or stills; eye contact breaks (e.g., slowly, eyes averted, body becoming still, "If you think so ...”).	Superficial buy-in. Disagrees with suggestion or intervention but unable to assert opinion clearly.
Strong negative feedback	Strong, clear, congruent negative message (e.g., shaking head while firmly saying, "No, I do not want to.").	Disagreement with interpretation or suggestion.

Note: Based on Thomas (2005)

when trying to encourage clients to discuss their feelings and experience them more deeply, while paraphrases are more useful for gaining an understanding of facts and ideas (Ivey & Ivey, 2003).

Encouragers

Encouragers are very brief summaries of the most central content or emotion. They are generally one to two words taken directly from the client's response and focus discussion on that particular idea. **Minimal encouragers**—"Uh huh," "Mmm," "Yup," a head nod, or an empathically appropriate facial expression—can quickly communicate understanding and encourage further discussion.

Sherman:	I just don't know what to do anymore. People keep going up to me, to Dion, and asking about the baby-making process. I don't want to have to answer any more questions. I don't want to feel anymore.
Clinician A:	More questions ... (encourager)
Clinician B:	Anymore? (encourager)
Clinician C:	Uh Huh. (minimal encourager)

Notice how encouragers can get people talking about either content or feelings, depending on the particular encourager used. Think about what Sherman might say to the responses "more questions" and "feel." Mimimal encouragers like "Uh huh" do not get in the way at all, although they still influence clients' direction. When used well, encouragers and minimal encouragers can quickly and elegantly get clients talking, gently nudging them in a particular direction, without focusing the attention on the clinician in the way that long, involved paraphrases, questions, or interpretations might.

Like any other therapeutic lead, minimal encouragers and encouragers can be overused. Clients can perceive clinicians who repeatedly nod their head and say "Uh huh" as stiff and disingenuous. Encouragers may also confuse some clients, especially those who are not used to people really listening to them.

Closed and Open Questions

A fool may ask more questions in an hour than a wise man can answer in seven years.

—English Proverb

Clinicians both gain their understanding and communicate it by asking questions, which is often an important way of gathering a lot of information quickly. Questions take two general forms: closed or open. Closed questions generally start with "is," "are," "do," "does," "would," "could," or "have" and can be answered with one or two words (e.g., "Are you tired today?"). They are good ways of gathering information quickly and efficiently. They are most appropriate in structured situations where a large amount of information must be gathered quickly or with overly talkative clients.

Teenagers often respond especially poorly to closed questions and may reply very briefly even to open questions (e.g., "How have you been doing this last week?" "Good."). Teenagers are not the only ones who respond poorly to questions, though. Think about Sgt. Mehl's style of questioning Andrea Yates in the next box. Could his questioning be appropriate in one setting but inappropriate in another?

Effective clinicians resist the tendency to ask more questions when they receive a poor response to their first question. Instead, depending on the setting, they either back off or move to a reflection of feeling or paraphrase of the session process (e.g., "It sounds like you're not ready to talk yet." or, "You look like it was very difficult to come here today."). Of course, reflecting the difficulty talking is only appropriate when that appears to be the problem (e.g., she is looking downward, sitting in a closed posture, struggling for words or holding strong emotions back). When a client is not talking because he or she thinks therapy is boring and a waste of time—that is, he or she is leaning back in the chair, not paying attention, and making flip or off-track comments—that should be the core of the reflection (e.g., "It seems like you don't want to be here today.").

Finally, some statements take the form of one microskill but perform a different function. "Could" is generally a closed question but can also serve as a **directive** (e.g., "Could you go to your 'safe place' now?"). Using a closed question as a directive can be an especially useful way to give clients a choice and a sense of control, both of which are often important in the course of treatment.

Open questions generally start with "what," "how," or "why" and, in contrast to closed questions, are often used to encourage discussion. Each prompt leads to a different sort of response (Ivey & Ivey, 2003). "What" questions lead to discussions of content (e.g., "What would you like to do after college?"). "How" questions lead to further discussion of feelings or processes (e.g., "How do you handle it when you start to get overwhelmed?"). "Why" questions focus on underlying purpose (e.g., "Why did you choose to take this course rather than the other one?"). Why questions should be used infrequently, because clients often perceive them as blaming and may become defensive in response to them (Ivey & Ivey, 2003). The function of Why questions can often be better met with How questions, which often make them feel less blaming (e.g., "How did you come to take this course rather than the other one?").

Here are several examples of open and closed questions. Paying attention to one's own emotional and cognitive responses to these can help clarify their function.

Sherman: I'm all over the place today. I'm tired of this. I just want to stop feeling.

Clinician A: What do you think might happen if you remained open to your feelings about this? (open question)

Clinician B: Could you try sitting with your feelings for a while and see what happens? (closed question functioning as a directive)

Clinician C: Why do you think you should stop feeling? (open question)

Clinician D: Are you feeling like you just cannot go on any longer? (closed question)

Open questions are often useful because they encourage people to talk, but they may not be useful with people who talk at length. With such clients, closed questions may slow the therapeutic process down enough so that both clinician and client have room to work together productively.

Finally, certain types of questions may be problematic in some types of settings, especially during forensic interviews (Gilstrap, 2004). Forced-choice questions can be leading ones and suggest that the correct choice is one of two options, even though neither is correct (e.g., "Did he touch you in the bedroom or the living room?"). The clinician's preferences can be further signaled by tag questions (e.g., "He was in the living room, wasn't he?"). Asking children to imagine certain types of events can also distort memory (e.g., "Could you imagine what he would say?").

Questions can also be problematic in more therapy-oriented settings. Asking closed questions can encourage dichotomous responses (e.g., "Are you feeling suicidal today?"). What degree of suicidality is enough to report? This sort of question could lead to either overestimates or underestimates of a client's suicidality. It might be more useful to ask, "On a scale from 1 to 10, how suicidal are you today?"

In assessment situations, especially with young children, forced-choice questions can be leading and problematic. However, in therapy settings, these questions can sometimes be useful. It can be helpful to give a child two choices (e.g., "Do you want to color or play a game?") rather than either a single one or an unlimited number of choices. Giving a single choice can increase oppositional behavior, while providing unlimited choices can increase indecisiveness and sometimes cause problems in clinical settings.

Transcript of Andrea Yates' Confession
Associated Press

This book started with a portion of the forensic interview between Andrea Yates and Dr. Phillip Resnick. This is about 5% of the interview between Andrea Yates and Houston Police Sgt. Eric Mehl, which led to her confession. The rest is readily available online (Associated Press, 2001). Although the murders are not described in this portion of the interview, the rest of the interview takes much the same form, with Ms. Yates responding very briefly to Sgt. Mehl's questions.

Sgt. Eric Mehl 1: Um, after you drew the bath water, what was your intent? What were you about to do?

Andrea Yates 1: Drown the children.

Sgt. Mehl 2: OK. Why were you going to drown your children? (15 seconds of silence) Was it, was it in reference to, or was it because the children had done something?

Yates 2: No.

Sgt. Mehl 3: You were not mad at the children?

Yates 3: No.

Sgt. Mehl 4: OK, um, you had thought of this prior to this day?

(continues)

Yates 4: Yes.

Sgt. Mehl 5: Um, how long have you been having thoughts about wanting, or not wanting to, but drowning your children?

Yates 5: Probably since I realized I have not been a good mother to them.

Sgt. Mehl 6: What makes you say that?

Yates 6: They weren't developing correctly.

Sgt. Mehl 7: Behavioral problems?

Yates 7: Yes.

Sgt. Mehl 8: Learning problems?

Yates 8: Yes. (Associated Press, 2002, para. 107–124)

- Think about Sgt. Mehl's interview. What were his goals? What did he do well? Not so well? Are these strengths and weaknesses consistent with his goals for the interview?
- Go back through the interview. What microskills did Sgt. Mehl use during the interview? What percentage of time did he use open questions? Closed Questions? Paraphrases? Reflections of feeling? Encouragers? Were there any other microskills that he used?
- What did you think of Sgt. Mehl's use of silence in his second response? Why?
- Compare this interview with Dr. Resnick's interview in Chapter 1. How do they differ? How are they similar? Consider how you would have interviewed Ms. Yates if this had been a clinical interview. How would you have approached it differently? What might you do in the same way?
- What did Ms. Yates "say" about herself and, parenthetically, her relationship with Sgt. Mehl in this interview segment?

Summarizations

Summarizations are like paraphrases, but they cover a longer time period. They are a way of helping clients organize a large amount of information and to see the forest rather than only trees. Like paraphrases, summarizations generally take a specific form: (a) a succinct summary of a longer segment of the session, followed by (b) a check-out, to check the client's understanding. In this case, however, check-outs take a somewhat different form than with paraphrases and reflections of feelings, but these questions still work to make sure that the clinician and client are on the same page.

Summarizations can be used at any point in a session, as in these two examples. They provide an effective bridge between two parts of a session or between two sessions or parts of treatment:

Clinician A: Last session we were talking about the difficulties you've been having since learning that Dion couldn't get pregnant. We were challenging your thinking about this. What have you been thinking since then? (summarization, open question; at the beginning of the session)

Clinician B: We've been talking about the ways that irrational thoughts cause our feelings. You've given examples of how your thinking patterns are directly related to your anger, frustration, and sadness about having to stop the infertility treatments. [nods] If you can cause these feelings, you can also control these. [nods] We discussed some ways that you could do this—and you did a great job! [pause] Is there anything else you'd want to add? (summarization, feedback, closed question; during the middle or at the end of the session)

Rather than the clinician telling clients what they got out of the session, they can be asked to describe their own experience. These client-generated summarizations can help them organize the session and, in addition, can be empowering for the client, who then "owns" what was taken from a session. Like a check-out, a client-generated summarization can ensure that the clinician and client are on the same page.

There are several ways that clinicians can help clients summarize their sessions. Clinicians can start sessions by asking, "What was really important *to you* from last week's session?" This open question can help clients organize material and draw something important from it. At the end of a session, clinicians might ask, "What was the most important thing you learned, thought about, or felt today?"

Clinicians can also ask, "What homework would you give yourself based on today's session?" This open question indirectly assesses what clients found important and lets them identify how they are going to act on the ideas from the session. Of course, when clients' homework assignments are too ambitious, clinicians can scale back assignments to something more manageable.

Pay attention to the way that Natalie Rogers uses these microskills in the next box. How does she match these to her probable treatment goals for Robin?

Do I Cope the Way Everybody Else Does?
Robin

Different therapeutic leads pull different responses from clients. Use them thoughtfully in ways that support your treatment plan. Notice how Natalie Rogers (b. 1928) does this with Robin in this brief transcript from a longer interview. Rogers describes herself as an expressive arts therapist, although she uses many of the basic listening skills of her more famous father.

Natalie Rogers 1: Well, Robin, it's nice to have you here, and I'm hoping to spend some time with you really getting to know you and anything you want to talk about, [Mhm] and as I mentioned just briefly earlier, I am an expressive arts therapist, so I will perhaps offer you the opportunity to use art as a way of communication, but that will be very much up to you. [Okay.] You can feel free to say yes or no, uh, I really mean that. But the way that I like to start with clients, if this is okay with you, is to spend just a minute quietly together with

(continues)

our eyes closed just to really try to get present, to really get here, be present at the moment. [Okay.] Would that be all right with you?

Robin 1: Yeah, that's fine.

Dr. Rogers 2: Well, let's just put our feet on the floor and close your eyes for a minute, take a big breath. Tell your body to relax. And as we take this minute in silence, if you can pay attention to any thoughts or feelings or sensations that are going on within you, that would be good. (20 second silence) And when you're ready, you can open your eyes. So, I'd like to start wherever you want to begin.

Robin 2: That was good.

Dr. Rogers 3: Was that good? [Yes.] Mhm. What went on?

Robin 3: Basically clearing my mind. [Mhm, mhm] Sometimes it takes, [Takes a while] yeah. Take ten seconds just to get away and get a break and clear my mind, releases tension and stress and things like that.

Dr. Rogers 4: So even just that little bit helped you? [Mhm.] Be here or just empty?

Robin 4: Empty.

Dr. Rogers 5: Empty, okay.

Robin 5: It's sort of like I sometimes have tons of things going in. If I close my eyes and just relax for a few minutes, it just clears it all away, you know, and I don't worry about things. It feels good.

Dr. Rogers 6: Good, so, it's nice to have a minute not to worry about things.

Robin 6: Right, right. But, um, it cleared everything out. I mean, just, so there's no stress, there's no worrying about things going on [Mhm] and things like that, so.....

Dr. Rogers 7: So there are things that you worry about, but at the moment that kind of cleared it away?

Robin 7: Mhm, yeah. I think I worry about what everybody else worries about, you know, um, where I am going to be five years down the road, you know. Is what I'm doing now the right thing? Um, just, just normal everyday life. Sometimes, I guess my biggest thing I think about sometimes is how does everybody else cope with the things that go on that are everyday life to other people. How do they cope as compared to me? Am I in that midstream, do I cope the way everybody else does, or...?

Dr. Rogers 8: So you have these things that are going on that you are concerned about the future somewhat. [Mhm.] How do you really compare yourself to others? How do others do it? (Carlson & Kjos, 1998, para 1–15)

- What do you think of Natalie Rogers' opening exercise and use of silence? Why? What do you think Robin thought of it? How do you know?
- What do you think of Dr. Rogers' ability to hear and understand Robin? What did Robin think? How do you know?
- Although we haven't talked about all of the skills that Dr. Rogers uses, she did use some minimal encouragers, paraphrases, reflections of feeling, and questions. Identify each of these. Pay attention to how Robin responds to different sorts of leads.

STRATEGIES FOR UNDERSTANDING OTHERS DEEPLY

I tell you everything that is really nothing, and nothing of what is everything, do not be fooled by what I am saying. Please listen carefully and try to hear what I am not saying.

—Charles C. Finn

Some people may be able to clearly and directly describe how they feel. Many people, however, have difficulty putting their thoughts and feelings directly into words. They may scream, "I'M NOT ANGRY!" They may avoid talking about the things that are most important to them, choosing to talk about superficial topics instead. They may talk about the issues that are pressing for them but may do so in a matter-of-fact manner, as though they are trivial. They may describe something as important one day and then deny its significance—even its existence—the next. They may simply be silent. These styles of self-expression—denial, evasion, revision, and silence—complicate therapy but can also be cues about clients' inner lives (Mozdrzierz et al., 2009; A. G. Rogers, 2001; A. G. Rogers et al., 1999).

Several authors have talked about the ways that some groups (e.g., women, trauma survivors, people with borderline personality disorder) have silenced themselves, even making self-reports that are directly contradictory to their inner experiences (L. M. Brown, 1998; Linehan, 1993; A. G. Rogers, 2001). Even these groups, however, "leak" how they think and feel (e.g., saying, "That's a great idea," while frowning, looking away and quickly changing the subject). This leakage is especially true when clients are feeling safe and believe that their clinician wants to understand them.

Learning to be empathic requires listening to the words that a person uses but can demand much more. Rothschild (2004), for example, suggests that clinicians should pay attention to their own body's responses to help them identify their own emotions and those of their clients. Mirroring a client's breathing and following their movements can build understanding, rapport, and prosocial behaviors (Lakin & Chartrand, 2003; May, 1967; van Baaren et al., 2004). The reverse is also true. Speaking quickly and loudly, for example, with someone who is speaking quietly and slowly can interfere with rapport.

It is important to note, however, that the client's behavior and clinician's feelings can be misleading. Clients may breathe rapidly due to anxiety or may be gasping for breath due to asthma. A clinician's anxiety during a client's discussion of her mother's illness, for example, may be more related to events in his own life than his client's anxiety. While gathering observations, clinicians are generating hypotheses rather than identifying facts; confidence about conclusions increases with additional consistent information.

A. G. Rogers (2001) describes four strategies for deepening empathy beyond the words clients use. She suggests that clinicians:

- **Approach the story from different viewpoints.** When working with a client with Alzheimer's, for example, pay attention to when his memory was good and when it was weaker. When and how was he compliant with staff and in which ways did he resist authorities? Finally, think about things that were hinted at but never fully described. Any new interpretation—thinking about racial issues, the role of gender in his life, age, ability, religion, and the like—broadens and deepens the picture told. This is one of the advantages of using multiple strategies like genograms, psychosocial histories, and timelines during the assessment process.

- **Listen for language cues and metaphors.** Pay attention to word and metaphor choice and what they say about the speaker. When people use active voice (e.g., "I am ...," "I did ..."), it suggests that they see themselves as a direct and active participant with an internal locus of control, while the use of passive voice (e.g., "... was done to me," "It happened to me ...") suggests an external locus of responsibility. Using past tense suggests that the client sees the problem as being in the past, while present tense suggests it is perceived as an ongoing problem. Metaphors can directly or indirectly describe things that may otherwise be unclear (e.g., "I trudged through an evening of work."), in this case suggesting that work was tedious, dirty, and perhaps even toxic.

   People use words for all sorts of different reasons. Poor word choice, such as "I *sludged* through an evening of work," could indicate having (mis)heard the idiom rather than seeing it spelled out, enjoying playing with words, or even having brain damage. In addition, the ways that people tell their stories are influenced by various contextual factors, including cultural and temporal factors, audience, mood, environment, and chance events (see Table 11.3). As suggested previously, conclusions about the meaning of someone's words should be drawn only after exploring the possible hypotheses.

   Often what clients talk about can be read on several levels. For example, in saying that today is a nice day (it being true), one is also saying that the weather is not always nice. When a client says, "I really trust you," she may also be saying that she did not expect to trust her counselor, that her sense of trust is increasing, or perhaps that this trust is still wobbly. People rarely notice or talk about the things that are stable or known in their lives; instead they focus on and talk about the gaps.

TABLE **11.3**
Factors Influencing the Quality of the "Story" Shared.

- **Temporal, cultural and situational contexts.** Some people share intimate information more readily with people they know well, others with people they know less well. They may emphasize some things at the expense of others, depending on their perceptions of the listener's intents. How strong is the therapeutic relationship? How does the person's past, present, or future context influence what and how the story is told?
- **Communication goals.** Most people's communications are purposeful (e.g., to get medicine, understanding, a diagnosis, or a "good report"). What does the client hope to gain?
- **Medium.** Some people communicate better orally, others in writing, artwork, or through play. Is the medium one in which this client communicates well?
- **Insight.** People cannot share what they do not have access to. Does the client observe and understand his or her thoughts, feelings, behaviors and motivation?
- **Personal, cultural and situational self-disclosure norms.** Stories take time to tell. Longer periods generally allow greater completeness and can develop the kind of relationship that encourages an honest, three-dimensional description. What rules govern the depth and content of self-disclosures? To what degree are these norms salient?

Caution is necessary when drawing conclusions about people from other cultures. Clients' language and nonverbal behaviors take different forms because of regional, ethnic, or age cohort differences that may not have the same meanings as in the clinician's culture.

- **Observe what gets omitted or muddied.** There are many different ways that sensitive information gets distorted or omitted. Clients may directly *deny* a problem: "I haven't cut this week" (when they did). They may change the subject to *evade* a problem: "You know, that's an important issue, but I really need to tell you about _____ first," hoping that they never get back to the problem subject. They may *revise* their story: "Well, yes, I told you that I didn't want to talk about that, but I really do." They may provide poorer descriptions than usual: "Yes, school is going well." Their story can be characterized by *silence*, thus actively or passively avoiding discussions of a problem.

  Even when not talking about a problem (by denying, evading, revising, becoming vague, or remaining silent), clients tell a story about both the problem and themselves. For example, the client who denied cutting may be saying that he or she is afraid of the consequences of sharing this knowledge with someone else (or, perhaps, of admitting it to him- or herself).

- **Track relational dynamics.** Relationships shift and change with time. As the relationship changes, what can be told and how, as well as what is not disclosed, is altered. These changes both reflect and cause changes in the relationship. Clients may disclose an intimate part of their past when they feel safe and understood; their disclosure may in turn cause the clinician to behave in ways that draw out more disclosures.

  These dynamics should be examined in the course of a particular relationship, however. Some people find it easier to disclose vulnerabilities to strangers, while others can only disclose in close relationships. For example, as the therapeutic alliance develops, it may become easier to disclose some feelings, but if the client believes her clinician sees her as strong and competent, it may become more difficult to disclose vulnerabilities.

With these ideas in mind, listen to Anna Michener's story.

My Worldview or Yours?
Anna J. Michener

When Tiffany (b. 1977) was 13, she was sent to a psychiatric hospital because her grandmother said she was "disobedient" and out of control. Over the next several years she was moved from institution to institution and then finally placed into a foster home shortly before she turned 16. There she took her foster parents' last name, Michener, to honor the people "who have been more of a family to me than any of my biological relations ever

(continues)

were." She took a new first name, Anna, to make a clear separation from her past life and "to symbolize the fact that I am my own person" (Michener, 1998, p. 253). She describes herself as White.

Although her memoir was written during the period between her 16th and 17th birthdays, you can hear how she is in transition about how she sees herself and her world. Pay attention both to how she had seen herself and her newer view.

> My grandmother claimed to love me forever.... Perhaps if she had not "loved" me so much I would have felt a little love for her. I was not even impressed by the times she made cookies with my brother and me, took us to the park to sail boats, or allowed us to play with her toys for an afternoon. We could only "earn" these things from her by doing whatever she said we had to do for them. Nothing came for free, in the true spirit of grandmotherly love. While my brother was easily controlled with bribes, I resented them more than the thin metal rod my grandmother kept at the top of the stairs.
>
> I was always the "willful" one. When my grandmother could no longer make me cry out when she whipped me, she whipped my little brother in my place. She knew I would rather die than see him hurt.
>
> Although I could never be bullied into anything, my grandmother could manipulate me with the large crocodile tears that spilled out of her eyes sometimes when she spoke of "loving me so and hating to see me on the road of a person with bad character," or whined about my "poor, weak mother" and my "callous treatment of her."
>
> She put it into my head that if I loved my mother I would have, from the age of six, kept the house clean and made dinner each night, done all the chores, and taken care of my brother, as well as maintaining perfect grades at school. I should have sacrificed everything for my mother, thought of her above all else. I should never have asked her for anything. I should never have even touched her. My grandmother called being touched by children "unnecessary stress."
>
> I felt completely responsible for my mother's physical health and emotional state. No one else even tried to help her. My grandmother sure didn't do the things for my mother that she always said I should be doing. In fact, my grandmother did the complete opposite of reducing stress for my mother. Around my grandmother, or even just when thinking about her, my mother got the look on her face of a prisoner who longs to climb a fence of barbed wire but never dares. (Michener, 1998, pp. 4–5)

Anna was in and out of psychiatric institutions before her 16th birthday, once for a year. She saw hospital staff as siding with her grandmother against her and objectifying her and the other children there. She reported that their behavior was pathologized, their basic rights and privileges were restricted, and that they were rarely treated, from her point of view, with kindness or consideration.

Although Anna has received accolades for her criticism of the mental health system, she has also been criticized.

> I have been accused of saying in my book that I and other children institutionalized with me are perfectly innocent and everyone who worked with us was evil.

(continues)

(continued)

But it is this interpretation, and not I who is so black and white. I do not believe anyone is perfectly innocent and I do not believe anyone is evil. I believe children become what they live and the only way to combat the violent, depressed, and anti-social behavior of abuse victims is with understanding, acceptance, and love. However, I also see how this is hard to do. Mental health and social workers who do not understand the roots of certain aberrant behaviors will naturally react with fear, ignorance, and cruelty even if they are not cruel people. I did not write this book for revenge, to point fingers, or to start fights. I hope simply that everyone who reads it puts him/herself in my place for a moment and asks-how would I feel if I had grown up this way? How would I have reacted? What would I have become? (Contemporary Authors Online, 2003, para. 2)

- How does Anna see her world? What does she value? What is she interested in? How would you identify her strengths and weaknesses? How do you know?
- How does her grandmother (at least through Anna's eyes) see her world? What does she value? What is she interested in? How would you identify her strengths and weaknesses? How do you know?
- Reread this passage, paying attention to the subtleties of Anna's language use. Line by line, pay attention to what she says without directly saying it (e.g., "My grandmother claimed to love me forever," *but didn't*).
- Go back and look at what you concluded about Anna and her grandmother. Would each have described *herself* in the way that you've written about them? If not, go back and consider how they would have written about themselves from their own point of view, keeping in mind that behavior generally makes sense to that person.
- Do you agree with Anna's assessment of the criticism of her book? Why or why not? How might your reactions influence your own work in the mental health field and with clients?
- Return to Annie Rogers' story in the beginning of the chapter, and listen for the nuances embedded in her statements. How does Dr. Blumenfeld respond to these? Are his responses effective? How do you know?

ACCURATE EMPATHY

He who does not understand your silence will probably not understand your words.
—**Elbert Hubbard**

Empathy is only effective in facilitating change when it is expressed either verbally or nonverbally. Words can accurately communicate empathy without adding anything else (**accurate empathy**), distort or lose the client's understanding (**subtractive empathy**), or capture the client's full meaning, both stated and not directly stated, helping a client to gain insight that may not have been recognized or understood previously (**additive empathy**; Carkhuff, 1969). Although each clinician in the following exchange uses a reflection of feeling, their responses illustrate these different levels of empathy.

Sherman: We have worked so hard to have a child. It's difficult to know how to go on from here. Should we just accept that we'll never have a child of our own? Should we look into adoption?

Clinician A: It sounds like you're feeling pretty hopeless about the future right now. (subtractive empathy)

Clinician B: It sounds like this has been a difficult process and that you're feeling pretty confused about what you should do next. (accurate empathy)

Clinician C: It sounds like this has been a difficult process and that you're feeling pretty confused about what you should do next, but that you are *also* beginning to think about the future and recognize that life will go on, that *you* will go on. (additive empathy)

The first clinician missed the mark. In doing so, Sherman would likely respond in confusion, perhaps feeling alienated, perhaps needing to help his clinician understand him. If his clinician was lucky, Sherman would have responded, "No, not really *hopeless*, but I am pretty confused about what we should do next" (see Table 11.2). All clinicians make occasional missteps. If these mistakes are relatively infrequent and small, they might not damage the therapeutic alliance (Strupp, 1996).

The second clinician was on track, which would probably cause Sherman to expand on what he had been saying, "Yes, it has been difficult and I'm really confused about where to go and what to do. What do I do next?" The third clinician, however, hit the nail squarely on the head, both recognizing how Sherman had been lost and also how he and his wife were beginning to think differently about the future. Empathic clinicians do more than just parrot their clients' words; "they understand overall goals as well as moment-to-moment experiences, both explicit and implicit. Empathy in part entails capturing the nuances and implications of what people say, ... reflecting this back to them for their consideration" (L. S. Greenberg et al., 2001, p. 383). As seen in this and other examples in this chapter, people's statements are multifaceted, with meanings extending beyond their words. Recognizing these nuances can help clients feel heard and understood. Because Sherman felt understood by Clinician C and free enough to explore other parts of himself, he responded:

Sherman   Yes, that's it! Over the last several years, we've been tossed back and forth between doctors, blindly doing whatever each doctor recommended. I didn't like it, but never recognized it at the time. Now I'm starting to feel that we have a choice and can take charge of our lives again. I feel like we can go on again.

His thoughtful expansion on this third clinician's statement suggests that he believed that he was deeply understood.

While words do communicate empathy, empathy must be expressed nonverbally as well as verbally; furthermore, verbal and nonverbal messages must be consistent and genuine. People are confused by conflicting verbal and nonverbal messages (Langton, O'Malley, & Bruce, 1996). Saying "It sounds like you are having a hard time" but yawning and failing to make eye contact will probably signal a lack of interest. Saying the same thing while fully attending signals an active commitment to the person and relationship.

Clients communicate that they feel misunderstood by blushing, fidgeting, or restlessly shifting position, avoiding eye contact or becoming silent, or making more speech disruptions, including hesitations, stammers, and very rapid speech (Mordecai, 1991). Clinicians may do the same things when they feel bored, impatient, or inadequate, disrupting the empathic connection without being aware of doing so.

Return to Dr. Blumenfeld's responses to Annie Rogers at the beginning of the chapter. At what level of empathy—additive, subtractive or accurate—would you describe his responses? How do you know?

EMPATHY: THE NEED FOR VALIDATION AND POSITIVITY

This is why unpleasant events are "news"; compassionate activities are so much a part of daily life that they are taken for granted and, therefore, largely ignored.

—The Dalai Lama

Pinel and Constantinou (2003) argue that people have two needs in relationships. People need to hear positive things about themselves, but they also need to have their viewpoint validated.

People with low self-esteem dismiss or reinterpret positive feedback. When they are given positive feedback by a credible source (e.g., from their clinician), they may be unable to dismiss it and therefore become anxious. They prefer negative to positive feedback (Pinel & Constantinou, 2003; Swann, Chang-Schneider, & Larsen McClarty, 2007)! However, people with low self-esteem (which characterizes many therapy clients) prefer feedback that validates their self-concept but that also includes small amounts of positive feedback (Pinel & Constantinou, 2003). Thus, rather than glibly saying that everything will be better in the morning, many people prefer feedback that both acknowledges the problem (**validation**) and that also hints at some hope (**positivity**). This type of feedback may at least partially match their own perception—otherwise why would they be in therapy? Notice how Clinician C's last response was validating while also being hopeful (i.e., "It sounds like this has been a difficult process and that you're feeling pretty confused about what you should do next, but you are *also* beginning to think about the future and recognize that life will go on, that *you* will go on.").

Because the need for validation is so strong, some writers argue that clinicians should address it very early during treatment (Finn & Tonsager, 1997; Ivey & Ivey, 2003; Pinel & Constantinou, 2003). In sharing their understanding of clients—from the client's own viewpoint—clinicians both confirm their clients' ability to be understood and demonstrate their own clinical competence.

Food for Thought

Did Anna Michener feel validated by the clinicians working with her? How did she respond to this perception? Did Dr. Blumenfeld respond to Annie Rogers' needs for validation and positivity? How did his responses to her needs for validation and positivity impact their relationship? What about Natalie Rogers' responses to Robin? Were they validating and positive?

SUMMARY

Empathy is expressed verbally using different therapeutic leads in order to meet different clinical goals. Paraphrases summarize the content from the client's last statement and encourage discussions of facts. Reflections of feeling summarize emotions and encourage continued focus on emotions. Encouragers, generally no more than a few words in length, get clients to expand their discussion of those ideas. Questions solicit information. Closed questions solicit specific information, often obtaining yes or no answers; open questions are less likely to be answered in a few words and are often used as the starting point of a discussion. The nature of the question (who, what, when, where, why, and how) pulls different types of client responses, focusing on different information. Summarizations succinctly pull together themes from part or all of a session.

Nonverbal and verbal responses, even when formed well, are not always on track. Those that paraphrase the client, without either diverting or adding to the client's understanding, are accurate empathy; most empathic responses used by effective clinicians belong to this category. Off-track responses (subtractive empathy) interfere with the relationship when they occur too frequently or when they are handled poorly. Additive empathy accurately identifies both the overt message and the underlying subtext of a client's statements, thus encouraging deeper thinking and experiencing.

There are numerous strategies for developing empathic understanding. A. G. Rogers (2001) suggests (a) approaching the client's story several times from different viewpoints; (b) listening closely to cues in the client's language and metaphors; (c) paying attention to what gets omitted or muddied in a discussion; and (d) tracking the changing emotions and relational dynamics in a session.

Generally, people respond best to messages that are both positive and validating of their self-concept. They must also be realistic and understandable from within the client's worldview. Positive and validating statements reflect clinicians' deep understanding of their clients, engage clients more effectively, and build the therapeutic relationship.

How Do These Issues Apply to Your Life and Work?

1. Pay attention to what good listeners and poor listeners do verbally. How do they demonstrate that they are listening well (or not so well)? How do others respond to them? Does the nature of the setting or their relationship seem to influence the reactions they receive?
2. Practice using the basic verbal listening skills (e.g., paraphrases, reflections of feeling, and summarization) without using questions, self-disclosures, or the verbal influencing skills. How does the other

(continues)

(continued)

person respond? How do you feel in doing this? If you feel awkward, remember that awkwardness is normal when learning a new skill.

3. Continue practicing with the verbal listening skills. What happens when you use them well? What happens when you use intentionally poor empathic responses (e.g., saying "It sounds like you had a really bad day!" when someone is happy and bouncing off the wall with joy.)? Debrief your "research participants" afterwards!

CHAPTER 12

Facilitating Change

WHERE ARE WE GOING?

1. What common strategies are generally shared across theoretical viewpoints?

2. Why is listening prior to intervening important in facilitating change?

3. What can clinicians do to help clients change behaviors, thoughts, and feelings?

4. What factors can serve as barriers to treatment and how can these be effectively addressed?

5. How can clinicians assess the success of their interventions?

I Don't Drink Every Single Day
Beth Schneider

Beth Schneider is an attractive, middle-class white woman in her 30s. She is eight months pregnant, described as healthy, active, fun-loving, and carefree. She has become more careful about her diet since becoming pregnant, but also made a controversial decision about drinking alcohol. "I don't drink every single day. It's probably four or five days a week that I enjoy a glass of wine. A beer. [sound of a cork popping from a wine bottle] Love that sound. [laughing] You know, when you get one glass a day, you milk the hell out of it."

She continued, "I've heard of Fetal Alcohol Syndrome, and of course, you know, everything scares you as a pregnant woman, and they put fear in you."

Her husband Jeff said, "There is a chance. How big of a chance? We don't know. It's not something to worry about or stress about."

Linda Murray, editor-in-chief of BabyCenter admitted, "We have quite a few women … who've told us that for the first time in their lives [now that they're pregnant], they really want beer. They love the smell of it, they love the taste of it."

A number of women reported that they drink, but never in public. One observed, "It's not really worth risking public ridicule or scorn or all the advice I'm sure I'd get."

Beth concluded, "I don't care. I'm a firm believer that anything in moderation is OK." (Chang, Chan, & Stern, 2008)

- Why does Ms. Schneider drink? Assuming her physician had recommended that she stop drinking for her child's health, but she continued to talk about her drinking in this way, in what stage of change would she be in? How do you know? What barriers are there to stopping drinking?
- If her obstetrician asked you to help her stop drinking during pregnancy, how would you approach this? Why?
- How do your feelings about drinking during pregnancy influence your reactions to her? How would they influence your ability to work with her?
- The *Good Morning America* video for this story is available at http://abcnews.go.com/video/playerindex?id=4232465. Does watching the interview with Ms. Schneider change your view of her? If so, how? What made the difference?

Although clinicians of diverse theoretical stripes do many different things in the course of treatment, they are alike in more ways than they are different. In this chapter, we begin by describing the commonalities across the diverse approaches to therapy in terms of treatment goals, factors facilitating change, clinician characteristics, and treatment strategies. We then outline a general approach to change, which involves first connecting empathically, and then introducing change. We detail specific strategies for facilitating change in behaviors, emotions, and beliefs. We describe a general approach to identifying and working with barriers to change. We conclude by describing a strategy for evaluating treatment.

COMMONALITIES ACROSS TREATMENT APPROACHES

Treatment Goals

The curious paradox is that when I accept myself just as I am, then I can change.
—**Carl Rogers**

An ultimate goal of treatment is to increase clients' ability to continue to be successful after termination from treatment; developing self-efficacy, assertiveness, a sense of hope, and problem-solving skills can be essential skills in this process (Curtis, 2002; Epston & White, 1995; Goldfried, 2002; L. S. Greenberg, 2002; Wachtel, 2002). Clinicians foster their clients' autonomy, so that after termination from treatment, clients are able to problem solve and use healthy and adaptive coping mechanisms. As much as possible, treatment should encourage clients to develop their personal resources and natural support systems. As a result, although clinicians may often brainstorm and evaluate options with clients, they generally give clients choices rather than advice (May, 1967).

Depending on the population, between 80% and 90% of clients are not yet ready to take action (Prochaska & Norcross, 2001). Therefore, a more proximal goal of treatment is to help clients identify a problem that they are willing to work on and increase their desire to change. In addition, many clients hope that their clinicians will be able to make their trauma and suffering magically disappear (May, 1967). Whenever possible, however, clinicians should help clients *own* their treatment—that is, take the initiative to explore ideas, make their own discoveries, and be as active in treatment as their clinician (Friedlander, Thibodeau, & Ward, 1985; Strupp, 1996).

Factors Facilitating Change

Clinicians generally agree that the therapeutic relationship is central and foundational to therapeutic growth (Goldfried, 2007; L. Greenberg, 2008; Lambert & Barley, 2001). Clinicians should develop a positive working relationship with clients, and together agree on specific treatment goals and methods. Both client and clinician need to be equally committed to and active in the change process, rather than one party taking the majority of the responsibility for the work (Friedlander et al., 1985; Prochaska, 1999; Prochaska & Norcross, 2001).

Most clinicians believe that unconditional acceptance and nonjudgmental attitudes facilitate the therapeutic alliance and clinical work and, conversely, agree that criticism and judgmental attitudes interfere with the therapeutic relationship and inhibit therapeutic growth (Goldfried, 2007; Linehan, 1993; May, 1967; C. R. Rogers, 1957/1992). In fact, Goldfried argues that when these qualities are not emphasized in writing about counseling and psychotherapy, it is because these "nonspecific factors" have been accepted in the profession as givens. Furthermore, most clinicians agree that their ability to be empathic, accepting, and **congruent** facilitates clients' awareness of emotions and their ability to label, understand, and communicate their emotions to others (Watson, 2007). Perhaps paradoxically, empathy and acceptance of clients just as they are facilitate clients' ability to change (Frankl, 1946/1984; May, 1967; Watzlawick et al., 1974).

Finally, a strong therapeutic relationship creates positive expectations and a sense of hope (Frank & Frank, 1993). It fosters clients' motivation to change and addresses their ambivalence about the change process (Prochaska, 1999; Prochaska & Norcross, 2001). Clients' experience of a different sort of relationship or outcome can create a **corrective experience**, which helps clients feel differently about themselves, their relationships, their past, and their future (Alexander & French, 1946; Goldfried & Davila, 2005).

Characteristics of Clinicians

Clinicians often share certain personal characteristics. As described earlier, clinicians are empathic, accepting, and genuine in their clinical work (C. R. Rogers, 1957/1992). They are patient, recognizing that clients change at their own pace and that rushing clients can be counterproductive (Goldfried, 2007; Strupp, 1996). They are nonjudgmental and not easily shocked or offended by the things that their clients expect to be shocking (May, 1967).

Effective clinicians aspire to be genuine, humble, and nondefensive (C. R. Rogers, 1957/1992; Strupp, 1996). They recognize that they make mistakes and are imperfect, but aim to learn from their mistakes. Clinicians are introspective and aware of how their needs, frustrations, goals, and values might influence their clinical decisions. Therefore, they wonder how these factors might be impinging on their ability to empathize and make productive decisions. When telling a story or making a decision, for example, effective clinicians wonder whether they are doing it with their client's best interests in mind (Strupp, 1996).

Treatment Strategies

Emotional and physical pain are givens in life, although people do not need to behave in ways that increase that pain. Instead, especially when the pain cannot be changed or removed, clinicians generally focus on understanding, coping with, transforming and using trauma and other stressors and hardships in more positive ways (Frankl, 1946/1984; May, 1967). Some writers have focused on how it can lead to growth and have identified ways of increasing the potential for growth (e.g., C. L. Park, 2004; C. L. Park, Aldwin, Fenster, & Snyder, 2008; C. L. Park, Lechner, Antoni, & Stanton, 2009).

Clinicians meet treatment goals by listening carefully to what clients say directly, what they allude to, and their juxtaposition of topics and ways of talking about them (Mozdrzierz et al., 2009; A. G. Rogers, 2001; A. G. Rogers et al., 1999). They listen to the themes that clients develop within a therapy hour and across treatment (Strupp, 1996). Clinicians also listen to their own emotional and cognitive reactions, recognizing these reactions as important cues about their clients' concerns, responses, and dynamics (Rothschild, 2004; Strupp, 1996).

Encouraging clients to become actively involved in treatment and curious about their lives engages clients in treatment, which is related to more positive outcomes (Friedlander et al., 1985). Furthermore, clients' active involvement demonstrates the clinician's deep respect for each client; this respect can provide a corrective experience that clients may not have previously experienced from other people (Strupp, 1996). Finally, this expectation that clients will be actively involved in treatment suggests that they can exercise control and make positive changes in response to trauma, rather than being buffeted about by life.

Making treatment active occurs on several levels. Both client and clinician should be actively engaged in treatment, with clinicians entering each session with enthusiasm and a fresh eye (Strupp, 1996). Rather than only talking about problems in the past, as much as possible they look for ways to make treatment active and bring concerns into the **here and now** (Goldfried, 2002; Yalom, 2003). They pay attention to how clients are relating to them at that very moment. What are they thinking now? How helpful or maladaptive are their client's current cognitions? Rather than only talking about problems, many clinicians will find ways of making treatment livelier, using metaphors, and stories and enactments, and by activating cognitive, affective, and behavioral realms (Goldfried, 2002). This can be done within a session or by assigning homework to be completed outside sessions.

Talking about divorce, trauma, grief, loss, and failures to connect for much of the workday can be grim work, yet many clinicians find that their ability to find joy and maintain their sense of humor can not only be helpful self-care strategies, but, more importantly, are ways of helping clients rediscover joy and reconnect with their sense of humor as well (Strupp, 1996). Effective clinicians look for ways to connect with their clients, using their clients' language and metaphors, while avoiding jargon. Good clinicians offer their comments as tentative rather than authoritarian.

These commonalities—treatment goals, factors facilitating change, clinician characteristics, and treatment strategies—exist across therapeutic modalities and theoretical orientations and give rise to a general way of approaching the change process. Below, we describe this general approach, which consists of first developing a shared understanding and then implementing specific change strategies. We identify more specific ways to intervene, which involve simultaneously attending to where the client is right now and developing treatment goals jointly with clients.

GENERAL THERAPEUTIC APPROACH TO CHANGE

First, Develop a Shared Understanding

So when you are listening to somebody, completely, attentively, then you are listening not only to the words, but also to the feeling of what is being conveyed, to the whole of it, not part of it.

—Jiddu Krishnamurti

Friends and family members often respond to clients' problems either by agreeing (e.g., "You're right, you should leave him") or dismissing their viewpoint (e.g., "You can't just sit around! Get up and do something!"). However, these responses can be nonproductive and nontherapeutic. Clients frequently perceive criticism as invalidating their experience; they tend to dig in their heels and resist changing (Beutler et al., 2001). Critical, judgmental, and blaming responses especially put people with a history of mental illness at increased risk of relapse (Hinrichsen & Pollack, 1997; Hooley & Hiller, 2000; Hooley & Teasdale, 1989; O'Farrell, Hooley, Fals-Stewart, & Cutter, 1998).

Ivey and Ivey (2003) describe a more helpful approach to facilitating change. They suggest that clinicians should listen, share their understanding, and intervene only after that understanding is recognized. Effective treatment begins with clinicians listening to clients deeply, holding the assumption that their clients' viewpoint is valid (Fraser & Solovey, 2007; Ivey & Ivey, 2003; Linehan, 1993). Rather than jumping in too quickly to intervene, they take the time to develop a strong empathic understanding of their clients and their worldview, becoming curious about how their clients see the world, their place in it, their problem and ability to change it. With suicidal clients, for example, listening can be essential to the engagement process, as family and friends may not have wanted to listen to their story (G. K. Brown et al., 2006). Listening carefully to their story can also help clinicians identify risk factors and create a strong case conceptualization.

Once clinicians believe they understand, they must share their understanding of the client and the problem from the *client's* point of view, which might differ from the viewpoint of the clinician or the client's family and friends. Clinicians undermine treatment when they prematurely put interventions into place, even when their interventions are "right." Only when clients recognize their clinician's empathic understanding can clinicians intervene to provide a new perspective and motivate change. See types of verbal influencing skills in Table 12.1. In the following case, pay attention to whether Antonia feels understood and how she signals her understanding.

TABLE **12.1**
Verbal Influencing Skills.

- **Reframe.** Provides a new way of looking at an old behavior. Can be either positive, making the behavior more desirable, or negative, making the behavior less desirable. "*Your 'helping behavior' enables him to continue using and getting high.*" "*Your 'enabling behavior' is a sign of your deep compassion for the people around you.*"
- **Interpretation.** Identifies a deeper, underlying meaning to client behavior. "*I wonder whether your lateness to sessions might indicate your ambivalence about being here.*"
- **Self-disclosure.** Discloses material that is somewhat personal to the clinician, including reactions, memories, dreams, actions, etc. "*I was thinking that we have been moving very quickly today.*" "*I had a very difficult time starting college and missed my parents something fierce.*"
- **Feedback.** A special case of self-disclosure that shares the clinician's perception of or reaction to the client or client's behavior. "*I get very annoyed when you are habitually late to your sessions.*" "*You say that others see you as distant and cold, but I don't see you that way.*"
- **Information giving.** Provides information to help the client understand the problem, symptoms, or others better. "*Many people with a history of child abuse have a difficult time with relationships and trusting other people.*"
- **Normalization.** Presents a behavior that client has perceived negatively as normal, at least under some circumstances. "*Everyone has both good days and bad. The problem occurs when the bad days are too frequent or severe.*"
- **Directives.** Tells client what to do, generally in a relatively circumscribed situation to help meet a treatment goal. "*Take three slow breaths and begin to center yourself.*" "*Monitor your thoughts over the next week, especially when you're having strong feelings.*"
- **Advice.** Tells client what to do, especially how to solve a problem that the client faces. "*If I were you, I would kick her out now.*"
- **Confrontation.** Identifies a discrepancy within or across realms, for example, between client's behavior and goal, or between behavior and values and paraphrases these discrepancies. "*You say that your children are everything to you, yet you've been out drinking each night this week.*" "*You want to have a closer relationship with your family, but you get angry every time we talk about them and change the subject.*"

Antonia 1:   [looking down, talking slowly] I've had a really difficult week. I keep struggling to stay on track with the things that we were talking about last week. It all seems like so much. Even getting out of bed seems like too much.

Clinician 1:   It sounds like you've been having a really difficult time, that you're struggling to stay on track with what we talked about last week, even getting out of bed. (paraphrase)

Antonia 2:   [nods] Yeah. I don't want to get out of bed, but I have some important things to do. I have to decide whether to fire someone at work. I have to choose a new day care for the twins. Mostly, though, Joel has been manicky lately and I have to decide whether I can continue living with him. [pause] It's all too much.

Clinician 2:   It's all too much. [nods and looks up] And, yet, you *have* gone on and have even begun to make some very difficult decisions at work and with your family. [Yeah.] (encourager, **feedback**)

Getting on Track with Clients

In her second comment, Antonia felt at least partially understood, "Yeah. I don't want to get out of bed" (A 2). Still, she signals that she has not felt completely understood when she continues, "… but I have some important things to do," (i.e., "I cannot afford to stay in bed."). When clients are feeling ambivalent and hopeless, there's a danger of falling into a "yeah, but …" game. When either the client or clinician responds with a "but" (unless the clinician is paraphrasing the client's ambivalence), there is a disruption in understanding. In this case, Antonia's clinician would be premature to follow up with a more action-oriented intervention and should instead focus on listening.

Sometimes, however, the "but" is only expressed nonverbally, through hesitations or breaks in eye contact (Thomas, 2005). As in the next example (A 3), hesitations and breaks indicate a failure to reach agreement and should be interpreted as a signal to slow down (see Table 11.2).

Antonia 3:   Uh … [pause, eyes drop] You're right. I really shouldn't stay in bed. I have important things to do. [posture becomes more closed and turns slightly away]

Antonia's hesitations and changes in body language (e.g., break in eye contact and change in body posture) signal that she is not on board yet, despite language that superficially suggests agreement. Her use of the word "should" also signals a possible problem. In this case, she suggests that she believes she *ought* to agree rather than that she does.

Empathic understanding is developed when clinicians hear the **discrepancy** between where clients are and where they believe they should be (Slattery & Park, in press a). Clinicians must validate both poles of the client's dilemma and experience (e.g., how a client is failing to meet her goals, yet sees these as essential, or is symptomatic, but wants to change; Fraser & Solovey, 2007; Slattery & Park, in press a). Without the former, clients may not feel understood, but without the latter, clients may not feel hopeful enough to begin to change.

Clinician 4:   You think you *should* do "important things" [Uh huh], yet you don't want to get out of bed. [Uh huh] It sounds like you want to do these things, but you are very ambivalent about them. How can you solve problems when you don't know what you want to do? (paraphrase, open question)

Antonia 4:   Exactly. [making eye contact, posture relaxing somewhat] How can I solve these
things when I don't know what I want to do?

In her fourth response, Antonia indicated both verbally and nonverbally
that she believed her clinician understood the nature of her problem (the discrepancy that needs to be closed). She said, "Exactly," while making eye contact and relaxing, then paraphrased her clinician, demonstrating that she
accepted that they were on the same page.

Food for Thought

The consequence of failing to listen well, of imposing views on clients, was
seen in Ms. Schneider's reaction to criticisms of her drinking in the opening
case material. Using this strategy of listening and intervening only after the
client indicates feeling heard, reevaluate your initial attempt at helping her
change. Did you use this process? If not, try reworking your response.

*****

How would you respond to the Lee family (Chapters 5 and 10), addressing
both Lia's specialness, as seen in the Hmong view of her epilepsy, but also
her parents' concerns for her physical health? How does this match what
her caseworkers and doctors did when working with the family? If the Lees
said they were willing to use a treatment to stop her seizures, how would
you handle their unstated ambivalence—both a willingness to try something
different, but also the barriers that prevented them from consistently
following through with medical care in the past?

*****

What if you were working with the young Malcolm X (Chapter 6) in the
period after his father's murder, when he was just starting to act out? How
could you acknowledge the feelings that motivated his acting out, while
also seeing the positive qualities that characterized this flowering activist? If
he talked about changing and following the school's rules, how could you
address both the part of him that wants to change and the part that might
be unwilling to do so? Why might this be important?

Then, Introduce Change

*God grant me the
serenity to accept
the people I cannot
change, the courage
to change the one I
can, and the wisdom
to know it's me.*

— **Anonymous**

Even after clinicians have convinced clients that they understand them and
their dilemma, clinicians must continue to work to maintain that relationship
while also, depending on their clients' stage of change, helping them recognize
the problem, resolving their ambivalence about changing, or identifying
strategies for changing or staying on track (Prochaska, 1999; Prochaska &
DiClemente, 1982; Prochaska & Norcross, 2001). Simply telling someone
what to do might not be helpful in the long term, because premature **advice**
can interfere with the therapeutic relationship, suggest that the listener is

incompetent and has not already considered an issue, or create dependency. Active interventions and advice can be very effective, however, when the intervention or advice is appropriate and timely, the client is receptive to it, and when both parties are approximately equally active in the interview (Friedlander et al., 1985; Ivey & Ivey, 2003; Santrock, 2006). As Bohart (2001) concludes

> [T]he client, not the therapist, is the engine that drives the therapy. The therapist provides structure, tools, and a good working atmosphere.... Clients who are openly involved and willing to participate will be much more likely to change than clients who are not. Contrary to medications, interventions have no power in themselves. Any power they have comes from the client's investment of energy, ingenuity, curiosity, willingness to learn, and intelligent participation. If a client does not actively "inhabit" a procedure (rather than merely comply and do it), the procedure will have no life to make anything happen. (p. 237)

How do clinicians identify what is appropriate and timely and what the client will be receptive to? How do they get clients to become "the engine" driving treatment? In part, this depends on the client's stage of change and treatment goals, but also partially on the quality of the therapeutic alliance, although receptivity may change across sessions and within a single one. As a result, before intervening, clinicians should listen to their clients and look for signs that they are receptive to further interventions (Ivey & Ivey, 2003). See Antonia's fourth response from above and Table 11.2 for examples of these signs of receptivity.

When clients signal that they have been understood and are receptive to interventions for meeting a goal, clinicians can begin planning ways of helping them change. As described in Chapter 9, clinicians need a clear picture of the "problem" and factors maintaining it as well as the research and theory on how to address it. Nonetheless, interventions must be grounded in an empathic understanding of the person, but be different enough from their current understanding to motivate change (Fraser & Solovey, 2007) (see Figure 12.1). Like Goldilocks's experience with the Three Bears, reframes, **interpretations** and other interventions that are too similar to the client's current viewpoint provide insufficient justification for change, while those that are too discrepant will be rejected as failures of empathy. Further, effective interventions must also be plausible and believable to both the client and clinician. Finally, interventions should not support maladaptive thinking and actions, but should motivate more benign self-perceptions and adaptive change (C. L. Park, Edmondson, & Mills, in press; Slattery & Park, in press a). Pay attention to how each of these clinicians responds to Antonia and how these fit within this model.

Antonia 5: Joel's moods are up and down and I never know what I'm going to walk into next. I'm feeling pretty hopeless about things ever getting better.

Clinician A: It's pretty unlikely that you'll ever get out of this. (a weak paraphrase that accepts Antonia's perception of the problem; subtractive empathy)

Clinician B: Oh, things will be easy, just wait and see! (groundless feedback that rejects Antonia's perception of the problem; subtractive empathy)

Clinician C: You're feeling pretty hopeless right now [Yeah ...], feeling stuck [Uh huh], but I also notice that you're saying that you're *feeling* hopeless rather than that the situation *is* hopeless. [Yes] I wonder if your moodiness and difficulties getting out of bed are signs of

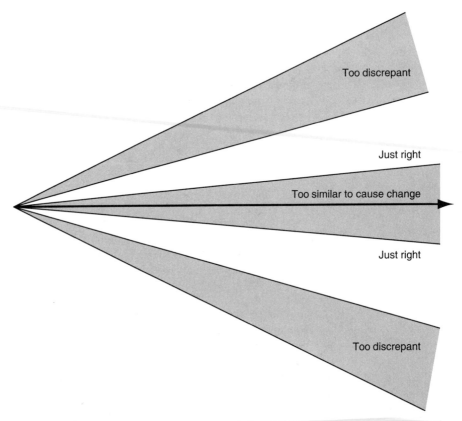

FIGURE **12.1** The Goldilocks view of interpretations: Interpretations can neither be too close nor too discrepant from the client's viewpoint (depicted as the bold line).

your deep ambivalence about very difficult jobs. You don't yet know what you can do to handle Joel better. (reflection of feeling, low-level interpretation; additive empathy)

Clinician A made a poor paraphrase that failed to catch Antonia's hesitancy—that she *feels* hopeless rather than that her situation *is* hopeless. Clinician B's glib response may be based on the clinician's own fears, anxiety, boredom, or restlessness, and is so far off the mark that Antonia is unlikely to feel heard. Notice that Clinician B's response could easily be framed as "yeah, but ..." (e.g., "Yes, but things will be easy, just wait and see!").

On the other hand, Clinician C empathizes with Antonia's feelings of hopelessness, while also noticing her hesitation. The additive empathy in this intervention can help Antonia feel listened to and, with some encouragement to explore her ambivalence further (e.g., "Could you tell me more about this?"), could develop her motivation for change. Finally, Clinician C framed the problem in a more hopeful way, that Antonia can find ways to "handle Joel better."

Timing is important to an intervention's effectiveness. If stated prematurely, the mild reframe in Clinician C's last sentence ("I wonder if your moodiness and difficulties getting out of bed are signs of your deep ambivalence about very

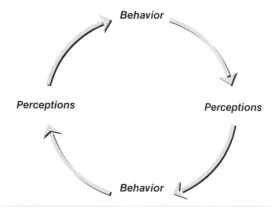

FIGURE **12.2** Reciprocal nature of changes in perceptions and behavior: Changing clients' perceptions changes their behavior, while changing their behavior changes their perspective on the problem.

difficult jobs...") will be rejected. However, when it was withheld until after Antonia accepted the reflection of feeling, Antonia was able to relax slightly, nod, and begin to consider other ways of seeing this problem.

Using the Goldilocks approach to developing interventions, interventions must be similar to a client's worldview, yet be different enough to introduce something that motivates change toward treatment goals. This intervention can offer a new way of seeing things (e.g., that Antonia's procrastination is her attempt to figure things out so that she can handle Joel better). It can be a different approach to an old problem, such as taking a breath before talking about a problem with a spouse. As seen in the following examples, changing clients' perceptions of themselves and the problem changes their behavior. Changing their behavior also changes the way they see the problem (see Figure 12.2).

- When Kerin begins to see her daughter as bright and curious rather than as having attention problems, instead of attempting to refocus her daughter, she may begin to support her daughter's curiosity. Her new assumptions change her behavior, which in turn changes the ways that she sees herself and her daughter. In addition, her daughter's behavior may also change in response to the new parenting style.
- Gib began by taking a breath before talking to his wife about problems and noticed that their discussions turned out better. This changed his view of their relationship (he was more hopeful), his wife (he saw her as more reasonable), and himself (he liked himself better when his reactions were more measured, reasonable, and empathic). With these changes in perspective and outcomes, he became more optimistic about their relationship and worked even harder to hear his wife's viewpoint.

Interventions should be underpinned by an empathic understanding that recognizes the person's potential and best motives, thus effective interventions are framed in an affirming, constructive, and hopeful manner rather than a cold, hostile, and rejecting one (May, 1967). Remembering exceptions to the problem and the client's strengths and positive intentions can make it easier to link empathy and interventions. Clinician C did this in two ways when responding to Antonia. First, Clinician C framed Antonia's "moodiness and difficulties getting out of bed" as "deep ambivalence," which might be an **ego-syntonic** self-perception that identifies a problem that they can work on (i.e., ambivalence). Second, Clinician C observed that Antonia doesn't "*yet* know what [she] can do to handle Joel better," implying that she will in the future. In addition, Antonia's use of "should" (in A 3) was reframed as "a want" by Clinician 4, thus as something she owned and desired (Ivey & Ivey, 2003). She accepted that frame of her problems in her next response, "How can I solve these things when I don't know what I *want* to do?"

STRATEGIES TO HELP CLIENTS CHANGE

We should remember that if a situation cannot be changed, there is no point in worrying about it. If it can be changed, then there is no need to worry about it either, we should simply go about changing it.
—**Dalai Lama (2009)**

As described earlier, changes in perceptions can lead to changes in behavior and vice versa, so dividing interventions between these two is arbitrary. Nonetheless, it can be useful to pay attention to how some styles of intervention lead to different ways of thinking, while others more directly address behavior, and still others focus specifically on emotions. Where and how to best intervene depends in part on the nature of the problem (C. L. Park, Folkman, & Bostrom, 2001; Prochaska & Norcross, 2001), but also clients' preferences based on individual or cultural expectations about change (Slattery, 2004).

Strategies for Changing Behaviors

As described in Chapter 8, many clients entering treatment have not yet identified a problem and committed to change. In fact, Prochaska and Norcross (2001) estimate that, depending on the population, only 10–20% of clients are in Action, another 30–40% are in Contemplation, and between 50 and 60% are in Precontemplation. Given this, they suggest that early in treatment clinicians should assess clients' stage of change and be cautious about assuming that all clients are ready to take action on the primary identified problem (e.g., quitting drinking).

Clinicians can move beyond dichotomous ways of thinking about change (e.g., drinking or not drinking) to thinking about change as a process, with many smaller steps on the way. With clients in Precontemplation, clinicians can empathize, accept, and validate clients' experience, gradually helping them to perceive the negative consequences of their behavior (Goldfried, 2007). Clinicians' ability to be patient and accepting when clients fail to move rapidly can be very helpful, especially when this patience is balanced by gentle encouragement. In fact, clinicians' frustration can interfere with treatment and may even lead to clients' deterioration.

Clients in Contemplation can be encouraged to explore the costs and benefits of changing, as well as to address barriers to change (Prochaska & Norcross, 2001). Even when clients may not be ready to take action on the primary identified problem, they may be ready to take smaller behavioral steps that prepare them for more challenging interventions, including identifying the situations in which they consider drinking, monitoring their stress levels, developing a more positive support system, and using positive coping strategies (G. K. Brown et al., 2006; Linehan, 1993). Identifying barriers to treatment and making small, positive steps towards the goal, rather than being insignificant, may be essential to treatment, in that doing so increases clients' hopefulness and significantly increases their probability of change on the primary identified problem (Prochaska & Norcross, 2001).

Effective treatment begins by performing a triage, addressing the most pressing issues first. For example, although it may be important to help people who are suicidal develop stronger coping mechanisms, it may be more important to first stabilize them by using more external supports like emergency services, then later to help them develop coping skills and natural supports to use during a crisis (G. K. Brown et al., 2006). These barriers can occur at all levels: environmental barriers, family and culture role expectations, and psychological issues stemming from the immediate stressor and from earlier history of abuse (Grigsby & Hartman, 1997). Grigsby and Hartman suggest that clinicians intervene first with the most external of these layers (environmental), as more "internal" interventions can feel blaming, especially when introduced prematurely.

As described previously, when clinicians are **solution-focused** and use **strength-based** approaches and interventions, they can help clients access the strengths and skills they already have to respond to the problems they are facing (Berg, 1994; O'Hanlon & Weiner-Davis, 1989). Clinicians can identify the positive intention behind the problem behavior (e.g., that "nagging" reflects the client's "caring" for the other person's needs). They can recognize the client's strengths and resources in other realms, which can be readily transferred to the problem realm. They can listen for exceptions to the problem and the times when their clients are already handling the problem successfully. They can notice evidence of change across sessions, even changes that might otherwise appear insignificant.

Antonia 6:   Joel's moods continue to be up and down. Today I just walked away from him when he got angry.

Clinician 5:   Hmm, that's interesting. [Huh?] One month ago, when he got angry, you got angry and in his face. What are you doing differently?

Antonia 7:   I hadn't thought about it in that way, but you're right. It *is* different. [pause] I've been meditating, like we've talked about, and so when he got angry, I was calmer and didn't take what he said so personally. I knew that I had to leave the room, though, as I still don't feel strong enough to handle his anger.

In recognizing and commenting on this change, Antonia was able to identify the skills and strengths that she has been developing. Her clinician could have identified these changes for her. However, because a general goal of treatment is to empower clients so they are able to continue the change process following termination from treatment, it is most helpful, when possible, to have clients take ownership for treatment and identify their own changes and what they are doing to make them (Curtis, 2002; Epston & White, 1995; Goldfried, 2002; L. S. Greenberg, 2002; Wachtel, 2002). In addition, note how Antonia's meditation practice affects the nature of her interactions with Joel and that this causes her to perceive herself differently.

Specific Areas to Attend to

In most cases, an important part of treatment includes helping clients develop good coping and problem-solving skills. Across time, clients should begin to recognize the ways that negative coping is both ineffective and makes problems worse (Aldwin, 2007). Clients should explore ways in which their coping strategies such as self-medicating; self-injuring; and engaging in minimization, denial, or rationalization are less adaptive, and begin to substitute more adaptive coping mechanisms. Clients can also explore more adaptive coping skills, including solving controllable problems using planful action and attempting to understand and accept problems outside their control. Clients with weak social networks can develop stronger ones and thus gain empathy, advice, and tangible support, and work through difficult or confusing feelings (Aldwin, 2007).

For example, people who are depressed are less likely to engage in basic health-promoting practices (e.g., Gonzalez et al., 2009; G. C. Jones, Rovner, Crews, & Danielson, 2009); therefore, paying attention to basic health care practices can be an important aspect of treatment. Creating a healthier lifestyle may include eating well, getting enough rest, exercising regularly, maintaining a healthy weight, using alcohol moderately or not at all, learning how to relax, pursuing hobbies and leisure activities, and taking vacations. Furthermore, a regular spiritual practice may be an important part of creating and maintaining a healthy mind and body.

In addition, people who are depressed often have both acute and more chronic social skill deficits (Petty, Sachs-Ericsson, & Joiner, 2004). People who are depressed and have a history of panic disorder are more likely to relapse when they are low in assertiveness (Ball, Otto, Pollack, & Rosenbaum, 1994). People with critical, blaming, and judgmental family members are at greater risk of relapse (Hinrichsen & Pollack, 1997; Hooley & Hiller, 2000; Hooley & Teasdale, 1989; O'Farrell et al., 1998). Addressing these and other skill deficits in both clients and their family members can be an important aspect of treatment and decrease the risk of relapse after termination from treatment.

Strategies for Changing Beliefs

Depression is the inability to construct a future.
—**Rollo May**

As described in Chapter 3, a person's beliefs, values and goals influence a wide variety of behaviors throughout the day, thus intervening at the level of worldview can have significant and wide-ranging ramifications throughout a person's life. When the underlying thoughts and perceptions are realistic and useful, emotional responses and behaviors will be more adaptive, whereas when perceptions and thoughts are maladaptive, emotional responses and behaviors will be more dysfunctional (Pretzer & Walsh, 2001).

Challenging Beliefs and Developing New Meanings

Most people face very difficult issues in life—rejecting parents, lost jobs, chronic illness, divorce, trauma, abuse, and death. They often treat the meanings they draw in response to these events as truisms rather than possible responses among many others (Gray et al., 2007). Although their interpretations seem designed to protect them, they often do so at an unacceptable cost: New meanings attached to events can often be too extreme and overgeneralized. Healthy strategies for creating adaptive meanings take a middle ground, noting the self-protective nature of the meaning, but making it more moderate and adaptive (e.g., recognizing when one is unsafe, but also identifying how one can stay safer).

For example, Drew was recently assaulted and raped at a party. He has been feeling increasingly paranoid and unsafe, sees the world as unpredictable and out of control, and expects to be hurt. A variety of different types of interventions can challenge his problematic beliefs and assumptions.

Drew 1: I never feel safe. I can't go anywhere or do anything without looking over my shoulder and wondering who is going to hurt me next.

Clinician A: You feel like you're never safe, that someone is going to hurt you. [Yeah.] "Never." [pause] That word seems awfully extreme to me. You, too? [pause] Are there times when you feel safer or less safe? (reflection of feeling, **self-disclosure**, closed questions)

Clinician B: It sounds like you feel small and helpless since the attack because you're afraid that someone will hurt you again. [Yeah.] It takes a lot of *courage* to keep trying even when you're afraid, to come here every week. (reflection of feeling, reframe)

Clinician C: You're feeling unsafe [uh huh], maybe even a little bit crazy. [Yeah.] Most people feel that way in the weeks following an attack—they feel like they're always looking over their shoulder. That's not crazy; it's a way of feeling safe again. (reflection of feeling, normalization, reframe)

Clinician D: You're feeling unsafe. [Yes.] Take a minute and close your eyes and breathe more slowly, like we've been practicing. [long pause] OK, how are you feeling now? [Calmer. More in control] Ah! You *felt* unsafe and out of control [uh huh], but you still have ways of regaining safety and control. (reflection of feeling, directive, open question, feedback)

Drew began with an extreme statement that was unlikely to match real experience (i.e., that he is *never* safe). Each clinician responded to his statement with a reflection of feeling, but then attacked his assumption in a different way. Clinician A addressed his extreme thinking, which is often indicated by language such as "always," "never," "none," "terrible," and "awful," and suggested more moderate and realistic language and thinking. It is not realistic to suggest that Drew will always be safe, especially since he has already been assaulted and raped, but it is realistic to believe that there will be times when he will feel safer. If Drew was unable to identify safer times, assuming that the therapeutic alliance is strong, his clinician could bring the discussion back into the here and now (e.g., "How do you feel right now?").

Clinician B addressed Drew's underlying assumption of personal weakness by presenting a reframe of the "problematic" behavior (i.e., "It takes a lot of *courage*..."). Drew assumed that his fears and anxiety were all-encompassing; his clinician suggested that they were part of his experience, but that he was also courageous. B might further suggest that it would be foolhardy *not* to be afraid. Reframes can be powerful interventions, but they should not be used to dismiss a client's feelings in a "yeah, but..." fashion. They should start with a validation of the client's feelings, with the reframe introduced only after the client feels understood.

Clinician C normalized Drew's reactions as part of a common process experienced by victims of an attack, then used a reframe where he suggested this common response is also a healthy one (i.e., "it's a way of feeling safe again"). Like Clinician B, C could suggest that it would be foolhardy *not* to be afraid after being raped and assaulted. Like Clinician A, Clinician C could ask whether Drew is *always* looking over his shoulder or whether there are times when he feels safer. The techniques of **normalizations** and **information giving** can be powerful ways to attack the client's self-perceptions of being crazy: "This is a normal reaction. Let's find a healthier way of responding to this, though."

Clinician D did something somewhat different than the other clinicians did by using a directive (i.e., "Take a minute and close your eyes and breathe more slowly..."). Rather than only thinking about when he feels safe or unsafe, Drew explored his experience in the here and now by trying things to regain his sense of safety and control. D could continue this exploration by having Drew practice his breathing in other settings and noticing how he felt afterwards. D could also encourage Drew to examine his behavior at other points to identify other behaviors that would challenge his belief that he was unsafe and out of control. Notice how this intervention also brings Drew's experience into the here and now and provides a new and corrective type of experience.

Treatment is an opportunity to reduce the size of discrepancies between life events and worldview, develop a coherent and positive life narrative, and make sense of life and experience in a hopeful and useful way (Neimeyer & Stewart, 2000; Slattery & Park, in press a). Notice how each clinician helped Drew to do this. In some instances, it may be also be adaptive to readjust goals; for example, clients may need to accept more realistic health and exercise goals when aging (Cheng, 2004).

Searching for new and more adaptive meanings is especially important when the problem cannot be repaired, such as after illness, loss, or trauma (Mattlin, Wethington, & Kessler, 1990). Asking clients to reframe their experience and identify some positive consequence or meaning is something that should only be done, however, after clients feel deeply heard and understood (Ivey & Ivey, 2003). If reframes are made prematurely, most people feel that their feelings have been dismissed.

Clinician 1: It sounds like you feel like you'll never be safe, that someone is going to hurt you. [Yeah.] That you and your world have been irretrievably damaged. (reflection of feeling, reflection of meaning)

Drew 2: [pause] Yeah. I often feel shattered.

Clinician 2: You often feel shattered. [Yeah.] No one would ever wish that something so terrible would happen to you or anyone else, but some people do find good things come from bad ones. I'm wondering what your experience has been. What positive things, even something small, have you seen come from this? (reflection of feeling, information giving, self-disclosure, open question to begin a search for a client-initiated reframe)

Drew 3: I usually think about the bad things, [pause] but you're right. Now I know who my real friends are. [pause] I know if I can get through this I can get through anything. [pause] My life was shattered, but I am also starting to think about what's really important in ways that I hadn't done before....

Helping clients find meaning and a more balanced perspective following a painful or negative situation can be really profound work, but clinicians need to be very careful not to negate the client's experience and suffering. By offering clients opportunities to begin thinking about potential positive outcomes as well as the more negative ones that they have focused on (e.g., stronger coping, better relationships, and deeper spirituality), they can begin to move beyond cycles of negativity. This strategy is most useful for events and circumstances that occurred in the past and that are not amenable to change or control. Being sensitive to issues of timing with this intervention is important. In addition, the clinician's focus on this discrepancy (e.g., both the loss and possible growth and advantages) should be only minimally ahead of the client's own awareness and readiness for recognizing positives resulting from the loss or trauma.

Developing More Adaptive Views of Themselves and Their Future

An ultimate goal of treatment is to leave clients with a sense of self that is more benign and hopeful. Rather than accepting all of the credit for changes made during treatment, they encourage clients to perceive their work as collaborative in nature, develop a stronger sense of self-efficacy, and own the changes they made in treatment (Curtis, 2002; Epston & White, 1995; Goldfried, 2002; L. S. Greenberg, 2002; Wachtel, 2002).

There are many different ways that clinicians can help clients reenvision themselves and their lives. In fact, they should look for opportunities to do so at all points in their clinical work and while working on other types of treatment goals. These four clinicians approached this same goal in different ways.

Clinician A: This was difficult work today, but you approached it openly and courageously. (feedback)

Clinician B: That's a good question. How do *you* see yourself doing at this point? (feedback, open question)

Clinician C: You've focused on the ways that you are "broken," but I also hear you describe the ways that you are using your anger in healthy and adaptive ways. (paraphrase, feedback)

Clinician D: I'm wondering what was most important for you today. What do you want to take from today's session and use throughout this next week? (self-disclosure, open question)

When identifying strengths and giving positive **feedback**, clinicians should be concrete and specific. They should be genuine and, rather than whitewashing problems, notice the healthy intention and adaptive nature of the client's behavior. They should not dismiss problems or play Pollyanna, but recognize, identify, and enlarge successes and exceptions to the presenting problem (Berg, 1994; de Shazer, 1988; O'Hanlon & Weiner-Davis, 1989).

Throughout treatment clinicians should listen to their clients' descriptions of people who have been supportive of them in either the past or present (e.g., parents, grandparents, a favorite teacher, neighbor, or pets). These supports can be accessed physically if they are still alive and available, but they can also be "accessed" through positive memories or images (e.g., "When your pain is at a 6 or 7 on a scale from 1 to 10, I want you to imagine your grandmother's warm hand on your shoulder and listen to whatever words of wisdom she might offer you."). Clinicians can supplement these natural supports with stories about contemporary or historical figures who are especially important to the client, including sports, religious, or cultural figures (Slattery, 2004).

Reducing Rumination and Avoidance

Following a loss or trauma, people often ruminate obsessively; they also experience more negative emotions and fewer positive emotions. When ruminating, they have lower levels of psychological well-being, report less life satisfaction, and are more likely to report feelings of anger, anxiety, and depression (Briñol, Petty, & Wheeler, 2006; Hardin, Weigold, Robitschek, & Nixon, 2007; Wade, Vogel, Liao, & Goldman, 2008). The tendency to ruminate may be either a temporary state or a style of approaching the world—some people tend to ruminate about a wide variety of situations—but it is related to perfectionism and difficulty forgiving (Wade et al., 2008).

Ruminations and **intrusive thoughts** may be attempts to reduce perceived discrepancies, for example, between a person's actual behavior and values (Briñol et al., 2006; Dalgleish & Power, 2004; Gray et al., 2007). Ruminations can be adaptive when they help a person resolve the discrepancy, but they are maladaptive when they do nothing to help solve the problem (Nolen-Hoeksema, Wisco, & Lyubomirsky, 2008). In fact, rumination typically interferes with problem solving.

Negative cycles of rumination, intrusive thoughts, and avoidance can be stopped in one of several ways. **Distraction** can be useful in the short-term, as it leads to greater amounts of positive affect, which can help people calm and, eventually, problem solve (Nolen-Hoeksema et al., 2008). When distraction leads to long-term avoidance, however, outcomes are more negative. Counterintuitively, **mindfulness** can also be helpful for people who obsessively ruminate. In mindfulness work, clients are encouraged to observe their thoughts, feelings, and sensations without judging them or becoming stuck in them. Becoming more mindful can increase hopefulness and self-efficacy as clients stop avoiding painful emotions and learn that they can control their thoughts. **Cognitive restructuring** can help clients challenge the validity of their maladaptive thoughts rather than accepting them as accurate. Finally, as described above, rumination often interferes with problem solving. Helping clients to problem solve and take appropriate action can sometimes reduce rumination (Nolen-Hoeksema et al., 2008).

Food for Thought

Consider Ms. Schneider's drinking. In what ways do her beliefs about herself, her relationships with others, and alcohol, maintain her drinking and prevent her from changing? If both she and her doctor identified her drinking as a problem and she was ready to begin working on it, how would you

(continues)

address the beliefs that serve as barriers to change? What if she is not seeing her drinking as a problem?

*****

Return to the story Dr. Corsini told about the impact of his feedback following an intelligence test (Chapter 6). How do you understand that story given the ideas raised in this chapter?

Bad Luck Followed Us From Place to Place
John Bul Dau

John Dau (b. 1974) lived in the south of the Sudan in the middle of a civil war. He was forced to flee his village in 1987 and walked with thousands of other Lost Boys to Ethiopia. When forced to leave there, he walked to the refugee camp in Kakuma, Kenya. He lived there for 10 years before being relocated to Syracuse, New York in August of 2001. In Syracuse he contacted aid agencies active in eastern Africa, searching for family members who were still in Sudan and Uganda, worked two to three jobs in order to raise money to send to his family, and saved enough money to bring his mother and sister to the United States. He founded the American Care for Sudan Foundation, which raises funds for the Duk Lost Boys Clinic in Sudan.

Mr. Dau's story is one of hope, guilt, and survival. He is unlikely to feel understood without understanding each pole of his story.

> I have witnessed my share of death and despair. I have seen the hyenas come at dusk to feed on the bodies of my friends. I have been so hungry and thirsty in the dusty plains of Africa that I consumed things I would rather forget. I have crossed a crocodile-infested river while being shelled and shot at. I have walked until I thought I could walk no more. I have wondered, more times than I can count, if my friends or I would live to see a new day. Those were the times I thought God had grown tired of us. (Dau & Sweeney, 2007, p. 7)

He continued,

> Some of the Lost Boys whom I knew in New York State blamed themselves for the [2001 terrorist] attacks, as if bad luck followed us from place to place. They reasoned that they had lived quietly in their villages in southern Sudan, only to have their homes attacked. They had fled to Ethiopia and lived peacefully, only to be attacked. Now they had come halfway around the world to find a better life than the one they left behind, only to have their new home attacked again. They thought the unluckiness of the Dinka had cursed America for taking them in. (Dau & Sweeney, 2007, p. 200)

His cultural and religious beliefs helped him. He recognized that bad things could happen, even to good people.

> Job [from the Old Testament] never did anything wrong, and he loved God. Yet Job lost his family and his property, and he almost died. Job realized that just

(continues)

(continued)

loving God did not mean that God would do good things in return. (Dau & Sweeney, 2007, p. 201).

I remembered my mother telling me when I was a young boy in Duk Payuel that everything in life goes around and comes around again. When times are very good, she said, remember that hardship always returns. When times are very bad, remember God will send you joy again, and so be patient. (Dau & Sweeney, 2007, p. 218)

- What is Mr. Dau's worldview?
- What contradictory messages and themes does he present?
- If you were seeing Mr. Dau in therapy, how would you paraphrase these contradictory messages and themes? Thinking about this in terms of Carkhuff's (1969) model assessing empathy accuracy, how accurate was your empathy? How would you know?
- How would you help Mr. Dau address his feelings of loss and guilt? Why? How would the ideas outlined in Table 12.2 inform your interventions?
- How was your response for him different than it might have been for someone else? Why?

Strategies for Changing Feelings

As previously discussed, people's perceptions influence their actions and their actions in turn influence their perceptions of themselves and the world. This description, while useful, overlooks the role of emotions. Emotions strongly influence how people behave, set into play ways of thinking about events, and are in turn influenced by behavior and thinking. Each of these three influences how people make meaning of their experience (L. Greenberg, 2008; Ivey & Ivey, 2003).

Many people avoid negative emotions and feel overwhelmed by them. Negative emotions can be disruptive to functioning and have been described as resulting from maladaptive and catastrophizing ways of interacting with the world. From this point of view, the cognitive style causing negative emotions need to be controlled or tempered (Beck, 1976).

Avoidance of emotions, even negative ones, is itself problematic, just as avoiding negative thoughts can be (L. Greenberg, 2008). Emotions are a normal and healthy part of experience, signaling an event's importance. When working with emotions, it is important to attend to the degree to which emotions are maladaptively expressed, regulated, or controlled. Even when clients are stressed, anxious, or depressed, clinicians consider whether these emotions are primarily signs of distress as opposed to normal reactions to working through difficult issues. They should also pay attention to when emotions are used for instrumental purposes like getting attention or diverting blame, and when they are used to avoid a deeper feeling (L. Greenberg, 2008; L. S. Greenberg & Safran, 1987). For example, anger may mask feelings of shame and loneliness after losing a relationship.

TABLE **12.2**
Cultural Factors, Coping Strategies, and Predictors of Resilience among Refugees from Sudan.

Cultural factors

1. Early experiences in normal separation (caring for cattle) and development of supportive peer communities.
2. Adults believe they are responsible for all children in community: "any child is everybody's child." (p. 208)
3. Low internal control, which allows them to cope with and accept loss: "When things want to happen you will not change them." (p. 209)
4. Respect for elders and their advice: "They saw the sun first." (p. 210)

Coping strategies and predictors of resilience

Feel parental guidance (through memories)

• "Although my parents were not physically present and I did not know if my parents were alive or dead, there was that connection—...the culture they had passed on to me and the advice they have given me when I was still at home." (p. 209)
• "I will find my parents one day, and if they find you as a person they don't like, that would not be good." (p. 209)

Develop supportive and guiding relationships with available caregivers

• "When I was crying, they would come and talk to me.... They would give me advice, so that it would calm me down, until I stop crying and forget about what was making me cry." (p. 208)

Have supportive peers who normalize their experience and help them

• "What helped me most was my friends." (p. 207)
• "I knew that I was not the only one in this situation." (p. 207)
• "When I am mad and don't want to talk to anyone... they come to me and ask me if I am ok. They try to involve you, even if you don't want to talk, they try to involve you in conversation." (p. 208)

Use healthy avoidance and acceptance, are optimistic

• Rather than succumbing to negative thoughts and depression: "make my heart strong" (p. 206)
• "So we need you to forget it for a second. We know it will be in your heart, but just focus on your life, what you are doing right now to manage it. If you think about it a lot, you will die." (p. 208)
• "And I said that if this is how life wants to be, then there is nothing I can do about it." (p. 207)
• "You have to think forward; don't think backward." (p. 207)
• "It is war, people get separated, those things happen. And God will help you, and one day you are going to find your parents." (p. 208)

Use religion to find meaning

• "I cannot say that I was the one taking care of myself. There was Someone taking care of me. And if there was no God, I would not be here today." (p. 207)
• "Every Sunday I would go to church, and I would hear the Bible. And somehow the Bible became like someone who is advising me in my life." (p. 207)
• "What made them not to die at that time? God not make their day to come. Maybe God has a purpose for them to do." (p. 207)

Note: From Luster, Qin, Bates, Johnson, and Rana (2009)

Leslie Greenberg (2008) concluded that clinicians have five emotion-focused tasks to work on with their clients: (a) becoming more aware and accepting of emotions, (b) expressing emotions more adaptively, (c) better regulating emotions, (d) reflecting on emotions and the events associated with them, and

(e) transforming negative emotions through their association with positive emotions. As many people avoid negative emotions and criticize both the emotions and themselves for having these emotions, an accepting, nonjudgmental experiencing in a supportive and empathic environment can be very helpful in reducing avoidance and increasing adaptive emotional regulation (L. Greenberg, 2008; Leahy, 2002; Linehan, 1993). Mindfulness, leading to an accepting and nonjudgmental attitude, and **meditation**, which strengthens skills in tolerating and regulating emotions, can be especially useful for people with depression or other poorly regulated emotions (Linehan, 1993; Teasdale et al., 2000).

Food for Thought

Reread the clinicians' responses to Antonia and Drew, paying attention to your own reactions and feelings while reading them. What do your reactions suggest about Antonia and Drew, their clinicians' responses, and you? Consider talking to someone else and comparing your reactions to those of that person.

IDENTIFYING AND ADDRESSING BARRIERS TO CHANGE

Teachers open the door but you must walk through it yourself.

—Chinese proverb

Strong clinicians anticipate that their clients will have some ambivalence about change and will investigate **barriers** even for people who appear ready to change (Fraser & Solovey, 2007). These barriers can be institutional, financial, environmental, cultural, relational, or intrapsychic (Grigsby & Hartman, 1997). Clients may not see treatment goals and methods as relevant, may feel alienated from the agencies providing treatment, or may believe that clinicians perceive them pejoratively and as unable to change (Caldwell, 2009; R. E. Lee, 2009). They may not have a reliable car, money for gas, or dependable childcare. They may perceive having problems as itself a problem or feel that asking for help and talking about problems is an indication of weakness. Clients and their partners, families, and friends may actively resist change, because it may destabilize the relationship, or they may even perceive the problem (e.g., corporal punishment, domestic violence, binge drinking) as normative and acceptable. They may feel hopeless, ambivalent about change, or unable to change. They may not have the skills to change or may not believe that they deserve good relationships, positive outcomes, or a hopeful future. Identifying and discussing possible barriers and reasons not to change can make treatment smoother and setbacks easier to anticipate and respond to.

A client's resistance to change can be seen in missed sessions, lateness to sessions, avoidance of topics, and refusal to discuss issues in depth. Clients can be passive or have a low level of motivation to change. Clinicians can respond to these challenging behaviors by becoming irritated, loud, or belligerent. Nonetheless, confrontational and conflict-laden responses further increase resistance and interfere with treatment, while supportive and empathic responses are more helpful (Beutler et al., 2001; Moos, 2003; Serran et al., 2003; Strupp, 1996).

Although the client may truly be resistant to the intervention *as framed*, Serran and colleagues (2003) suggest that clinicians should perceive the "resistant behavior" as a signal to change goals, strategies, or approaches. Rather than becoming irritated, angry or frustrated or, worse, becoming belligerent or combative with a client, it is generally more effective to listen and supportively but firmly challenge clients. Clinicians should remain calm and empathic when challenging clients about discrepancies between, for example, what clients say and what they do (Serran et al., 2003). They might say, "You say that you want to be a better parent, but you haven't done your homework in the last four sessions. I wonder what that's about?" When clients are very resistant with regard to a topic, clinicians can step back and work with clients on a less challenging issue until the therapeutic alliance is stronger and resistance is lower (Beutler et al., 2001; Serran et al., 2003). Treatment is not done *to* clients, but *with* them (Bohart, 2001).

Although it is tempting to focus on a client's symptoms, problems, and weaknesses as well as the barriers to treatment, it is equally important to recognize exceptions to problems and nurture a client's strengths (Berg, 1994; O'Hanlon & Weiner-Davis, 1989). In fact, even a client's "resistance" can be adaptive and may suggest that the client does not have the necessary skills, has significant reasons not to change, or is not confident enough in the clinician and change process (Beutler et al., 2001).

Food for Thought

What barriers made it difficult for Lil Loco (a.k.a. Reymundo Sanchez, Chapter 3) to change? What might make it difficult for John Bul Dau (this chapter) to work toward individual goals in counseling? What made it difficult for Andrea Yates (Chapter 2) or Ruthie Schlimgen (Chapter 9) to stay on their medications? What would you do to address these barriers? What are the adaptive parts of their resistance to change?

EVALUATING TREATMENT

You seldom listen to me, and when you do you don't hear, and when you do hear you hear wrong, and even when you hear right you change it so fast that it's never the same.

—Marjorie Kellogg

As described in Chapter 11, rating the empathy of clinicians' responses can be useful in determining whether the clinician is accurately hearing the client's surface and deeper meanings (Carkhuff, 1969). However, for any of a number of reasons, either psychological or environmental (or both), a client may miss the clinician's otherwise brilliantly framed empathic response or intervention.

Therefore, although it is helpful to think about the accuracy of the clinician's responses, it may be even more useful to consider the effectiveness of a session from the *client's* point of view. To what degree is the client accepting of or denying the reframe or intervention (Ivey & Ivey, 2003)? The rating system in Table 12.3, based in part on L. Seligman's description (2004), can be useful in this regard. To what degree do the clinician's responses and interventions lead to greater or lesser insight and behavioral change and advance

TABLE **12.3**
Rating the Effectiveness of a Session or Intervention

5	Listening is accurate and insightful. Moves treatment in a productive direction. Promotes greater self-awareness, helpful ways of thinking about the "problem," or positive changes in behavior.
4	Listening is generally accurate. Moves treatment in a productive direction, but leads to limited self-awareness, helpful ways of thinking about the "problem," or positive changes in behavior.
3	Neither contributes to nor detracts from treatment goals, therapeutic process, and therapeutic alliance. Client accepts the reframe, although it does not lead to change.
2	Detracts somewhat from treatment goals, therapeutic process, and therapeutic alliance. Clinician's responses suggest poor listening or lack of interest. Client may hear and accept part of the message, but not other parts.
1	Damaging to movement on treatment goals and interferes with the therapeutic process and therapeutic alliance. Clinician's responses sound blaming, judgmental, and critical. Client may deny or reject the intervention.

Note: Adapted from Carkhuff (1969), Ivey & Ivey (2003), L. Seligman (2004)

treatment goals? To what degree do they either strengthen or weaken the therapeutic alliance? These questions can be asked both at the end of a session and throughout it. As discussed in earlier parts of this book, paying attention to clients' nonverbal cues, the ways they develop themes in treatment (or fail to), and verbal indicators of disagreement can signal whether the therapeutic alliance is strong and whether the client is accepting of the clinician's interventions (Thomas, 2005).

Food for Thought

Review transcripts of interviews from earlier parts of the book (Andrea Yates, Chapters 1 and 11; Claire, Chapter 7; Annie Rogers, Chapter 11; Robin, Chapter 11). How would you rate their responses in terms of empathy (Carkhuff, 1969)? How would you rate these short transcripts in terms of their productivity using the scale in Table 12.3? What did you conclude from this process?

SUMMARY

Regardless of the particular treatment goals that clients and clinicians negotiate, effective clinicians want their clients to continue to be successful after termination from treatment, and they help develop their clients' self-efficacy, assertiveness, hope, and problem-solving skills. Because many clients are initially unready to change, paying attention to their readiness is an important aspect of treatment. Motivating clients to change depends on a strong therapeutic alliance, characterized by unconditional acceptance and empathic, genuine, and nonjudgmental attitudes.

Before clinicians ask clients to change, particularly those who are more highly resistant, clients need to feel understood and accepted. Clients who feel understood are generally more receptive to clinical interventions. In general, these interventions should require a shift in perspective, although not one that is so large as to be unacceptable.

Changes in behavior often lead to changes in perspective and vice versa. Further, emotions influence actions and ways of thinking about issues, and along with thinking, influence how people make meaning of their experience. This chapter described a number of strategies to create clinical change in the behavioral, cognitive, and emotional realms.

Effective treatment recognizes and addresses barriers to changes. These occur at the institutional, financial, environmental, cultural, relational, or intrapsychic levels and may manifest in passivity, low motivation for change, or resistance. As treatment is done with clients rather than to them, it is important to work on the therapeutic alliance at stuck points and to consider the ways that this "resistance" is adaptive.

Rather than paying attention to the quality of the intervention alone, effective clinicians evaluate the effectiveness of their work, especially how it strengthens the therapeutic alliance, causes clients to become more insightful, and leads to positive behavioral change.

How Do These Issues Apply to Your Life and Work?

1. What happens when you do not believe that your viewpoint was heard before someone asks you to change? How do you feel about and react in this situation?
2. In what ways have you noticed that changing your behavior in some way (e.g., quitting smoking, getting a new job) also changed the way that you perceived yourself and others differently? In what ways have you noticed that changing your thinking and perceptions (e.g., understanding someone), also changed your behavior?
3. If you have been "resistant" to change at some point, consider the adaptive nature of this resistance. What were you trying to accomplish?
4. Pay attention to your own clinical work using the scale in Table 12.3. How do you respond when you recognize that you are off track (lower on the scale)? To what degree is this sort of response helpful?

CHAPTER 13

Ending Treatment Well

WHERE ARE WE GOING?

1. What differentiates normal from premature terminations?

2. How can clinicians assess risk of ethical or legal complaint?

3. What strategies can clinicians use to decrease risk during termination from treatment?

4. What goals do clinicians generally hold for the termination process?

5. What feelings do clients and clinicians frequently report at termination? How might these affect the termination process?

6. What characterizes good terminations from treatment?

7. What factors should be addressed in the course of planning discharge from treatment?

I Felt Like I'd Been Beaten Up
Elyn Saks

Elyn Saks, an attorney who graduated from Yale University, specializes in mental health law, and a dean at the University of Southern California, had her first psychotic break when she was doing graduate work at Oxford University. She had three extended hospitalizations and has been in psychoanalysis and on antipsychotics for much of her adult life. She did analytic work with Dr. Kaplan for 13 years, although eventually became unhappy with how it was going.

> I'd accomplished many successful life changes during that time. But he'd often been hard on me, and over time (Kaplan's many strengths and his humanity as an analyst notwithstanding) it had come to feel too hard, even punishing. He'd become more restrictive somehow—for example, he didn't want me moving around the office; he didn't want me to cover my face with my hands during our sessions, something I'd done with all my analysts to help me feel safe and contained. He kept saying that if things didn't change, he'd "terminate" me. "I'm going to terminate you." It was brutal to hear that, brutal for him to keep saying it. Was he doing it to elicit some kind of response from me? I didn't feel safe with him anymore; he was unpredictable, mercurial, even angry. Some days, I'd walk out of session feeling like I'd been beaten up.
> "We're not getting anywhere," he'd say. "This isn't even therapy we're doing." It had been going badly for two years, he said—since around my diagnosis with cancer and my engagement to Will. (Saks, 2007, pp. 331–322)

She asked for a consult with Dr. Freed, an analyst who had provided backup during Dr. Kaplan's vacations.

"You've done years of good work with him, Elyn," Freed said. "Relationships go through transitions; perhaps this is one. You really should try to work it out with Kaplan. It's vital that you do" (Saks, 2007, p. 322). Per his suggestion, she reconsidered her decision to quit working with Dr. Kaplan, although "I wasn't sure I could; I wasn't sure I wanted to even try" (p. 322).

> I went to my office to draw up a plan, some kind of negotiation. What had to change, I wondered, in order for me to stay with Kaplan? I made a list: I needed him to stop saying we weren't getting anywhere. I needed him to stop threatening "termination." I needed a lessening of the physical restrictions. None of these seemed onerous....
> Kaplan flat-out refused to change a thing.
> I was stunned. (Saks, 2007, p. 323)

That was their last session together, although Dr. Kaplan later called Ms. Saks in order to work things out. Ms. Saks began seeing Dr. Freed, but observed

> Dr. Kaplan probably helped me more than anyone else in my life, and I love him today as much as I have ever loved anyone. For a long time, I carried inside me

(continues)

(continued)

a palpable sense of loss. The decision to leave him was so awful, but I couldn't see any way around it; besides, it always felt like he'd made that decision first. By refusing to negotiate with me, by threatening me and pushing me, he had in fact fired me. He'd rejected me, he'd betrayed me. (Saks, 2007, p. 324)

- What did you think about Ms. Saks's requests and Dr. Kaplan's reaction? What, if anything, would you do differently if you were in his shoes? Why?
- How might Ms. Saks's worldview have influenced her decision to end her work with Dr. Kaplan?
- Were you surprised that Ms. Saks felt so many positive feelings about Dr. Kaplan given her decision to leave analysis with him?

NORMAL AND PREMATURE TERMINATIONS

Death ends a life, not a relationship.

—Robert Benchley

Treatment can end in any of a number of different ways: when both clinician and client agree that goals have been met; when a clinician makes a unilateral decision to end treatment because progress is not being made or the client is being actively harmed by treatment, due to unavoidable clinician-related factors (e.g., illness, maternity leave, moves, job changes, or personal difficulties impacting competency); or when a managed care company denies payment (Bennett et al., 2006; Younggren & Gottlieb, 2008). Clinicians may end treatment due to a potentially harmful multiple relationship, a conflict of interest, or a loss of objectivity (Younggren & Gottlieb, 2008). As seen in the opening case (Elyn Saks), clients can also end treatment for any number of reasons, including feeling disrespected in treatment or believing that they are no longer making progress.

Normal Termination

Normal termination is "the ethically and clinically appropriate process by which a professional relationship is ended" (Younggren & Gottlieb, 2008, p. 500). This does not necessarily mean that all goals have been met, but that clinician and client together discussed ending treatment and agreed to do so. Curtis (2002) summarized the criteria for normal termination identified in the literature. These included the capacity for enjoyment, ability to love and work, structural personality changes, and decreased symptoms.

One obvious criterion for termination is when treatment goals are met. Despite the apparent clarity of this criterion, treatment goals can change across time. Sometimes clients and clinicians set more modest treatment goals later in treatment, which may be more appropriate than initial, overly ambitious goals (Goldfried, 2002). In addition, the plan to end treatment when goals have been met assumes that movement on treatment goals only occurs during treatment. It is arguably valid to assume that the goal of treatment is to give clients the skills to make change, although the change might not be seen in part or in toto until after treatment is ended.

Most clinicians work on the goals that clients identify and end treatment when their clients are ready to end treatment or are not motivated to continue (Curtis, 2002; Goldfried, 2002; L. S. Greenberg, 2002). Termination is often a collaborative process: clients and clinicians discuss treatment, its successes and failures, the themes that developed over the course of treatment, and the ways that clients are now handling problems more successfully. Depending on the length and type of treatment, sessions are often tapered as termination approaches (Curtis, 2002; Goldfried, 2002). For clients with recurrent depressive episodes, however, Goldfried recommends maintaining ongoing, albeit infrequent, sessions, although he perceives the therapist's role under these conditions as like that of a lifeguard, intervening only "when absolutely necessary" (p. 371).

Premature Termination

For a variety of reasons, some people do not meet all of their treatment goals before ending treatment. Sometimes, as described in Chapter 8, they end treatment because clinician and client disagree on the goals of the treatment (Hawley & Weisz, 2003). Sometimes the client has done all that he or she is able or willing to do at the time (Curtis, 2002; Goldfried, 2002; L. S. Greenberg, 2002). Sometimes, leaving treatment early reflects a problem in the therapeutic alliance: for example, like Ms. Saks, the client does not feel accepted or understood by the clinician. At other times, the benefits of continuing in therapy do not balance positively against its financial or psychological costs (Brogan, Prochaska, & Prochaska, 1999; Curtis, 2002).

Sometimes determining whether a client has left treatment early is a matter of definition, about which reasonable people disagree. For example, Hatchett and Park (2003) looked at **premature termination** using four different commonly used **operational definitions:** the clinician's judgment, the client's failure to attend the last scheduled appointment and the client's attendance at fewer than the median number of appointments for the population. Depending on the definition used, between 17% and 53% of their population were identified as premature terminators. Hatchett and Park reported relatively high agreements between therapist judgments of premature termination and the client missing the last scheduled appointment, although the other measures were less helpful and may be measuring something else altogether.

When defining premature termination in terms of length of treatment, Brogan and her colleagues (1999) concluded that clients who ended treatment in fewer than 10 sessions could be identified based on their stage of change. In particular, premature terminators were more likely to be in Precontemplation (not identifying a problem) and to identify costs but few benefits of changing. These findings suggest that one important aspect of treatment is helping clients to identify a problem they want to work on and recognize real benefits in changing.

When clients and clinicians disagree about when it is time to end treatment, it can be helpful for clinicians to describe their viewpoint (e.g., what can still be accomplished, what barriers may be discouraging clients or causing anxiety, what can be done to meet specified goals). However, feedback should be offered in ways that are respectful and empowering and that increase the client's self-efficacy. It can often be useful to respond like this:

> You know your own experience better than anyone else can, and I think we should trust your conviction that it's time to stop. We've discussed a number of issues that I think it would still be useful for you to work on, but you can do that on your own. If you do find—even if all in all you're doing fine—that some things come up occasionally that you think it would be useful for us to talk about together, I'll be available. And if, at some later point, you feel it might be useful for us to resume more regular work together again, just let me know. (Wachtel, 2002, p. 381)

Notice that Wachtel clearly identified his concerns while also supporting the client's autonomy, as well as other end-of-treatment goals. His statement briefly addressed **relapse prevention**, opened the door for future treatment, supported the client's self-determination, and was empowering.

Abandonment

When clinicians end treatment in ways that are not ethically or clinically appropriate, licensure and ethics boards, courts, and clients perceive this action as **abandonment** (Younggren & Gottlieb, 2008). Failing to do any of a number of actions that are part of normal, competent practice—to discuss the end of treatment and factors related to this end (when appropriate), to facilitate transfer to step-down services, or to inform clients of coverage and emergency services when out of town—could be perceived by clients as abandonment and puts clinicians at increased risk of lawsuit or disciplinary action (Bennett et al., 2006). Similarly, ending treatment against a client's wishes while the client is actively suicidal or homicidal is likely to be reasonably perceived as abandonment (Bennett et al., 2006).

The best-case scenario for termination is one where clients feel understood and well-treated, goals have been met, and termination is discussed with and understood by the client. However, these ideal circumstances are not always possible. Sometimes managed care organizations are unwilling to continue to pay for treatment or clients are unwilling or unable to pay co-payments. Clinicians have the right to end treatment under such circumstances: Although they must refer clients to other services, if appropriate, and stabilize clients in crisis, clinicians are not obligated to offer long-term **pro bono** treatment (Younggren & Gottlieb, 2008).

Even relatively abrupt terminations can be appropriate and ethical. Clinicians have the right to be treated respectfully by their clients. In fact, Younggren and Gottlieb (2008) argued that clients who have violated their clinicians' rights, threatened them in any way, or engaged in significant boundary violations (e.g., the inappropriate client in the movie *What about Bob?*) have "actually terminated the relationship already" (p. 502). Similarly, clients who do not adhere to reasonable expectations for treatment, including showing up to sessions intoxicated or frequently missing appointments, indicate that they are not actively committed to treatment. Of course, Younggren and Gottlieb's argument could also be made in reverse: Clinicians sometimes show their lack of commitment relative to working with their clients. In these cases, clinical risk is increased.

Food for Thought

Review the description of Ms. Saks's termination from treatment from Dr. Kaplan. If you see problems in this case, what were they? Although the clinical risk in this case is more subtle than that incurred by Dr. Helper or Dr. Dietz (Chapter 2), what does Dr. Kaplan do that increases his risk of ethical complaint or legal action? What if anything could he have done to decrease this risk, short of severely limiting his practice?

Clinical Practice

Charlene has been actively suicidal for several months. She frequently calls and e-mails her therapist, Martin, throughout the day. Martin had expected that Charlene would require a much less intensive level of service when he conducted the initial intake. As Martin works full time at a university, he does not feel able to provide the level of care that he believes Charlene needs. Charlene was just involuntarily hospitalized and Martin is considering terminating Charlene's treatment. What recommendations would you give Martin about his current risk level and ways for reducing future risk?

CLINICIANS' AND CLIENTS' FEELINGS DURING TERMINATION

Many of us spend our whole lives running from feeling with the mistaken belief that you cannot bear the pain. But you have already borne the pain. What you have not done is feel all you are beyond the pain.

—**St. Bartholomew**

The end of treatment can be associated with many confusing feelings for both clients and clinicians. Clinicians who monitor their own feelings and handle them well can make the termination process easier for their clients.

Clinicians' Reactions

People entering the mental health fields differ in the strengths and weaknesses that they bring to the table. In many settings, treatment demands patience, a sense of commitment, a willingness to persevere through difficult periods, and an ability to recognize and work with intrapsychic dynamics (Noy-Sharav, 1998). These skills may be especially important during termination, when treatment may raise difficult issues for both clients and clinicians. Furthermore, having a worldview that allows clinicians to handle endings and loss well, and to end treatment despite some goals being less than complete, can be helpful.

Some clinicians may work in settings or under reimbursement plans that set firm session limits. For example, university counseling centers and other treatment settings are increasingly limiting the number of sessions that clients are allowed (Uffelman & Hardin, 2002). Similarly, some **managed care** plans and **employee assistance programs** may cap the number of sessions for which they will pay. Terminations that are triggered by these structural considerations are called **forced terminations.** Forced terminations can intersect with the clinician's issues about loss and abandonment and their needs for perfection and control. Forced terminations can challenge clinicians' comfort with their **professional identity** and cause them to doubt the value of their work.

Normal terminations can also bring up feelings of loss, guilt, shame, and abandonment, or pride, omnipotence, and excitement, depending on the clinician's worldview. Clinicians who approach terminations in a negative manner, however, are more likely to experience burnout (Noy-Sharav, 1998). Clinicians who adopt positive views of termination—seeing it as recognizing a client's ability to continue to change or even as a healthy aspect of treatment—handle termination more positively, as do their clients (Noy-Sharav, 1998).

Although we've been talking about individual dynamics and how these influence the termination process, termination can also be influenced by dynamics related to the clinician's gender or culture, as in the following example:

> [A female therapist may] positively reinforce expressions of transference feelings toward her; she will be more vulnerable to the male patient's needs to act independently without showing concern for her ideas and her needs. The therapist may encourage prolonged relations even after termination, for instance, by frequent follow-up interviews. If the discrepancy between the therapist's and patient's needs is great ... termination may "abort," with the patient leaving in rebellion before the planned date of termination. (Noy-Sharav, 1998, p. 73)

Conversely, clinicians with high autonomy needs and expectations for independence—in the United States, often males—may perceive a client's desire to extend treatment as evidence of continuing dependency needs and react with irritation or annoyance. In each of these examples, the problem is not that clinicians are struggling with these feelings, but when they act without awareness. At such points, they are more likely to project their own feelings and needs on their clients, lose the ability to use feelings in therapeutic ways, and act in ways that cause or increase their clients' anxiety, dependency, and guilt.

Clients' Reactions

Similarly, clients differ in their reactions towards termination depending on their worldview, especially their attitudes about connections and loss. Some clients experience positive emotions during termination and use this period as an opportunity to explore and come to terms with other losses. Others are able to internalize feelings of competence and transfer these feelings to other parts of their lives. Conversely, some clients feel abandoned or rejected and may leave treatment prematurely and abruptly rather than facing the pain that may arise during termination. Others regress to earlier, maladaptive strategies for handling problems. These reactions may be caused when the client—and sometimes the clinician—thinks dichotomously and fails to remember that the physical separation between client and clinician that occurs following termination does not necessarily cause a psychological loss of the clinician by the client (Schafer, 2002). In fact, clinicians may continue to "comfort" and "coach" their clients years after termination from treatment by means of the internalized messages that clients created during treatment. Clinicians can even help clients develop and use these messages during treatment so that this skill will be more accessible at later points.

In some cases, client reactions may reflect clinicians' own attitudes about endings in general and termination from therapy in particular (Noy-Sharav, 1998; Schafer, 2002). Clinicians' unresolved feelings can interfere with their clients' ability to process feelings at the end of treatment or transfer positive skills from treatment to other settings. Perhaps Dr. Kaplan's own personal needs, dynamics, and attitudes about treatment influenced his reactions to Ms. Saks's decision to leave treatment. Clinicians may also inadvertently or unconsciously undermine their clients' positive reactions to termination by perceiving these reactions as resistance or avoidance of therapeutic issues. Empathic clinicians recognize both their clients' fears and hopes and use their assessment of dynamics raised during this period to guide their development of interventions during this stage of treatment.

Clinical Practice

During a consultation with a colleague, Martin recognized that his client Charlene's suicidal feelings had increased as they approached termination. He also observed that he had become more anxious and pessimistic and less hopeful as she had become increasingly suicidal. Furthermore, he recognized that some of his reactions may be due to unprocessed feelings about his mother's suicide. What recommendations would you give him at this point?

GOALS FOR THE END OF TREATMENT

What you get by achieving your goals is not as important as what you become by achieving your goals.
—**Zig Ziglar**

As described in Chapters 10 and 12, the treatment process has a pattern, with the beginning of treatment focusing more on joining and assessment, the middle more on putting the treatment plan into action, and later parts focusing more on **transfer** and **generalization** of skills across settings (Ivey & Ivey, 2003). Generalizing and transferring skills from treatment to the real world is often an essential part of the therapy process, although not emphasized in every theoretical approach (Ivey & Ivey, 2003; Prochaska & Norcross, 2001). Clients need to identify ways of being able to be assertive with their friends and family as well as with their clinicians. They need to see themselves as competent and capable rather than as dependent on their clinician's expertise and brilliance (Curtis, 2002; Epston & White, 1995; Goldfried, 2002; L. S. Greenberg, 2002; Wachtel, 2002). They must be able to self-disclose

TABLE **13.1**
Principles Guiding Termination from Treatment.

1. Change is an ongoing process, neither beginning nor ending in the therapy room.
2. The client is an autonomous being who should be active in guiding the process of termination.
3. Termination should be a planful process, although the length and depth of these plans depend on the clinician's theoretical stance. In particular, clinician and client should
a. Identify ways of consolidating gains incurred during treatment, develop stories about treatment and termination that leave the client in a confident position, and review the mechanisms by which these gains were met.
b. Prepare for ending treatment, including discussing the difficult (and often normal) feelings associated with termination, including loss, anxiety, and fears about the future. Sessions should be tapered, when appropriate to the length and depth of treatment.
c. Anticipate problems that often follow ending therapy, including lapses and ways of responding to these lapses.
d. Leave the door open for future consultations without building dependency.
4. Treatment and the termination processes should empower clients and build their self-efficacy. Gains should be attributed primarily to the client's efforts rather than to the clinician's skill or brilliance.

Note: Modified from L. S. Greenberg (2002)

safely and challenge their negative cognitions both inside and outside of therapy. Furthermore, they need to be able to continue using these skills long after therapy has ended (Prochaska & Norcross, 2001). Some approaches to change, including Alcoholics Anonymous and other substance abuse treatments, emphasize the importance of transferring and maintaining skills (e.g., staying sober one day at a time).

In general, clinicians from different theoretical orientations often share similar goals for the end of treatment (see Table 13.1 for an overview). As described in this table, many clinicians attempt to empower their clients so that they feel able to continue their work following the end of treatment. They equalize the power in the relationship to empower their clients, increase their clients' self-efficacy, and help them become their own therapists (Curtis, 2002; Epston & White, 1995; Goldfried, 2002; L. S. Greenberg, 2002; Wachtel, 2002). Rather than accepting all the credit for changes made during treatment, they acknowledge that their work was collaborative in nature, and they encourage clients to own these changes.

Balancing Opposing Reactions to Termination

As discussed earlier, termination can be an exciting process, but also one characterized by feelings of loss and even abandonment. Empathic approaches to termination from treatment recognize both of these poles: the gains and increasing competency developed across treatment but also the dependency, fears about relapsing, and anxiety about losing an important relationship. Some clients and clinicians may emphasize one pole over the other. For example, they may assume that a particular client is incompetent and will have difficulty continuing on his or her own, or collude to agree that a client is doing very well, has no concerns about termination, and will have no difficulty staying on track. In most cases, both sets of concerns are present and should be addressed: that the client is strong and capable, but, like other people, will have better and worse periods in the future.

Discussing these mixed and confusing feelings can help clients consolidate the changes they made during treatment and develop positive stories about treatment, their work in it, and their relationship with their clinician (Epston & White, 1995; Wachtel, 2002). It can help them identify positive and growth-promoting ways of perceiving "negative" feelings.

Food for Thought

To further understand these ideas, review how in case material presented earlier in the chapter, Wachtel (2002) and Dr. Kaplan balanced these opposing feelings and end-of-treatment tasks. How did they respond to these tasks? What did they do well or not so well?

Relapse Prevention

Everyone has ups and downs, good days and bad; therefore an especially important task of treatment is relapse prevention. Relapse prevention includes transferring skills to other situations, identifying strategies for maintaining skills across time, and preventing lapses (Prochaska, 1999; Prochaska & DiClemente, 1982). As described in Chapter 8, there are two essential aspects to reducing the frequency and impact of lapses: (a) eliminating triggers to the problem behavior (e.g., boredom, loneliness, stress, and environmental stimuli associated with the behavior), and (b) challenging negative cognitive and emotional reactions to lapses. People with high self-efficacy and positive self-attributions following a lapse are less likely to have a second one, thus these self-perceptions should be promoted during treatment (Shiffman et al., 1996).

In some cases, it can be useful to help a client's family reframe the meaning of lapses, as they may also believe that a lapse signals a return to the full-blown syndrome that brought the client into treatment. In general, when family members are critical, high in expressed emotion, or distressed, clients with a wide variety of serious mental illnesses are at higher risk of relapse (Hinrichsen & Pollack, 1997; Hooley & Hiller, 2000; Hooley & Teasdale, 1989; O'Farrell, Hooley, Fals-Stewart, & Cutter, 1998). Although criticism and other negative emotions predict relapse, familial warmth decreases the probability of relapse (López et al., 2004). Furthermore, the relative importance of warmth and criticism depends on culture. For example, one study of people with schizophrenia found that low familial warmth predicted relapse for

Mexican Americans, while for Euro Americans, high criticism better predicted relapse (López et al., 2004).

Clinical Practice

Amber has had a history of heavy binge drinking throughout her adult life. Her husband and daughters are frustrated by her drinking and, although she has been abstinent for the last 15 months and has been handling cues that could trigger her drinking, are afraid that she is never going to be able to stay dry. What messages would you give her and her family at the end of treatment? How would you frame these messages? Would the fact that her mother is a Latina and her father is German American influence your intervention?

GOOD CLINICAL PRACTICE DURING TERMINATION

This life is yours. Take the power to choose what you want to do and do it well.

—Susan Polis Schutz

Although clinicians do not need to continue seeing their clients forever, and Dr. Kaplan did not need to continue seeing Ms. Saks, clinicians should balance their duty to their clients, their right to terminate treatment under some circumstances, and their clients' right to avoid being abandoned (Younggren & Gottlieb, 2008). Wise clinicians do a number of things to manage their risk in the infrequent case of abrupt or unilateral terminations (Knapp & VandeCreek, 2006; Younggren & Gottlieb, 2008), some of which are listed in Table 13.2. Rather than jumping to conclusions about the meaning of their clients' problematic behavior, they discuss their concerns with their clients. For example, it is possible that a clinician could have misunderstood his or her

TABLE **13.2**
Questions for Clinicians to Consider in the Course of Both Normal and Abrupt Terminations.

1. Have I discussed the proposed termination process with my client and any concerns that were raised? Did I offer reasonable options for aftercare?
2. Is the termination process respectful of my client's presenting problems and ongoing needs?
3. Is the proposed termination process consistent with my theoretical model?
4. Is the proposed termination process consistent with that described during discussions during the initial informed consent process?
5. If there were problems raised by the end of treatment, did I discuss these in consultations or supervision? Did consults conclude that the proposed termination process was appropriate and consistent with ethical guidelines and the standard of care?
6. Have I carefully documented my termination process, especially the process for abrupt terminations?
7. Having identified an appropriate decision and termination process, am I following it in a consistent, yet respectful manner?

Note: From Knapp & VandeCreek, 2005; Younggren & Gottlieb, 2008 client's behavior (e.g., what the clinician thought might reflect the client's "stalking behavior" might be due to the fact that the client has business down the street from the clinician's office). Furthermore, clients' problematic behavior can be a reflection of the very issues that brought them into treatment (e.g., agoraphobia, chronic suicidality, or disorganization).

As discussed previously, risk of legal action or ethical complaint is low when clinicians have engaged in good clinical practice. As described in Table 13.1, clinicians decrease risk when they give reasonable notice of the interruption or end of services, make good faith efforts to facilitate their clients' transfer to other appropriate services, and are thoughtful and respectful of their clients' needs (Bennett et al., 2006). Providing a careful informed consent process and describing the clients' rights and responsibilities at the beginning of treatment—as well as the consequences of failing to meet reasonable expectations—can make clinical decisions more understandable to clients and a decision to terminate treatment less problematic (Younggren & Gottlieb, 2008). Depending on the population with whom one works and one's theoretical orientation, an informed consent process might include discussions of financial responsibilities, missed appointments, and phone coverage during vacations. Good clinical practice may include appropriately tapering the frequency of treatment, providing reasonable aftercare recommendations, and assessing potential harm to self and others. Good clinical practice varies with theoretical orientation, but should be justifiable within it. For example, clinicians offering long-term depth therapies who regularly terminate treatment abruptly without examining the issues of loss raised by termination are not practicing within the profession's standard of care.

Strategies for Helping Clients to Own Their Change

Epston and White (1995) suggested that clinicians often overemphasize loss in therapy, which "subtly reinforces the dependency of the person seeking assistance on the 'expert knowledge' of the therapist" (pp. 339–340). Instead, the end of treatment can be seen as an important period in which clients can explore the ways in which they have solved and overcome problems both in and out of therapy, a period where they begin seeing themselves as the expert on their own lives and change process. Of course, attributing the change process to the client requires the clinician to have a certain amount of confidence (Noy-Sharav, 1998). As described in Chapter 12, clinicians can use questioning as an integral part of the change process, helping their clients be curious about the change process, own their change rather than attributing it to another person or a force beyond their control, and feel more empowered and in control of where they are (Epston & White, 1995). To help clients identify their role in the change process, clinicians may ask questions such as:

- "Imagine that I have a client with problems similar to the ones you used to have. What advice would you give this person given what you know now?"
- "If I'd met you at an earlier point in your life, what would I have seen that would have let me know that you would have broken free of this problem?"

- "As you think about the work we've done together, what are the most important things you've learned about yourself and your relationships?"
- "How will what you've learned here continue to influence the decisions you make in life and how you see yourself? Using these skills, where will you be in five years?"

Many clients enter treatment assuming that change is done *to* them rather than *by* them. Sometimes they believe that their clinicians have a magic wand (or crystal ball or time machine). Notice how these questions undermine these assumptions and firmly postulate that the client (with the aid of the clinician) made the change, had the necessary skills to change, and will be able to continue to expand this change process.

Handling Difficult Terminations

Most terminations from treatment are easy and straightforward. When they are not, however, the clinician should discuss the process in supervision or consultations (Bennett et al., 2006; Knapp & VandeCreek, 2006; Younggren & Gottlieb, 2008). Furthermore, factors influencing the decision to terminate, recommendations made during consultations, the client's mental status during the termination process, and the nature of aftercare recommendations should all be carefully documented.

After careful consideration and consultation, clinicians may ultimately make a decision about termination with which their clients may disagree. Clinicians may believe, for example, that they do not have the appropriate level of competence to work with the client and the presenting problem, while their client may argue that does not matter. Younggren and Gottlieb (2008) very clearly concluded that it is unwise to waver about termination in response to clients' badgering or concerns. Doing so can undermine treatment and reinforce manipulative or self-defeating behavior. Even in such situations, the process should not be mean-spirited or disrespectful; instead, it should be empathic, considerate, and warm, yet firm.

THE DISCHARGE PROCESS AND DISCHARGE SUMMARY

I wanted a perfect ending. Now I've learned, the hard way, that some poems don't rhyme, and some stories don't have a clear beginning, middle and end.

—**Gilda Radner**

As described earlier, even during normal termination, there are a number of concrete issues that need to be addressed before treatment ends. These include consolidating emotional, cognitive, and behavioral skills developed during treatment; developing strategies to prevent lapses and respond well to them when they occur; ensuring that the client has a strong social support system in place; and identifying appropriate step-down services, when appropriate. Step-down services might include less frequent therapy sessions, a less intensive treatment modality (e.g., outpatient treatment after inpatient treatment), self-help groups, or the use of a crisis line.

Whether or not discharge from treatment was mutually agreed upon, clinicians should write a **discharge summary**. This summary can be relatively short, but should briefly describe progress, as well as issues that remain outstanding (Younggren & Gottlieb, 2008). Reports should include posttermination recommendations, including **referrals** for step-down services. A sample discharge summary for Jayne (Chapter 9) is included in Table 13.3. As with other clinical writing, discharge summaries should be clear and respectful and should draw appropriate conclusions while remaining tentative about aspects of the client's situation that continue to be unclear. Because discharge summaries are sometimes requested at a later date by a third party (e.g., attorneys, physicians, other clinicians), they should not include gratuitous information. For example, the mother's history of incest as a child would probably be inappropriate for a child's discharge summary from treatment for an autism spectrum disorder—unless the mother's poor psychological status impacted implementation of treatment goals.

TABLE **13.3**
Discharge Summary for Jayne Romero (sample).

Sofie Catawnee, MSW

Licensed Clinical Social Worker

1467 Vine St., Ste. 232

New York, NY 10037

Discharge Summary

Name: Jayne Romero

DOB: 3/30/1995

Dates of treatment (inclusive): 1/15/2008-5/4/2009

Background Information: Jayne is an attractive 14-year-old Latina who is in the ninth grade. She lives with her parents, both born and raised in Puerto Rico, her two younger sisters (12 and 9), and her maternal grandmother, all of whom are in good health. Jayne was referred for outpatient psychotherapy after accusing an adult neighbor of having molested her, frequently missing school, and being briefly hospitalized with suicidal ideation. During the inpatient stay she reported a recent history of mild depressive symptoms, frequent intrusive thoughts, and occasional flashbacks and nightmares. During outpatient treatment she additionally reported occasional mild self-injurious behavior and moderate suicidality, significant social withdrawal, an inability to concentrate during school and while doing homework, and distrust of family and friends, with rocky relationships with same. Throughout elementary school Jayne's grades had been good. She was active in the community, had a number of good friends, and strong relationships with her family. She excelled in organized sports (softball, volleyball) and music (piano).

During the course of therapy, Jayne made a contract to decrease depressive symptoms, cope with feelings in positive ways, and develop more positive relationships with herself and others. She was seen approximately weekly, 42 times as of this report, although she had been seen by another outpatient therapist for three months before transferring services. She had been hospitalized four times before her transfer to this therapist and three times since then, most recently in October 2008. She is currently taking Lexapro (20 mg) to decrease depressive symptoms, as prescribed by her psychiatrist Dr. Samson, and uses an albuterol inhaler as prescribed by her PCP, Dr. Garcia.

Diagnosis at Discharge
I.   309.81 Posttraumatic Stress Disorder
     300.4 Dysthymic Disorder
II. 799.9 Diagnosis Deferred
III. Exercise-induced asthma

(continues)

TABLE **13.3**
Discharge Summary for Jayne Romero (sample) (Continued)

> IV. Severe: Problems with school, primary support system
> V. GAF (current) 60 (at start of treatment) 45

Assessment: Jayne is presumed to be of average to above average intelligence, although was failing eighth grade when first seen. She is superficially pleasant and cooperative, has good social skills, and makes good eye contact, although admits having difficulties self-disclosing to others and being assertive with them. Her judgment and impulse control are generally fair, although poor when she is with peers. While she appears to have been truly suicidal in her first two to three psychiatric hospital admissions, she has tended to overreport symptoms since then in order to avoid large tests, projects, or papers at school. When there are no stressors at home or school, she has denied symptoms. This has made progress inconsistent. She can be psychologically minded, but also seems to tell therapists and other service providers what she thinks they want to hear. She is very avoidant of situations with a possibility for negative judgment (her own and others'), and withdraws in treatment when she fears judgment, even when passivity and noninvolvement are inappropriate.

Status at Discharge

Jayne's symptoms have not completely disappeared, although they have decreased to a manageable level at this point in time. She is attending school regularly, passing her courses, and has not been hospitalized in almost seven months. Her attendance in therapy, while once regular, has become inconsistent and she has been more distractible in sessions. As she is currently stable, all parties have agreed to take a break from psychotherapy at the present point in time. Treatment in the last month has focused on strengthening her support system at school, in the community, and at home, and to prevent relapses. She has agreed to continue seeing her psychiatrist regularly and to take her medications as prescribed.

Recommendations to Client

1. Continue using positive coping strategies (e.g., running, talking to grandmother and guidance counselor, challenging negative self-talk, writing in diary), as discussed during treatment.
2. Continue appointments with psychiatrist and taking medications, as prescribed.
3. Use relapse-prevention strategies on a regular basis. In particular, Jayne should (a) monitor levels of stress and depression regularly throughout the day, (b) avoid triggers, and (c) challenge her thinking about "slips," framing these as lapses rather than relapses.
4. Should additional services be required, Jayne and her family should contact this agency or other providers, as needed, to set up additional appointments.

Respectfully submitted,

Sofie Catawnee, MSW

Licensed Clinical Social Worker

As described throughout this book, responding respectfully and empathically to clients, recognizing and handling risk factors well, obtaining appropriate consultations, and documenting decisions well are important aspects of a strong risk-management strategy. The more problematic the termination process, the clearer the documentation of that process should be (Bennett et al., 2006; Younggren & Gottlieb, 2008). Such documentation should include information that allows the reader to understand the rationale for ending treatment, the names of clinicians and other resources consulted about the termination process, the steps the clinician took to end treatment in a competent and ethical manner, and recommendations made for aftercare.

Clinical Practice

Although Martin acknowledged that his feelings of stress and anxiety were only partially related to Charlene, he recognized that he did not have the time or psychological resources at this point in time to continue working with her, especially since, while in the hospital, she had disclosed that she experienced frequent dissociation, extensive self-injurious behavior, and chronic suicidality. What issues should he consider as he prepares to transfer Charlene to a more appropriate level of outpatient care? What issues might he consider as he makes his referrals and recommendations?

SUMMARY

Treatment follows a pattern, with different issues addressed at the end of treatment than in either its beginning or middle. In particular, these include transferring skills to other settings, increasing client ownership of the change process, and preventing a relapse. These tasks may occur in the midst of confusing feelings of both excitement and hopefulness and also loss and abandonment for both clients and clinicians. These feelings and tasks should be addressed in such a way that clients are aware of the potential pitfalls they will face, yet also remain hopeful about continuing the change process begun in therapy.

All clinical interventions are associated with some risk. Clinician-initiated terminations, although sometimes necessary, can sometimes be perceived by clients as abandonment. Clinicians can, however, do some things to decrease their risk of ethical complaint or legal action at these points. This includes responding respectfully and empathically to the clients' needs and concerns, requesting consultations, and documenting their decisions and decision-making process well. Careful discharge summaries are one part of this risk management process.

How Do These Issues Apply to Your Life and Work?

1. If you've been in therapy before, think about the range of feelings you had when it ended. If you have not been in therapy, how did you feel during an important transition in your life (e.g., a move, graduation, end of a relationship)? How did you handle these feelings?
2. If you've been in therapy before, how did your clinician handle the end of treatment? Were the concerns raised by L. S. Greenberg (2002) and

(continues)

(continued)

summarized in Table 13.1 addressed well? If you have not been in therapy, think about another type of transition. If that transition was relatively difficult, what could have made it work better?

3. Pay attention to your feelings about perfection, control, and "complete-ness" over the next week. When do you have or want these? When are you able to give them up? What might this mean for your clinical work?

PART V

Continuing Growth and Effectiveness

In the closing section of the book, we discuss many practical issues that clinicians are bound to face in their professional lives. First, Chapter 14 discusses the tensions that exist for clinicians who are striving to be ethical, effective, and empathic when balancing the demands imposed by real-world considerations. Our final chapter, Chapter 15, discusses the importance of regular self-care in maintaining effectiveness in working with others and offers many concrete ways to take care of oneself. We emphasize the importance of engaging in good self-care practices and having effective safety mechanisms, which enable clinicians to remain respectful and empathic even when under stress.

CHAPTER 14

Ethical Work in the Real World

WHERE ARE WE GOING?

1. What strategies help clinicians remain ethical, empathic, and effective in challenging situations?

2. What common challenges to ethical behavior arise as a result of other competing demands on clinical practice?

3. How do one's personal identity and ethics support behaving ethically in professional situations?

That's Our Average Stay
Rosie Jacasum

Rosie Jacasum (age 28) was recently admitted to a **halfway house** after she had become increasingly suicidal following the deaths of her twin sons, who were hit and killed by a drunk driver. She generally perceived her stay in positive ways and saw the staff's behavior as within ethical limits and legal restrictions, yet her experience also highlighted the difficulties clinicians may experience balancing ethical standards, legal requirements, workplace expectations, and empathic and effective care.

Rosie was very suicidal when she entered the program. After several days, some distance from life stressors, and a new antidepressant, she was able to think more clearly about her sons' deaths and make decisions about her future without immediately considering suicide. She felt comfortable with her new medications, had appointments with her outpatient therapist and psychiatrist, and was ready to begin making the changes in her life that she recognized she needed; however, she did not believe that the program's group counseling sessions matched her current level of functioning or her needs. She talked to the director of the program and asked that she be released, but was told that she had been enrolled in the program for 2 weeks because "that's our average stay."

Most clinical settings have requirements for **productivity** and **census**, but clearly keeping her for 2 weeks solely because "that's our average stay" is unethical (consider the aspirational principles of beneficence, nonmaleficence, fidelity, and autonomy described by Kitchener, 1984). If Rosie was otherwise ready for release, it does not appear that she was being maintained in the **least restrictive environment**. Extending her stay might also be insurance fraud if unnecessary services were being provided and billed to an insurance company. What are more ethical ways of maintaining clients enrolled in the program? Perhaps census could be better maintained by strengthening the program's reputation in the community or by providing a type of service that was otherwise unavailable regionally.

Rosie had been involuntarily hospitalized on three previous occasions, but at this point was generally compliant with services and wanting to do better—things that were significantly different than at previous points in her life. Given these differences, although talking about an "average stay" might be a way of thinking about how long she *might* stay, the program director might also think about other ways of presenting his thinking that might be more effective at engaging her as a healthy consumer. He might have opened a discussion about her goals for her time in treatment, what she hoped to accomplish there, and how she would know when she was ready to leave. Rosie has a tendency to be impulsive and had problems with alcohol in the past, so this conversation might be especially important in terms of helping her develop skills to get her through future crises.

(continues)

Furthermore, the process of this discussion could promote her autonomy and her positive involvement and investment in her treatment.

The program's psychiatrist changed Rosie's antidepressant without discussing his reasons for doing this. She was also given a sleeping pill, although had not been having difficulties sleeping and had not requested one. How do these actions promote her autonomy and positive involvement in treatment? Would she understand his decisions and be compliant under these circumstances? Was he attempting to engage her effectively in treatment? Was he seeing and fostering her growth motivation?

For the most part, this program and psychiatrist were acting within acceptable limits and their decisions were probably not unethical or insurance fraud. However, with just slight changes in their interventions, this program and psychiatrist could have become much more effective and decreased their risk for a complaint. As Younggren and Gottlieb (2008) observed, satisfied consumers are less likely to file complaints.

- What ethical concerns are raised by the program's and psychiatrist's actions? How would you have handled this instead?
- Although you have limited information, evaluate the program's and psychiatrist's risk given the model described in Chapter 2 (Bennett et al., 2006). What could you do to decrease their risk in this situation? What could you do to decrease risk *and* maintain a high standard of care?
- Ms. Jacasum's father was a traditional Cree Indian. She is living in an urban area and attempting to get in greater touch with her Cree roots and values. To what degree did the program respond to her in a manner consistent with her Native American culture, as described in Table 14.1? How might this be an ethical issue? How could her psychiatrist and the program have done a better job?
- To what degree are the principles outlined in Table 14.1 similar to those described by other models of psychotherapy? How are they different?

TABLE **14.1**

Healing Conditions Identified by Native American Clients and Healers.

Foundational conditions
- The healer's ability to understand the client and the client's ability to feel the healer's empathy are significant to the healing process.
- Healers accept and respect clients unconditionally and do not judge or reject their clients based on their history of mistakes.
- Through their attitude and way they live, healers show that a good life is possible despite hardships and difficulties in life.
- A healer's genuineness fosters his or her credibility and legitimacy.
- Healers create an atmosphere of safety and trust, which is essential to the healing process.

(continues)

TABLE **14.1**

Healing Conditions Identified by Native American Clients and Healers. (Continued)

The healing process
- People must be open to change and healing in order to change.
- Healing comes from paying attention to and understanding one's inner life and conflicts, which can be significant influences on problematic thinking, feeling, and behaving.
- Healers recognize that daily living offers a rich source of opportunities from which to learn and heal and offer direction and guidance to help clients use these opportunities well.
- Healers challenge their clients to be more self-evaluative and deliberative in their thoughts and actions. They encourage change, mobilize positive forces, and help their clients evaluate their decisions and lifestyle.

Spiritual foundation to native healing
- Healers provide the sacred teachings; clients receive and honor these teachings, which they use to guide their lives.
- Healers use rituals and ceremonies to clearly demark the healing journey and create a sense of community to support growth and change.
- Healing depends on believing and accepting spiritual guidance from the Creator.

Note: McCabe (2007).

THE THREE Es: ETHICS, EMPATHY, AND EFFECTIVENESS

The best and safest thing is to keep a balance in your life, acknowledge the great powers around us and in us. If you can do that, and live that way, you are really a wise man.

—Euripedes

Throughout this book, we have discussed ethics, people, and the professional challenges that may arise in working with them. In Chapter 2, we presented five important ethical standards that guide clinicians throughout their work (informed consent, competence, confidentiality, dual relationships and sensitivity to differences). When the ethics code is clear, clinicians are likely to make good, ethical choices, especially when the decision is reinforced by legal precedent (Jennings, Sovereign, Botorff, Mussell, & Vye, 2005). Codes of ethics, however, are by necessity incomplete and do not address the nuanced ethical issues that may arise, such as those seen in the case of Rosie. Furthermore, when the ethical considerations of a situation are less clear-cut, clinicians are less likely to "do the right thing," relying more on their own personal values and interpretation of the ethics code. The five aspirational principles toward which all clinicians must strive—beneficence, nonmaleficence, fidelity, autonomy, and social justice—help address these gaps in the ethics code, although they alone are insufficient to resolve the inherent contradictions and tensions involved in acting ethically (Kitchener, 1984; Knapp & VandeCreek, 2007).

This question of how to identify and choose the right thing in ambiguous or complicated situations underlies the discussions throughout this chapter. How does one choose between an individual's welfare and the community's, for example? What if the short term involves perceived harm, although there is a good probability of benefit in the long term? What if a client is unable to make fully competent decisions? Extending the basic information on ethics presented in Chapter 2, we discuss the clinician's role as negotiator of the ethical demands and practical challenges presented on a daily basis in clinical work and recommend strategies for maintaining an ethical practice.

Although, ideally, enacting ethical principles and standards would be clear and obvious in every situation, in fact, remaining an ethical, effective and empathic clinician involves continuous negotiation of multiple competing demands. Professional ideals and practical considerations may be at cross purposes in the context of specific treatment goals and one's own theoretical orientation. In this chapter, we describe a number of different domains of clinical work in which clinicians may encounter situations that will raise competing demands. In the process of our discussion, we will raise as many questions as we answer, but we will also provide a framework to help clinicians identify these competing demands and begin to resolve them in ways that are good for the client, clinician, profession, and community.

The partner of one of us argues that when you want food, you can get food with at most two of the following qualities: cheap, fast, and good. That is, you can get inexpensive food quickly and good food inexpensively, but you cannot get good food inexpensively and rapidly. While we can disagree about the validity of his argument, the underlying assumption is clear: We must give up some things that we want in order to get others.

Is this is a good assumption for work in the mental health professions? In navigating issues raised during clinical work, we believe it can be useful to think about striving for the Three Es: Ethics, Empathy, and Effectiveness. We maintain that it is not only possible but essential to be ethical and empathic in order to be effective; however, doing so is not easy and requires continual attention and self-awareness.

STRATEGIES FOR REMAINING ETHICAL, EMPATHIC, AND EFFECTIVE

Tenderness and kindness are not signs of weakness and despair, but manifestations of strength and resolution.

—Kahlil Gibran

It can be easy to get into a day-to-day routine, performing one's usual duties almost automatically. One's calendar can be heavily scheduled, leaving little room for reflection. It can be easy to fail to identify a situation as an ethical dilemma or correctly identify its nature (Kitchener, 1986). Having sex with a current client is clearly unethical, because it has a high potential for harming the client, clinician, and profession; but is giving a client an apple ethical? If so, under what circumstances? A colleague argued that giving a child client an apple without asking her parent can undermine the parent's authority, thus potentially harming both the parent and child and undermining their relationship (T. Bean, personal communication, 2000).

Time pressure, routine, and lack of time for consultation and reflection can pull clinicians toward one of the Three Es at the expense of the other two. Without a strategy for identifying and responding to clinical dilemmas as they arise, it is very easy to justify clinical decisions rather than draw unbiased ethical conclusions and to overlook information essential to the case conceptualization (Gollan & Witte, 2008). Both of these errors decrease competency and effectiveness.

Ethical decision making is not simple; as we noted in Chapter 2, "reasonable differences of opinion can and do exist" regarding the resolution of conflicts among aspirational principles, ethical standards, and legal rulings (ACA, 2005, p. 2). When conflicts are identified, clinicians should clearly indicate their

TABLE **14.2**
Goals of Learning to Practice Ethically and Tasks for Meeting These Goals.

Goals	Tasks
Recognize and identify the ethical dimensions of a situation	• Recognize that actions have moral overtones that can either help or hurt others • Read and discuss ethics code, applying it to cases • Identify particular situations as having ethical implications
Formulate a course of action integrating diverse factors	• Learn to use moral thinking that views situations in complex manners • Recognize the range of factors impacting a decision • Perceive the situation from both the client's and others' points of view • Anticipate possible positive and negative outcomes of action
Choose an ethical plan of action	• Identify and address obstacles (e.g., social, financial, time, ambition) to behaving ethically
Implement that plan	• Develop ego strength, courage, perseverance, and assertiveness in order to "do the right thing" despite pressures to do otherwise

Note: From Kitchener (1986).

commitment to their ethics code and "take steps to resolve the conflict" (APA, 2002, p. 1062). The appropriate resolution of these conflicts is less clear, yet somehow clinicians must find a way of resolving them. The ACA (2005) concludes, "[N]o specific ethical decision-making model … is most effective, [but] counselors are expected to be familiar with [and use] a credible model of decision making that can bear public scrutiny" (ACA, 2005, p. 2). Having such a strategy, consulting with colleagues about concerns, and documenting this process carefully are central to behaving ethically and reducing risk (Bennett et al., 2006).

Ethics codes, ethical principles, and ethical theory all should be brought to bear on ethical decisions (Kitchener, 1984), but learning to make ethical decisions depends on four tasks: learning to recognize and identify the ethical dimensions of a situation, coming to view ethical decisions in complex manners that are influenced by diverse factors, committing to ethical actions despite factors that might make this difficult or unpleasant, and building the personal and moral fortitude that allows one to "do the right thing" despite pressures to do otherwise (Kitchener, 1986) (see Table 14.2). These tasks depend on and build intellectual, empathic, moral, and personal strengths for ethical and effective practice. Asking and considering questions raised by case examples is an important aspect of learning and applying ethics well (Eberlein, 1987; Gawthrop & Uhlemann, 1992; Kitchener, 1986).

When facing a difficult or problematic situation, we recommend that clinicians step back and take some time to think clearly in order to be able to identify the ethical dilemmas raised by that situation, hear the client's viewpoint while also being sensitive to those of others, and contextualize these dilemmas with an understanding of the client's personal strengths and weaknesses, the nature of treatment goals, the research findings relevant to the

TABLE **14.3**

A Process for Making Ethical Decisions.

1. Describe the situation and factors influencing a decision, both from the client's viewpoint and that of an outside observer.
2. Identify all parties affected by this situation and consider their rights, responsibilities, and welfare.
3. What ethical principles, standards, and theory might be raised by this case?
4. What other factors including agency policy, legal statutes and rulings, theoretical framework, and research might also influence this decision?
5. What personal biases, values, stressors, and self-interests may influence this decision?
6. Enlarge the frame beyond the initial options presented. What other ways of approaching this problem are possible?
7. Evaluate options. What are the short-term and long-term consequences of these proposed actions? How does each proposed intervention fit within the case conceptualization, treatment plan, and available research? How does it meet ethical, legal, agency, personal, and other demands? How does it meet the client's preferences, values, and goals?
8. Choose a plan of action taking into account the ethical principles, standards, and theory, as well as other factors that may impact the decision.
9. Take action in a respectful and empathic manner.
10. Monitor outcomes and correct these if necessary.

Note: Modified from Canadian Psychological Association, 2000; Eberlein, 1987; Knapp & Vandecreek, 2006.

problem and population, and the clinician's theoretical framework and case conceptualization (see Table 14.3). Clinicians should further examine the legal, agency, personal, and other demands that bear on that situation. As Kitchener (1986) suggested, clinicians should identify a range of responses, evaluate these responses, and put them into action. When there is a conflict between two ethical principles or between ethical principles and some other demand, Knapp and VandeCreek (2007) suggest evaluating ethical decisions based on the presence of a rationale for trumping one ethical principle over another, the action's probability of success, considerations of other options, and efforts to reduce harm. Because the effectiveness of an intervention is determined as much by its presentation as by the intervention itself (see the opening case, Rosie Jacasum), acting in a compassionate and empathic manner increases the probability of an ethical and effective outcome.

For example, with Lou, a man who is actively suicidal, refusing to identify and agree to a safety plan and unwilling to go to the hospital, a clinician's first step might be to step back and breathe. Doing so could provide the necessary calmness to recognize and identify ethical dilemmas, hear Lou's perspective well, and also see the big picture. A clinician's history of ongoing continuing education, regular self-care, and personal therapy can make this process easier and decrease the probability of making impulsive decisions. Setting goals to guide clinical work (e.g., ethical, empathic, effective) can also help clinicians maintain a calm, stable, core during crises. Prior to intervening, Lou's clinician should reflect Lou's feelings and concerns (Ivey & Ivey, 2003). Lou must feel heard and understood before he is likely to be receptive to any intervention.

A number of apparently competing factors are raised in this case. Some clinicians might conclude that fostering a client's autonomy might mean allowing him to decide to commit suicide. Doing so, however, ignores how his

284 CHAPTER 14 • Ethical Work in the Real World

suicidality varies significantly across time and how the welfare of his family, friends, and acquaintances would also be affected by his suicide (Knapp & VandeCreek, 2007). Furthermore, the reputation of Lou's clinician's profession and practice may also be negatively impacted if the community were to discover that his therapist had been aware that he was suicidal and had not intervened. Other factors might include agency policies requiring case consultations of actively suicidal clients, questions about his dangerousness to others and whether there is a duty to warn, and perhaps the clinician's welfare given her health, life stressors, and current resources. In addition, Lou's clinician may want to inform him about her agency's policy on responding to suicidal clients, yet also want to choose a strategy for intervening that strengthens his engagement in treatment. What this case indicates is that a clinician cannot focus on only a particular ethical principle or even a single person, but instead must simultaneously balance a number of different factors.

Clinical work should not be a solely rational, cold, objective, and impersonal process, but one informed by a strong empathic understanding of an individual client that is grounded in the research and theory on the problem and population (Orlinsky et al., 2005). Returning to our example, Lou has generally been a pessimist, but his negative outlook increased further with his recent job loss and ensuing mortgage foreclosure. He has been withdrawing more and feeling judged by friends and acquaintances, but feels safe and accepted in the counseling setting. His disclosures have not been manipulative, he has been low in reactance, and he has previously been cooperative with recommendations. His disclosure of suicidality may signal his ambivalence about suicide—both wanting things to be different, yet not knowing how to accomplish this in a positive way. Appropriate interventions will depend on his degree of suicidality, history of suicide attempts, lethality of plan, impulsivity, substance use, social support, and other factors (Bennett et al., 2006) (see Table 14.4). In this case, his usual slow, deliberate approach to decisions and strong connection to his clinician are strengths, while his tendency to binge drink, history of previous serious suicide attempts, recent losses with associated shame, inability to identify a support system, and possession of guns increase his risk.

Clinicians should avoid a false dichotomy, that one either allows Lou to commit suicide or involuntarily hospitalizes him. During a period of immediate crisis, clients are unwilling to be involved with developing or agreeing to a reasonable safety plan, and the threat of suicide continues to be imminent, clinicians may have few choices but to act in ways that counter their clients' decisions (Knapp & VandeCreek, 2007). Although they may privilege some goals over others—in this case beneficence over autonomy—effective clinicians aim to infringe on the violated principle as little as possible. How can Lou's therapist do that in this situation? She could actively listen to his fears and concerns, giving him as many choices as possible and keeping his preferences in mind to the degree possible (e.g., developing a safety plan with him, allowing him to decide whether and when he would enter the hospital and which one, whom he will inform, and so on). In such a way, Lou's clinician can maintain apparently contradictory treatment goals in mind throughout her work. As this can be difficult during periods of crisis, it is often helpful to learn ethical and legal requirements as well as consider treatment options

TABLE **14.4**
Factors to Consider in the Course of Assessments of Suicidality.

Predisposing factors—Factors putting client at risk, including psychiatric diagnoses, history of childhood abuse or punitive parenting, presence of family violence, and specific risk factors (e.g., unmarried, male, Euro American or Native American, unreligious, homosexuals, or adolescents, young adults, and older adults)

Precipitants—The nature and severity of stressors, especially those that involve shame or loss (e.g., loss of relationship or job, being sent to jail, becoming a victim of a crime), but also "background stressors," that could have a cumulative impact (e.g., unpleasant work environment, problems with partner or child, financial problems)

Symptomatic presentation (past and present)—Diagnostic presentation, including Axis I and II disorders related to suicidality. Also consider feelings of anger and agitation and positive and negative coping mechanisms, including self-injury and substance abuse

Feelings of hopelessness—Perception that the situation is bleak and that nothing can or will change; extreme pessimism

Level of suicidality—Frequency, intensity, and duration of suicidal thoughts, presence of a plan, lethality of the plan, access to means to enact the plan

Previous suicidal behavior—Number and nature of previous attempts, including the client's perception of lethality and outcomes and the opportunity for rescue

Impulsivity—This includes both background impulsivity and also changes in impulsivity that might be produced by substance use or perception of recent stressor

Protective factors—Nature and breadth of social support system, nature and use of coping skills, cognitive skills, ability to identify reasons to live or recognize negative outcomes accruing from suicide, relationship with therapist

Note: Modified from Bennett et al., 2006.

in the abstract, before a problem reaches crisis point. In addition, work with suicidal or otherwise dangerous clients should include consultations with supervisors or colleagues as a normal part of this process.

As this discussion suggests, remaining true to the three Es means being self-aware and knowledgeable about the competing tensions among them and the practical realities one may encounter. However, vigilance and attention are essential, and monitoring one's emotions and evaluating one's behavior in terms of ethics, empathy, and effectiveness must be ongoing. Once Lou and his therapist have identified a plan, they must implement it. As she goes through the implementation process, she should make observations that will help her assess whether the plan is on track and effective (e.g., does he feel understood, is he becoming more unstable, is he experiencing additional major stressors?). When she identifies a problem, she should take further action to stabilize the situation.

CHALLENGES FOR ETHICAL, EMPATHIC, EFFECTIVE THERAPISTS

Below, we describe some common domains in which therapists often find themselves facing competing demands. These domains include legal considerations, worksite requirements, financial considerations, supervisory issues, risk management, and competing priorities for and limitations of the therapist's time and energy.

Legal Considerations

The most important human endeavor is the striving for morality in our actions. Our inner balance and even our very existence depend on it.
—**Albert Einstein**

Ethical standards and legal requirements often address the same situations. However, conflicts between our Three Es and legal considerations frequently arise; as a result, decision making in clinical settings often involves many shades of gray. While ethical principles are derived from moral decisions about "right" and "wrong," legal considerations are based on a complex mix of historical precedents, social norms, and moral decisions that have evolved over many years through legislation and court cases.

For example, confidentiality is clearly an ethical standard that must be diligently maintained except under certain mandated situations, such as reporting child abuse, or when the client voluntarily gives up confidentiality. These limitations are generally clearly outlined in informed consents. However, this quickly becomes messy. Consider three examples:

Clinical Practice

While working in a prison, an inmate in counseling, Ralph, who was an alcoholic, told his therapist that he had been "clean" (abstinent) for months; however, another client told the therapist that not only was Ralph still drinking but he was also making and selling alcohol. Now that his therapist knew this information, could she use it in therapy and, if so, in what ways? Should she confront the client? Should she protect or divulge the source of her information? The informed consent said that the therapist would not share information with the prison administration, but it did not address these more mundane (and important) questions. What factors might influence these decisions?

* * * * *

Marci (age 15) was brought to treatment because she was being "disrespectful" at home and her grades were falling at school. Her mother wanted to know from the counselor whether Marci was doing anything "dangerous," although Marci wanted her privacy and forbade her therapist from disclosing any information. Further muddying this discussion, children, their parents, and clinicians may differ in their identification of "dangerous" behaviors (Hawley & Weisz, 2003; Steinberg, 2001). As family dynamics often underlie children's symptoms, helping children and teens learn to communicate with parents in safe and effective ways is often important. How can one be ethical, empathic, and effective under these circumstances?

* * * * *

Tiona was referred for treatment by Child Protective Services after she left bruises on her two daughters. Tiona accused the agency of being racist (she's African American), noting that this style of parenting was the way that she, as well as her family and friends, were raised—"It worked for me!" What ethical issues are raised by this case? How would you work with her on these issues?

Even in situations where the need to violate confidentiality is legally mandated, such as reporting abuse or ensuring the safety of a suicidal client, making such determinations is often unclear. For example, clients often talk about wanting to hurt themselves or someone else. When is such talk "letting off steam" and when is it to be taken as an urgent conveyance that the client intends harm? Some clinicians may discourage such discussions, fearing that if they know too much, they will have to act to hospitalize their client. Remaining effective and empathic requires allowing clients to fully express and explore their thoughts and feelings while remaining vigilant for signs that they may need to take some action, such as hospitalizing a particular client, based on what they are hearing (see Table 14.4). Regardless, rather than only considering *whether* suicidality and other kinds of dangerous behaviors should be disclosed, answering this question should always include considerations of *when* and *how* to disclose (Meichenbaum, 2005; Sullivan, Ramirez, Rae, Razo, & George, 2002). Disclosures should be discussed with clients first whenever possible, giving them an appropriate sense of control and choice during a difficult period.

Laws and legal precedents covering mandated reporting of child and elder abuse differ across states, as does the duty to protect, duty to warn (i.e., *Tarasoff*), requirements to report dangerous driving, and confidentiality afforded children and teenagers. Outlining these variations in state law is beyond the scope of this book, although more detail is provided in state publications and websites. Clinicians should learn the rules in their state and maintain ongoing competence on changing interpretations of these issues.

Worksite Requirements

The particular workplace in which a therapist practices comes with a unique set of considerations. Each setting will have its own intake system and strategies for managing treatment and making and documenting clinical decisions. The specifics of each setting place particular constraints and expectations on clinicians, some of which may, at times, put them in difficult situations, taxing their empathy, compromising their effectiveness, or testing their ethical decision making.

Clinical Practice

Mae (age 10) entered treatment because she was tantrumming and oppositional at home, although not at school. Her therapist, Soozie, believed that the problems were related to marital issues and the pattern of triangles and alliances occurring in the family. However, her agency does not provide family therapy—although Soozie has had considerable training and expertise in it—and her supervisor suggested individual treatment instead. Should Soozie compromise the type of treatment she offers or refer Mae's family to another facility? Does it matter if referral to another agency negatively affects Soozie's ability to maintain productivity, which is another agency

(continues)

(continued)

requirement? What if the family's ability to pay for services requires them to remain at this agency?

* * * * *

College counseling centers often limit treatment to six or eight sessions (Uffelman & Hardin, 2002). Frances begins treating a student, Leon, using a brief treatment model, but discovers that Leon's problems are much more substantial than were apparent in initial assessments and are likely to require longer-term interventions. What options should be considered?

* * * * *

Bubb hates doing paperwork and frequently gets behind in it in order to maintain the high levels of productivity required at his agency and to do the clinical work that he loves (and is gifted in doing). When Bubb's supervisor discovers that he is behind in his documentation, she pulls him off his caseload for a week and asks him to complete his back paperwork. This requires him to complete SOAP notes for sessions from as far back as several months ago, which he does not remember. What should Bubb do? Why?

Financial Considerations

Although usually related to one's workplace, financial considerations can be so problematic that they are worth highlighting on their own. The introduction of money into the therapeutic context makes many clinicians uncomfortable, yet for most practitioners, clinical work is their livelihood, making financial considerations a central part of all of their clinical involvement. Further complicating matters, many graduate programs do not discuss financial issues or only do so to a minimal extent (Bishop & Eppolito, 1992). Most graduate training programs provide insufficient training and preparation for private practice; most students do not receive any type of business management training and, even if they did, many of their faculty would not have private practice experience.

Balancing ethical standards while remaining empathic and effective can introduce financial complexities. Both clinicians in private practice and those working for agencies and nonprofits need to pay attention to how they will maintain productivity and **billable hours** while also being ethical, empathic, and effective. For many clinicians, that may mean focusing on those services where their work is reimbursed by managed care or **private pay clients** rather than those that are not. They may choose to see additional clients rather than developing client handouts, reading professional journals, or obtaining consults from other providers working with a client. They may need to think about when they will see pro bono clients and under what circumstances.

In fact, clinicians with heavy managed care involvement work longer, provide more direct contact hours, report less satisfaction with their work, and are more likely to use cognitive-behavioral approaches than clinicians with less involvement in managed care (Cantor & Fuentes, 2008; Rupert & Baird, 2004). Both articles concluded that this is a situation that increases the risk of burnout.

Financial issues can have many impacts. Small or poorly funded agencies may have such tight budgets that they are unable to purchase the most current versions of psychological assessments (but see Turchik, Karpenko, Hammers, & McNamara, 2007). Time and money may prohibit adequate supervision of sufficient length to meet licensure requirements or, when clinicians live in rural areas, good supervision may be unavailable. Budgetary restrictions may require high levels of productivity that are manageable for some clinicians, yet impossible for an otherwise strong clinician—at least if he or she is going to retain his or her ability to be empathic and competent.

Furthermore, how does one maintain productivity and remain competent given the changing research and theory in the field? Each profession and state has its own standards for continuing education for licensed professionals. Still, one could argue that these are minimal competencies and that if one only performed the required continuing education, but did not do additional reading, discuss professional issues with colleagues on an ongoing basis, or consult about issues as they arose, one would be minimally prepared. These activities are not reimbursed by managed care and clinicians may or may not be paid by employers to attend continuing education workshops. Nonetheless, clinicians who bring a broad array of conceptual perspectives to their clinical work are more likely to perceive it as successful and rewarding (Orlinsky & Ronnestad, 2005b).

Clinical Practice

Fees and client **co-payments (copays)** should be specified early in the provision of service and a discussion of them should be a normal part of the informed consent process (Pomerantz & Handelsman, 2004). The Basset family readily agreed to the fees charged by their family therapists, but became reluctant to continuing paying them when Mr. Basset lost his job and health insurance and the family faced bankruptcy. Although they were highly motivated and more stable than when they first entered treatment, their fighting still escalated into violence about twice a month. What should their family therapy team do? When, if ever, should clients' financial situations influence the type or length of services they receive?

* * * * *

Insurance companies will not cover treatment unless clients have a psychiatric diagnosis, or even a diagnosis from a particular set of diagnoses (perhaps major depressive disorder, but not ADHD). Zane, in his initial assessment of Todd (age 6), recognized that Todd's problems at home and school were related to his mother's recent diagnosis of breast cancer. He did not believe that Todd had an Axis I disorder, but does believe that

(continues)

(continued)

without early intervention, Todd may fail first grade or be placed in an Emotional Support classroom. To what degree should Zane assign diagnoses with an eye toward allowing Todd and other clients better access to treatment? What else should he consider?

* * * * *

Under normal circumstances, D'Jon is able to maintain satisfactory levels of billable hours; however, since his partner's health status has declined, D'Jon is more distracted and feels unable to handle his normal caseload. His supervisor is threatening to cut him back to part-time status if he is unable to maintain productivity, although D'Jon and his partner would then lose their health care benefits, which are vital. Further, D'Jon wonders whether his supervisor's decision is related to the significant cost of his partner's treatment for end-stage AIDS. What are his options? What should he do?

Priorities and Limitations of Time and Energy

Problems arise in that one has to find a balance between what people need from you and what you need for yourself.

—**Jessye Norman**

A clinician's work is never completely finished: There is always more that can be done, more time and attention that might be extended to clients, more people who might be helped, more preparation clinicians can do for their clients, more reading and training needed to be more fully competent at the job. Maintaining the ability to continue performing clinical work competently depends on ongoing professional development. In fact, Orlinsky and Ronnestad (2005a) reported that 86% of their multiprofessional, international sample reported being "highly motivated" to further their development as a clinician. Nonetheless, this development requires time (which might not be reimbursed) and a willingness to identify professional development as an ongoing priority.

Furthermore, clinicians are human; they have their own needs to which they must attend, their own lives to live. This becomes an ethical issue for clinicians as they struggle in balancing their own needs with their involvement with their clients, ensuring that they are functioning competently. As further discussed in Chapter 15, regular and ongoing self-awareness and self-care are essential aspects of maintaining competency (Pope & Brown, 1996). All clinicians should consider how they are going to maintain their competency and expertise while also meeting their individual and family needs.

Clinical Practice

A number of writers have argued that under some circumstances, deviations from standard professional boundaries can be helpful, but that such deviations should be thoughtfully considered and discussed with colleagues, supervisors, or clients before the fact or as soon after the fact as

(continues)

possible (Barnett, Lazarus, et al., 2007; Knapp & Slattery, 2004; Slattery, 2005; Zur, 2001). What factors would you use to evaluate whether attending a client's wedding would be ethical, empathic, and effective? Would thinking about your own stress levels and time constraints be part of this picture? Why or why not?

* * * * *

There are a number of ways to think about the problems that Lia Lee's doctors had in working with the Lee family (Chapters 8 and 10). One way, though, is that her doctors were overextended and in a hurry to get things done. Because they did not recognize their limits, they did not listen to the family as well as they might have otherwise. What could you do to maintain a competent practice even when you are busy?

Supervisory Issues

Supervisors need to balance a number of different concerns, some of which may be of greater or lesser importance depending on whether they are working in a setting focused primarily on training or one that focuses on offering clinical services and only secondarily offers training and supervision. As a result, supervisors may emphasize, to differing degrees, training and development or service quality and productivity.

A multiprofessional, international research project examining correlates of clinical development and career satisfaction found that clinicians who were most satisfied with their career development reported both greater support and autonomy in the workplace (Orlinsky & Ronnestad, 2005b). Perhaps surprisingly, clinicians who described greater breadth and depth of case experience also reported greater career development. Satisfied clinicians also reported more client growth and perceived their clinical work as promoting client healing. Conversely, clinicians who experienced greater work-related frustrations (e.g., cancellations, slow client growth, client suicides) were least satisfied with their careers.

Given these findings, Ronnestad and Orlinsky (2005) made a number of recommendations for training clinicians at all levels (see Table 14.5). In particular, they suggested that supervisors who were concerned with their supervisees' growth and career development should give them direct clinical training from early on in their careers and provide opportunities to work with a diversity of clinical problems and a range of treatment modalities, including individual, relational, family, and group. Supervisors should assign cases so that supervisees experience clinical work as positive and healing, while limiting probable stressful experiences when possible. Furthermore, supervision should be provided in a positive and supportive atmosphere, with ample social support, in the context of a good working alliance.

TABLE **14.5**

Factors to Consider in Promoting Positive Career Development in New Clinicians.

1. **Interpersonal skills.** Should have well-developed interpersonal skills at the entry to training program. New clinicians should perceive themselves as having well-developed skills and the ability to develop warm relationships.
2. **Theoretical and technical training.** Training should be pragmatic rather than ideological in spirit, encouraging theoretical breadth, flexible application, and openness to learning.
3. **Direct clinical work.** Clinical work should begin early in clinical training, after students have received an orientation to the theory and technique relevant to their field.
4. **Case selection.** Cases offered should consider interns' skill levels and probable client challenges, in order to maximize their experience of clinical work as positive and healing, while limiting or buffering probable stressful experiences. Cases should include diversity in problems and treatment modalities (i.e., individual, group, relational, and family).
5. **Supervision and ample social support.** Supervision should provide ample social support, emphasizing the development of a good working alliance with trainees.
6. **Self-monitoring.** New clinicians should monitor their emotional reactions both during and out of clinical work, their caseload composition, and level of social support.

Note: Modified from Ronnestad and Orlinsky (2005).

Clinical Practice

Theo, a newly hired supervisor, is considering what tasks to assign to his new interns. On the one hand, he knows that the training process will be most successful if he assigns interns a range of client problems and modalities of treatment, but on the other hand, he wants his interns to have a positive experience (also correlated with career development). Furthermore, he wants his clinic to provide high-quality care. How could Theo approach thinking about these tensions between the needs of his interns, those of the clinic's clients, and the clinic's reputation? What other factors should he think about?

* * * * *

Fernanda is supervising Bubb, who is several months behind in his casework. She recognizes that Bubb is a talented therapist, but is also highly worried that they have no documentation for hundreds of billable hours. She is concerned that they may get audited and be unable to document their provision of services. She is also worried about what might happen in the admittedly infrequent case of a client suicide and how this might leave Bubb, her, and the agency open to a lawsuit. Furthermore, she is hesitant to continuing supervising someone who is willing to cut such corners in his work. What might she consider as she attempts to resolve this situation well?

TOWARD A POSITIVE APPROACH TO ETHICS

A man who has committed a mistake and doesn't correct it is committing another mistake.

—Confucious

Codes of ethics have historically been approached from a defensive posture—that is, what should not be done (Handelsman, Knapp & Gottlieb, 2002). The standards in the ethics codes, however, only describe minimal expectations and identify the behaviors that can lead to disciplinary action when violated. Rather than only meeting minimal qualifications, a more positive approach to competency, for example, includes an ongoing striving for the highest standards of competence (Knapp & Vandecreek, 2006). Clinicians should look for ways to enhance the nature of their relationships with clients, supervisees, and colleagues rather than only avoiding boundary violations and exploitive relationships. They should involve clients in decisions throughout treatment rather than only at its beginning; these decisions could include identifying treatment goals and interventions and discussing when and how therapy will end. They develop trustworthy relationships rather than only avoiding making prohibited disclosures. Instead of only avoiding being prejudiced or discriminating, they are open-minded, learn about other cultural viewpoints, develop their case conceptualizations using this knowledge, and promote fairness throughout their work (Knapp & Vandecreek, 2006; D. W. Sue & Sue, 2003). Consider how Ms. Jacasum and the other cases presented in this chapter might be handled differently using a positive approach to ethics rather than only following the defensive posture of the ethical standards.

When treated individually and in isolation, the aspirational principles and ethical standards can lead to an overly simplistic and caretaking approach to practice. For example, avoiding collecting information on child abuse in order to not further traumatize a client can itself be harmful, because avoiding these discussions suggests that abuse—and the people who were abused—are shameful (Becker-Blease & Freyd, 2006). Treating clients as though they were fragile or incompetent can be harmful, as it can create a self-fulfilling prophecy. On the other hand, openly discussing abuse, violence, loss, and oppression can be both distressing *and* helpful.

When balanced by each other and by the aspirational principles, the ethical standards provide a rich, thoughtful, and respectful way of doing clinical work. Clinicians can foster autonomy in decisions about end-of-life care, for example, while also recognizing that clients from another culture may perceive the process of decision making differently than they do. For many middle- and upper-class Euro Americans, responding to a cancer diagnosis is often primarily an individual decision; however, clinicians working with other ethnic groups, classes, and cultures might consider how treatment and other end-of-life decisions will impact the family as a whole (Candib, 2002). Nondisclosure of a cancer diagnosis might be seen as a paternalistic act in the United States, although in other countries (e.g., Italy, Vietnam, and Russia) such nondisclosure might be seen as an act that maintains hope and an ongoing sense of aliveness and connection in the patient (Candib, 2002).

PERSONAL AND PROFESSIONAL IDENTITIES

For many people, clinical work is "not only a job but also a calling, or vocation, a worthy profession that is chosen at least in part to provide a sense of meaningful activity and personal fulfillment" (Orlinsky et al., 2005, p. 11).

I now know myself to be a person of weakness and strength, liability and giftedness, darkness and light. I now know that to be whole means to reject none of it but to embrace all of it.

—Parker Palmer

How one sees oneself as a person and as a professional influences the nature of this calling and whether and how one grows.

We suggest that clinicians must develop clear personal and professional identities that foster ethical, empathic, and effective clinical work. One's personal identity frames one's ethics, values, goals, sources of meaning, and choices about how to spend one's time. Clinicians who identify as fair, honest, trusting, and open-minded will make different personal and professional decisions than those who hold other types of self-concepts. One's personal and professional worldview and values frame the nature of one's practice and work and its quality (Fowers & Davidov, 2006; Jennings et al., 2005). In fact, Jennings and his colleagues concluded that master therapists tended to share a common set of specific personal and professional values, which are outlined in Table 14.6.

Clinicians should assess their strengths and weaknesses, skills, and emotional resources on an ongoing basis (Bennett et al., 2006). A careful personal skill inventory also acknowledges that all characteristics are a double-edged sword: One's strengths can also be weaknesses, and one's weaknesses can serve as strengths (Bashe et al., 2007). A clinician may be proud of his empathy, for example, but should also be aware of how it sometimes interferes with his ability to be objective in assessing his clients. Another clinician may recognize that she sets strong personal boundaries and engages in regular self-care, yet find it difficult to work with crisis calls when they occur outside of regular work hours. Recognizing these strengths and weaknesses can be a proactive strategy for maintaining an effective practice.

Professional identity includes the centrality of one's identification as a clinician in one's chosen field and the meaning of that membership, one's perception of the tasks and goals that are central to that identity, and the ethical principles guiding that work. Professional identity influences not only what is done but also *how* it is done. Given their client population, work setting, theoretical orientation, agency policies, and so on, clinicians should develop a solid sense of the goals, values, beliefs, and theoretical assumptions that will guide their resolution of the clinical decisions that they must make throughout the day.

TABLE **14.6**
Values Strongly Endorsed by Master Therapists.

Building and maintaining interpersonal attachments
1. Relational connection
2. Autonomy
3. Beneficence
4. Nonmaleficence

Building and maintaining expertise
1. Competence
2. Humility
3. Professional growth
4. Openness to complexity and ambiguity
5. Self-awareness

Note: From Jennings et al. (2005).

In the best of all possible worlds, personal and professional identities will work together and support each other. For example, if a clinician's personal identity is that she is a "caring person," but she defines that in terms of giving hugs and gifts and being available at all hours in ways that are incompatible with her work with sex offenders, she is likely to become frustrated and is at greater risk of burning out (Baker, 2003). A clinician who believes that poor people live in poverty due to their own poor work ethic, yet is working in a community counseling center populated by the working poor, may have difficulty believing that his clients can change—even though he may be very effective in another setting. Clinicians who act in an open-minded and accepting manner but who do not think and feel that way are unlikely to be seen as genuine, and their interventions are likely to be less effective. Finding a setting, a population, and a way of being a clinician that is consistent with and supported by one's personal identity (e.g., strengths, weaknesses, skills, values, goals) is likely to lead to the greatest feelings of satisfaction and the fewest frustrations and stressors that increase the risk of burnout (Baker, 2003; Handelsman et al., 2005; Ronnestad & Orlinsky, 2005).

ALIGNING PERSONAL AND PROFESSIONAL ETHICS

The value of identity of course is that so often with it comes purpose.
—**Robert R. Grant**

Ethics and morals are important aspects of personal and professional identity. In the best-case scenario, one's professional and personal ethics enrich each other (Fowers & Davidov, 2006; Handelsman et al., 2005; Kitchener, 1984). Unfortunately, as illustrated by descriptions of various professional dilemmas throughout this book, this is not always the case. Dr. Helper (Chapter 2) crossed a number of professional boundaries in order to "help" a dead client's wife. Would he have made different decisions if his professional ethics had informed his decisions to a greater degree? Dr. Saeed's (Chapter 2) decision to discharge Andrea Yates from the hospital appeared to be primarily motivated by his perception of demands from managed care and limited time and less by his personal and professional ethics.

When clinicians are working from both their own spiritual or cultural values as well as their field's professional code and they actively search for ways to integrate both sets of values (Integration), they have a richer and more sophisticated decision-making process to access during treatment (Handelsman et al., 2005) (see Table 14.7). Rather than choosing between these two

TABLE **14.7**
An Ethical Acculturation Model.

		Personal Ethics	
		Low	High
Identification with professional ethics	Low	Marginalization	Separation
	High	Assimilation	Integration

Note: Adapted from Handelsman et al. (2005).

apparently competing sets of ethics, they should use both to inform decisions and help them navigate difficult decisions.

Relative to clinicians in Integration, clinicians working from only their personal or professional values (respectively, Separation or Assimilation) have a more difficult time responding to ethical problems, are more likely to feel alienated from either their personal values or their profession, and be at greater risk of burning out (Handelsman et al., 2005). Clinicians who adopt an Assimilation approach may apply state law and their profession's ethical standards in a rote manner without understanding the standard's underlying principles or recognizing that they are an insufficient guide to practice. Handelsman and his colleagues note that this is like "building a strong structure on a shaky foundation, and it may lead to empty, legalistic, and overly simplistic applications of our ethical principles" (p. 61). On the other hand, clinicians who have adopted a Separation stance do not use their ethical standards to guide their decision making. They may make "kind" gestures at the expense of their clients' autonomy or confidentiality, be frustrated by the limitations of the ethics code (without seeing its strengths), or believe that their personal values are stronger and more useful than those of their profession.

Clinicians adopting a Marginalization stance may be at even greater risk of an ethical infraction because they are rudderless, without the guide of a personal moral code or professional ethics (Handelsman et al., 2005). Even good and ethical clinicians may be marginalized from personal and professional ethics during a personal crisis. More effective clinicians can see clinical issues, including informed consent, confidentiality, dual relationships, and other issues, from the point of view of friendship, while also seeing them from their profession's ethical standards and principles. Furthermore, understanding one's implicit moral code and values may make it easier to appreciate the underlying principles governing the ethics codes.

SUMMARY

A positive ethical practice should be more than a defensive application of ethical standards in a rote manner (Handelsman et al., 2005); it should instead be directed by larger personal and professional aspirations. Other factors that should affect and inform clinicians' decisions include paying attention to the aspirational standards, legal statutes, state laws, court rulings, their personal moral code and theoretical approach, agency requirements, and client diagnosis and treatment plan. These can occasionally be at odds with each other. These dilemmas can be negotiated by aiming for clinical work that is empathic, ethical, and effective.

We provide a framework within which to make ethical decisions. This includes (a) developing a broad perspective that considers multiple factors (e.g., ethical standards, aspirational principles, laws and rulings, agency policies, theoretical orientation, the client's viewpoint, clinical self-interest), (b) identifying and evaluating multiple options, (c) choosing a plan, (d) taking action, and (e) monitoring feedback about the plan's effectiveness. Examples of the real-world challenges that one might face during clinical work are presented, including legal considerations, worksite requirements, financial considerations, priorities and limitations of time and energy, and supervisory issues.

A positive ethics is informed by one's clinical goals and aspirations, but is also supported by one's personal morals, values, and sense of identity. Under the best possible circumstances one's personal and professional identities and one's personal and professional ethics will inform and be supportive of each other.

How Do These Issues Apply to Your Life and Work?

1. Perform a personal skill inventory, including your current skill levels across a wide variety of realms, competencies, attitudes, and personal strengths and weaknesses, especially as they might impact your clinical practice (Bashe et al., 2007; Bennett et al., 2006). What are your strengths and weaknesses? How can your strengths serve as weaknesses? How can your weaknesses serve as strengths? What does this assessment suggest you should do to continue to develop as an ethical clinician?

2. Return to the "ethics autobiography" (Bashe et al., 2007) you wrote in Chapter 2. Consider how these experiences might intersect with and either support or challenge your new discipline's ethical standards and principles. What does it suggest about your ethical acculturation? (see Table 14.7).

3. What ethical challenges have you encountered in the course of your practice thus far? What were the competing factors and demands that you experienced in these situations? As you outline strategies for resolving these challenges, what are the short-term and long-term costs and benefits of each option?

4. Consider what your experience would have been if you had been the client in the previously described situations (Kitchener, 1986). Does this reflection change your perception of the situation? Would it change your behavior and, if so, how?

CHAPTER 15

Professional and Personal Self-Care

WHERE ARE WE GOING?

1. What is self-care? Why is it important?

2. What dangers do empathic clinicians face in their work?

3. How can clinicians remain vigilant to these dangers?

4. What other stresses do clinicians face?

5. What types of coping strategies are best for dealing with stress?

6. Rather than just learning to deal effectively with stress, how can we prevent it?

How Do You Do It?

Sheila Carluccio

As posted on a listserv for psychologists:

I'm tossing this out for discussion as I have recently returned part-time to private practice after a long medical leave. Currently, I find myself trying to carefully balance client care, with personal care, with caring for my mother who is in the hospital after undergoing open heart surgery.

One year ago my mother had a stroke which left her partially blind. At the time, I queried the listserv for psychologists in our area who might provide specialty treatment for medical issues in the geriatric population. I received not only recommendations for referrals but also a flood of warm, supportive responses from this list; many shared the difficulties they too faced caring for ill and elderly relatives. It was a difficult time, and my focus was about obtaining the best possible referrals for her.

But that's not why I am writing now. This time it's about *me*. This post is about balancing caretaking with self-care. About struggling to advocate for a hospitalized relative when you believe you see medical mishaps that may not endanger life but impact the quality of care they are receiving, struggling with feeling your emotions without acting out in such emotionally charged medical situations, struggling to be present to clients when an ill family member is on your mind, struggling with guilt watching family members pour out their caretaking 24/7 because you're struggling with feeling *selfish* if you include self-care in that equation. Struggling with the ever-evolving personal awareness that life is fragile and short and should not be wasted.

I hope I do not come across as *whining.* I know others here have been through much worse. I'd like to hear how they worked their way through self-care while remaining caring to personal and professional others. (S. Carluccio, personal communication, March, 2009)

- What barriers to self-care does Ms. Carluccio identify? What impact does she see this situation as having on her work as a psychologist?
- What do you think of a clinician who, like Ms. Carluccio, asks these questions? Why? What about one who is stressed and distressed, but who does not ask such questions?
- If you've asked similar questions about yourself, how did you feel about doing so? When were you most likely to ask these questions?

SELF-AWARENESS AND SELF-CARE

Life shrinks or expands in proportion to one's courage.
—Anais Nin

Treatment can be reactive, responsive to every gust of wind, or proactive, with a structure that guides the course of treatment and prevents problems. In the course of this book we have outlined several strategies for remaining proactive and forward-thinking in treatment, including using the therapeutic alliance, ethical guidelines, assessments, and treatment plan to set and guide the course of treatment. In this chapter we suggest two additional guides for treatment: self-awareness and self-care.

As discussed in Chapter 2, an important part of being ethical is regularly assessing one's skills, competencies, attitudes, strengths, and weaknesses, especially as they impact clinical practice (Bennett et al., 2006). However, *remaining* ethical requires ongoing self-monitoring and self-care, which includes attending to factors in the past or present that may negatively impact clinical skills, competencies, and attitudes about treatment and clients, even recognizing the ways that strengths can sometimes serve as weaknesses (Bashe et al., 2007). Remaining ethical includes being vigilant to signs within and across sessions, including blurred boundaries, increased cynicism and boredom, failures in being empathic, and vicarious traumatization.

DANGERS IN PROVIDING EMPATHIC THERAPY

As soon as there is life, there is danger.
—**Ralph Waldo Emerson**

As we have discussed throughout this book, empathy is key to working effectively with a range of clients and issues. Being an empathic clinician means allowing oneself to be emotionally open and receptive to the feelings of one's clients and striving to understand how one's clients perceive the world and themselves. However, continuously providing empathic treatment can be quite demanding for clinicians, and maintaining a balance between healthy emotional availability and respectful distance and objectivity is an ongoing challenge for all empathic clinicians (Wicks, 2008). Good self-care is particularly essential when empathy is an important value.

Self-care involves attending to one's own needs, which are basic to all human beings; these needs include paying attention to the health of one's physical, cognitive, emotional, and spiritual self (Carroll, Gilroy, & Murra, 1999). Taking good care of oneself, both personally and professionally, is critically important in becoming and remaining an effective clinician. In addition, good self-care increases clinicians' chances of remaining mentally and physically healthy and whole.

Self-care serves multiple functions in providing effective therapy. First, it allows clinicians to be more empathic and engaged while minimizing dangers such as burnout, as discussed below (Coster & Schwebel, 1997; Schwebel & Coster, 1998). Second, modeling a healthful lifestyle powerfully enhances the effectiveness of any therapeutic intervention. Finally, good self-care protects clients by reducing the risk of ethical violations on the part of the clinician (Carroll et al., 1999). In fact, some clinicians have termed self-care an "an ethical imperative" in that they consider it essential for avoiding harming clients (Barnett, Baker, Elman, & Schoener, 2007; Carroll et al., 1999).

Most practicing clinicians recognize that self-care is important, and they also well know many of the strategies for good self-care (Wicks, 2008). In fact, clinicians generally encourage and emphasize self-care with their clients (Carroll et al., 1999). Yet, when it comes to their own practice of self-care, clinicians are generally not very good at it (Baker, 2003). Why would this be so? Many clinicians give the same reasons for their inadequate self-care as anyone else would—lack of time, competing priorities, and lack of energy. In addition, clinicians often place the care of others ahead of the care of themselves, deny their own needs, and feel "selfish" or guilty when attending to their own care (Carroll et al., 1999; Wicks, 2008).

Nonetheless, providing effective treatment requires maintaining clear interpersonal boundaries between self and clients, remaining healthy and emotionally present and engaged in clinical work, and helping clients deal with traumatic issues without vicariously experiencing trauma oneself. Empathic clinicians who do not maintain a healthy balance in their lives are at greater risk of blurred boundaries, burnout, and vicarious traumatization (Bennett et al., 2006). Furthermore, stressed clinicians who are out of balance in their personal lives may react impulsively toward clients whom they perceive as demanding, manipulative, or irritating. They may also engage in enabling behaviors that do not meet the client's long-term needs because they are unable to step back and see the big picture for treatment.

Blurred Boundaries

In the context of therapy, **boundaries** involve frames, or a shared understanding, that define the roles for the clinician and client. The frame provides the "ground rules of therapy," including both the structure (e.g., time, place, and money) and the content (what actually transpires between clinician and client) of session time (Smith & Fitzpatrick, 1995).

As discussed in Chapter 2, it is useful to distinguish between boundary crossings and boundary violations. A boundary crossing is a nonpejorative term describing departures from commonly accepted practice, which may or may not benefit the client (Guthiel & Gabbard, 1993; Smith & Fitzpatrick, 1995). Boundary violations are departures that most clinicians would see as dangerous, with a high probability of a negative outcome for clients. These include dual relationships, such as sexual relationships and bartering.

Most clinicians would not intentionally engage in boundary violations, or other behaviors that they see as potentially harming their clients. Few newly licensed psychologists would report expecting to have sex with a client over the course of their career; yet in one now-dated study, about 9.4% of men and 2.5% of women reported having had a sexual relationship with at least one client over the course of their career (Pope, Keith-Spiegel, & Tabachnik, 1986). In addition, many reported having had romantic or sexual feelings toward a client at least occasionally over the course of their career. Ethical and competent clinicians recognize sexual feelings, engage in regular self-care in order to reduce the risk of engaging in boundary violations, request consultations to prevent harm to clients, and keep current on ethical guidelines through readings, supervision, and trainings (Bennett et al., 1996).

Ethical clinicians monitor when they engage in boundary crossings which, although they are less serious behaviors, put clinicians at greater risk of engaging in a boundary violation (Guthiel & Gabbard, 1993; Lamb & Catanzaro, 1998). One study found that clinicians reporting having made some types of boundary crossings (e.g., disclosing details of a personal stressor, crying in front of a client, giving the client unused sports or theatre tickets) were more likely to report engaging in sexual relationships with clients (Lamb & Catanzaro, 1998). This conclusion can be interpreted in at least two ways—either that boundary crossings increase clinicians' risk for boundary violations or that clinicians engaging in boundary violations also engage in boundary crossings. In any case, clinicians should acknowledge when they are considering engaging in boundary crossings, recognize their motivations for the behavior and the suspected costs and benefits of engaging in the behavior, and thoughtfully discuss deviations from professional norms with colleagues, supervisors, or the clients themselves as soon as possible (Barnett, Lazarus et al., 2007; Bennett et al., 2006).

Although ethical and competent clinicians can readily agree in theory that setting healthy boundaries is an essential part of good clinical work, what this means in practice can often be unclear because of the wide range of accepted theoretical models, interventions, and settings used in the field (Epstein & Simon, 1990; Knapp & Slattery, 2004; Slattery, 2005). Psychoanalytically oriented therapists may see self-disclosure and supportive work as ineffective, inappropriate, and outside acceptable boundaries. However, clinicians working in community settings, visiting clients who are seriously ill or have transportation problems, or doing in vivo generalization of skills in the community draw effective and helpful boundaries differently (Epstein & Simon, 1990; Knapp & Slattery, 2004; Slattery, 2005; Zur, 2001).

Clinical Practice

Phyllis has been having difficulty with her teenaged sons (ages 14 and 15), who violate family rules and reject parental opinions. She has been thinking a lot about her client, Charlie (age 13), whose parents are critical and neglectful of his needs. He has been in crisis recently and their sessions have frequently been extending beyond their normal limits. How would she know whether these boundary crossings are helpful or problematic? What actions should she be thinking about at this point?

Burnout

Burnout in health care providers, sometimes called compassion fatigue, refers to a progressive loss of idealism, energy, and sense of purpose for the work of therapy. Burnout is characterized by emotional exhaustion, an increased depersonalization of clients, and a decreased sense of personal accomplishment (Jenaro, Flores, & Arias, 2007; Rupert & Kent, 2007). Clinicians who are burning out may feel hopeless, disengage from their clients, and experience symptoms of stress, depression, and anxiety (Wicks, 2008). Burnout is caused by both work-related factors, such as excessive workload and lack of control, and personal factors, such as unmet needs (Baker, 2003). Several studies of clinicians found that those with high self-efficacy, a sense of personal accomplishment, job satisfaction, and positive coping strategies were less likely to report feelings of burnout (Jenaro et al., 2007; Kramen-Kahn & Hansen, 1998). Consider how Michael Partie describes this process of burnout for both clients and clinicians.

How Can We Avoid Being "Institutionalized"?
Michael Partie

Michael Partie (2005) suggests that mental health treatment can either enlarge or shrink people's view of themselves and the world. He did not stop there, however, noting that we ourselves experience moral decay working in some settings and with some people—unless we act to prevent this from happening.

> The people we support live in very small worlds, worlds often kept small by the manner in which we deliver services. Helping people expand the size of their worlds—socially, vocationally, physically, emotionally, recreationally, and existentially—must be a top priority. Institutionalization isn't about the kind of buildings or real estate one occupies, it's about the loss of power, movement, freedom, and vision.
>
> But how do we keep ourselves from becoming institutionalized?
>
> [In *A leg to stand on*, the neurologist] Oliver Sack points out that the process [of institutionalization] is often unseen and unheard, and can overtake any of us unaware. Awareness and the will to resist institutionalizing influences in ourselves and in others is a good start. Reflecting on our own practices and questioning our assumptions can keep us from becoming lazy or lapsing into superstition. Celebrating successes—individual and group—can keep us positively focused. Practicing honesty and individual integrity, honoring the good work of others, courageously confronting our colleagues when needed, receiving praise with grace and correction with gratitude, and perhaps most importantly of all, approaching the lives of others with humility, are all ways we can keep our humanity as we help others to live full lives. (para 9–11)

- Have there been some settings or periods of time when you have felt yourself becoming "institutionalized"? If so, how did you recognize this? What helped you break free? Or, if you are feeling stuck now, what helped you stay positively focused during better periods?

Vicarious Traumatization

When clinicians work with clients who are victims or survivors of violence and other traumatic events, they are at risk for vicarious traumatization, also called secondary victimization. **Vicarious traumatization** is a cumulative process "through which the therapist's inner experience is negatively transformed through empathic engagement with clients' trauma material" (Sabin-Farrell & Turpin, 2003, p. 279). Vicarious traumatization can also lead to clinicians' distancing, becoming insensitive or losing trust in others, as their clients' experiences and worldview begin to influence their own views (Baker, 2003).

Importantly, by definition, vicarious traumatization results from engaging empathically with clients' traumatic material (Sabin-Farrell & Turpin, 2003). That is, by being open to clients' pain, empathic clinicians risk absorbing that pain into themselves. For example, clinicians may incorporate their clients' painful stories into their own memory, which may lead to clinicians' experiencing flashbacks, trauma dreams, or intrusive thoughts, all symptoms of posttraumatic stress (Dunkley & Whelan, 2006). One study found that new clinicians and those with their own trauma histories were most likely to report psychological difficulties in the course of doing trauma work (Pearlman & Mac Ian, 1995).

Clinical Practice

Sam is a second-year graduate student who has recently been working with a client with a history of child abuse. Since beginning this work he has been irritable and having more problems sleeping. He is wondering whether he should tell his supervisor and what, if anything else, he should do.

REMAINING VIGILANT TO DANGERS IN PROVIDING EMPATHIC THERAPY

In dealing with those who are undergoing great suffering, if you feel "burnout" setting in, if you feel demoralized and exhausted, it is best, for the sake of everyone, to withdraw and restore yourself. The point is to have a long-term perspective.

—**Dalai Lama**

Because these dangers are ever-present for empathic clinicians, it is critical that clinicians learn about and understand them and remain vigilant in their own work for signs of these problems. This vigilance requires a commitment to honest and ongoing self-evaluation and a willingness to make changes in one's work when signals of these problems are detected (Baker, 2003). Many useful resources have been developed to help clinicians remain on their toes and prevent problems proactively—or at least as early as possible.

Clinicians should learn to recognize blurred boundaries and symptoms of burnout and vicarious traumatization. Clinicians may recognize blurred boundaries when they have moved into nontherapeutic roles or are engaging in behaviors that are at cross-purposes with clinical work (Pope et al., 1988; Slattery, 2005). Symptoms of burnout include feeling particularly cranky and irritable, resentful of time spent on others, relief when clients cancel, bored or apathetic about one's work or clients, exhausted, cynical, or isolated on a regular rather than occasional basis (Jenaro et al., 2007; Weiss, 2004).

It is likely that most, if not all clinicians, occasionally feel bored, exhausted, cynical, and unempathic (Pope & Vasquez, 2005) (see Table 15.1). Ideally, however, clinicians will recognize these early signs and intervene quickly. Clinicians should use supervision, peer supervision, and formal and informal consultation to help them objectively appraise their management of these ever-present dangers. A number of books provide checklists and questions for reflection (Baker, 2003; Pope & Vasquez, 2005; Wicks, 2008). These resources can be quite useful in facilitating this ongoing self-evaluation, but, of course, are only useful when used regularly!

Finally, as described in Chapter 2, clinical risk can be thought of as a function of four variables (i.e., client factors, clinician factors, intervention,

TABLE **15.1**
Problems That May Signal a Need for More Regular or Stronger Self-Care.

- **Holding negative attitudes about clients.** Focusing on clients' diagnoses, weaknesses, problems in motivation, and labels (e.g., "That borderline"), telling jokes about clients, ridiculing them.
- **Holding negative attitudes about clinical work.** Seeing their own work as meaningless, useless, and insufficient, or counseling and psychotherapy in general as a charade or fraud.
- **Making mistakes.** Although everyone makes mistakes, may make more mistakes than usual.
- **Lacking energy.** May wake up tired, be fatigued during the day, and be too exhausted at the end of the day to spend with family, friends, or do the things that would normally be fun.
- **Becoming more anxious and afraid at work.** Having difficulty negotiating the pressures, uncertainties, ambiguity, challenges, and stress of clinical practice. Clinical work requires optimism, hopefulness, and self-efficacy.
- **Using work to avoid negative feelings.** Work can produce feelings of joy, accomplishment, meaning, and purpose, but can also be used to avoid unhappiness and discontent in the rest of one's life.
- **Losing interest.** Going through the motions, being numb, losing interest in work, clients, and other parts of life.

Note: Modified from Pope & Vasquez (2005).

and context; Bennett et al., 2006). Being aware of these factors—especially the clinician factors—can guide one's regular assessment of skills, knowledge, emotional resources, and experience; moderate ongoing risk factors; manage stressors proactively; and reduce cognitive demands during crises. Although this practice does not have the same sort of allure as suggesting regular bubble baths and massages, maintaining a healthy clinical life and preventing problems can be an important tool in managing work-related stress well.

OTHER STRESSORS IN THE LIFE OF A CLINICIAN

Although these empathy-related dangers have been identified as particularly problematic for clinicians endeavoring to remain empathic and balanced, it is important to note that clinicians face many other stressors. These stressors also have the potential to take their toll on clinicians' own well-being as well as reducing their effectiveness in helping others. Some of these stressors are specific to the work of helping professionals while others are more ubiquitous in human life. Regardless of their nature, stressors can have a cumulative deleterious impact on clinicians' well-being. Dealing effectively with these stressors begins with recognizing them. Weiss (2004) identified four domains of stressors particularly relevant to counselors and therapists: client-induced stress, stress due to the work environment, self-induced internal stress, and stress related to events in one's own personal life.

Client-induced stress derives from the nature of clinical work. Clinicians encounter angry clients who throw tantrums or have outbursts; clients whose intense depression, suicidal ideation, or threats are frightening; clients who make accusations of incompetence or lack of caring; and clients who leave treatment prematurely (Weiss, 2004). Connecting empathically with these clients can create stress and distress for clinicians. Furthermore, each of these types of clients raises difficult questions.

- What is a realistic assessment of the clinician's role, if any, in current problems? To what degree are the client's accusations accurate?
- Are assessments and interventions on track? Do they reflect the quality care that this client deserves?
- Is this client receiving the appropriate type and level of care? Does this client require a higher level of care than can be realistically offered in this setting?
- What changes, if any, would help better stabilize this client?

Work environment stress comes from aspects of the settings in which clinicians work, including time pressure, excessive caseload size, organizational politics, nonsupportive colleagues, incompetent supervision, and excessive paperwork (Weiss, 2004). In one study, clinicians in agency settings reported lower levels of accomplishment and satisfaction and more stress than those in solo or group independent practice (Rupert & Kent, 2007), perhaps because those working in agencies have less control over their workloads, more exposure to managed care issues, greater time pressures, and more paperwork. Beginning clinicians may also experience additional stressors, including the pressures of obtaining licensure while also mastering clinical skills and obtaining the breadth and depth of experience needed to perform with adequate levels of competence (Baker, 2003; Weiss, 2004).

Self-induced stress involves clinicians' expectations for themselves, which may be unrealistic, as well as their fears of failure, self-doubt, feelings of perfectionism, need for approval, and emotional depletion (Weiss, 2004). Normal worry and fears can be adaptive, as they can serve as signposts, helping clinicians identify and prevent potential problems in treatment; nonetheless, excessive, unrealistic, and continuing fears and negative self-evaluations are problematic. Of course, clinicians are not the only ones who experience such self-induced stress, but they may face particular struggles with emotional depletion due to both their own expectations and those that others hold for them.

Event-related stress comes from many sources, including major life transitions, physical or medical problems, money pressures, and family issues (Weiss, 2004). Everyone is prone to these stressors, clinicians probably no more so than average. However, because stress is cumulative, these stressors add to the burden of stress posed by the other types of stress.

Clinical Practice

Harley is a supervisor of a small department in an urban community mental health center. Her staff has high caseloads and is paid poorly, things that she cannot control. She is wondering what she can do in order to reduce their stress, increase their job satisfaction, and prevent burnout.

COPING EFFECTIVELY WITH EMPATHIC HAZARDS AND LIFE STRESSORS

Our greatest glory is not in never falling, but in rising every time we fall.

—**Confucius**

Even though clinicians are trained to help others deal more adaptively with stress, as we noted above, they are often not particularly good at applying what they know about effective coping to the issues arising in their own lives (Gilroy, Carroll, & Murra, 2002; Radeke & Mahoney, 2000). Levels of distress, anxiety, and depression are high among clinicians (Gilroy et al., 2002; Radeke & Mahoney, 2000), leading to much misery for clinicians in their personal lives as well as impaired effectiveness in their professional lives.

Effective coping begins with thorough self-knowledge, gained through an ongoing process of self-assessment and self-awareness (Bennett et al., 2006; Gilroy et al., 2002). Self-assessments should attend to personal risk factors and warning signs. Personal risk factors include work with certain types of clients, the presence of increased challenges or stresses in one's personal life, and health or mental health difficulties. Warning signs include increased feelings of frustration, impatience, or anger toward clients; increased boredom or lack of focus; hope that certain clients will cancel their appointments; increased fatigue; decreased motivation; and decreased fulfillment and enjoyment from one's work (Barnett, Baker et al., 2007; Pope & Vasquez, 2005). During this process of self-assessment, Coster and Schwebel (1997) recommend asking questions like the following:

1. When clients have symptoms like mine, what would I look for? What actions would I propose?
2. What is happening when I am feeling depressed or like a failure? Am I forgetting to take care of myself? Have I been working with difficult clients without increasing my self-care? Has my client load decreased, causing me to worry about my income and job security?
3. When I am attracted to a client, how is this related to problems with my partner or in other parts of my personal life?
4. When I am feeling disillusioned, how is this related to having to focus on the less rewarding parts of work, including paperwork and corresponding with insurance companies?

When self-assessment and self-awareness are not sufficient, Coster and Schwebel (1997) recommend seeking help from a trusted colleague or peer, which may sufficiently help to normalize reactions, gather psychological support, change perspectives, increase resources, or decrease stressors. For some people, this process of self-assessment may include sporadic or ongoing psychotherapy, which can provide additional objectivity and resources, deepen self-awareness, identify ways of handling difficult issues raised in the course of treating others, and ascertain when work is a way of avoiding issues in one's personal life.

Clinicians face a number of barriers to self-care beyond that of the general population (Baker, 2003). Although some educators of clinicians-in-training advocate that personal therapy be a requirement of training (Schwebel & Coster, 1998), many clinicians are reluctant to seek psychotherapy for themselves, seeing a need for it as a sign of professional inadequacy and weakness.

They may hold problematic beliefs, including that they should be self-reliant and in control, and a paragon of mental health. They may have a difficult time shifting roles to become a client, with its associated vulnerabilities and decreased perceptions of control. While they may accept that one's personal psychotherapy is important to being effective as a psychotherapist, they may have a difficult time seeing how they can be helpful to others while they are themselves struggling.

BEING PROACTIVE: PREVENTION OF EMPATHY AND STRESS-RELATED PROBLEMS

You will make mistakes. You cannot help everyone. You will not know everything. You cannot go it alone.

— Bennett et al., 2006, p. 5

The helping professions focus extensively on helping people heal from damage they have already sustained. While healing is necessary, clinicians must remain mindful that the preferred approach is to actually *prevent* damage and promote health and well-being (Keyes & Haidt, 2003). This is true not only for clients but also for clinicians themselves. There are many ways that clinicians can be proactive and create conditions in their work and in their lives that minimize exposure to stressors and equip them with effective resources to minimize the impact of the stressors that they do encounter (Schwarzer, 2001) (see Table 15.2).

Probably the most important proactive stress deterrent is having strong interpersonal bonds. Maintaining strong relationships with family and friends is critically important not only for living a healthy, happy life but also for building a system of social support that can provide instrumental, tangible, and emotional support if and when the need arises (Kramen-Kahn & Hansen, 1998). Such social support is the most reliable and powerful buffer when people encounter difficulties in life (Aldwin, 2007; Folkman & Moskowitz, 2004). Having strong relationships outside of the therapy room also reduces the need to turn to clients to meet needs for respect, admiration, and support (Guy, 2000).

Another proactive strategy is to structure one's life in such a way as to minimize stress. For example, regarding work stresses, clinicians can assess and then address the areas that are particular hassles and drains on their energy. They can schedule breaks during the day, attend continuing education seminars to stay fresh, monitor the size and make-up of their caseloads, and

TABLE **15.2**
Strategies for Preventing Burnout and Other Problems in Clinical Practice

1. Being self-aware and maintaining one's psychological resources
2. Using one's personal values and principles to guide one's personal and professional lives
3. Balancing personal and professional lives, giving quality focus to each
4. Developing a strong support system at work and in personal life

Note: Modified from Coster & Schwebel (1997).

set realistic expectations for themselves (Faunce, 1990; Gilroy et al., 2002; Kramen-Kahn & Hansen, 1998; Pope & Vasquez, 2005; Sherman & Thelen, 1998). Having good role models at work can be quite helpful, but having models outside of work also provides broad opportunities for learning about a range of health-promoting behaviors, including being assertive, nurturing emotional sensitivity, balancing work and personal lives, maintaining boundaries with difficult people, and integrating spiritual ideals in daily life (Baker, 2003).

Like their clients, clinicians can develop good coping and problem-solving skills. Adaptive coping skills involve applying effort to solve problems that are controllable through planful action and applying efforts to understand and accept those problems that are beyond their control. Good coping often involves relying on one's social network for understanding and advice as well as tangible support and working through one's own difficult or confusing feelings (Aldwin, 2007). Clinicians should avoid relying on negative coping strategies, including self-medicating with various substances and engaging in minimization, denial, or rationalization. Negative coping is not only ineffective but can even make problems worse (Aldwin, 2007).

As discussed in Chapter 12, staying in top physical and mental shape goes a long way toward warding off stress and staying resilient and is as important for clinicians as for their clients (Wicks, 2008). This entails living a healthy lifestyle, which includes at least eating well, getting enough rest, exercising on a regular basis, maintaining one's healthy weight, using alcohol moderately or not at all, taking time out to pursue hobbies and leisure, and taking vacations (Carroll et al., 1999; Norcross, 2000). Given how basic and ubiquitous these elements of a healthy lifestyle are, it is remarkable how few clinicians implement them (Baker, 2003).

A healthy mind and body can also be cultivated through regular spiritual practices. For some, this might involve traditional religious engagement. For others, spirituality might entail appreciating nature, actively promoting community change, practicing mindfulness, doing yoga, or meditating (Schure, Christopher, & Christopher, 2008; Wicks, 2008). Finding purpose, meaning, and joy, despite being surrounded by pain at work, can be an especially important spiritual practice.

Above all, clinicians can proactively counter stress by working on their own perspective toward their work and their lives. They should recognize that striking a balance is a lifelong challenge and approach life with a sense of humor (Rupert & Kent, 2007). Recognizing and appreciating their ultimate reasons for engaging in therapeutic work in the first place is essential (see Table 15.3). Being a witness to the core struggles and triumphs of other human beings is a privilege. Clinicians should focus on the inherent rewards of this work, celebrating their successes and, like the clinician in the next case material, learn from their mistakes and less than satisfactory work (Jennings & Skovholt, 1999). Clinicians gain self-knowledge and, through their careers, have many opportunities to expand themselves, continue to learn, grow personally and professionally, and be a role model and mentor (Weiss, 2004). Furthermore, many appreciate the diversity in clients and presenting problems and tasks and find the constant variety rewarding.

TABLE **15.3**
Frequently Reported Rewards of Clinical Practice.

- Promoting client growth
- Enjoyment of work
- Opportunity to continue to learn
- Experiencing work as challenging
- Autonomy and independence
- Flexible hours
- Opportunity to gain increased self-knowledge
- Variety in work and clients
- Personal growth
- Sense of emotional intimacy
- Serving as a role model and mentor

Note: From Kramen-Kahn & Hansen (1998).

For many clinicians, having a sense of meaning and purpose can be an important part of preventing burnout and other practice-related problems. Some decide that being an effective clinician goes beyond simply maintaining the status quo to actively working to make things better (e.g., Brabeck & Brown, 1997; D. W. Sue, 2004). In fact, Coster and Schwebel (1997) argue that professional and community activism and involvement characterize well-functioning clinicians.

Ongoing professional development is another important strategy for helping clinicians deal with work-related stressors (Norcross, 2000). Professional development comprises a variety of different activities, including workshops, formal education or training, and supervision or consultation (Gilroy et al., 2002). It can also comprise setting up a practice that incorporates other types of intellectually rewarding activities such as teaching, writing, service on professional boards, and consulting. These broaden one's viewpoint and experience and can enliven one's mind and spirit.

Finally, as seen in the next case, clinicians do well in adopting a perspective of openness to their work and learning to view their mistakes as well as their successes as part of their own journey toward becoming an increasingly strong clinician. They set healthy goals for themselves, making reasonable and appropriate comparisons (relative to where they are rather than to the master clinicians they may have observed during training). They are open to learning from all sources—professors, mentors, books, movies, and clients—and accept and learn from their mistakes.

Regardless of the nature of self-care, it should be tailored to the person and the person's stage of life (Pope & Vasquez, 2005). What works for one person may not work well for another.

> Goodness of fit is as important in self-care strategies as it is in clothes.... Few of us would consider advising a person who has found happiness, significance, and contentment in a solitary monastic life with vows of silence and poverty, "You know, you really ought to get out and socialize more, and find ways to earn some money so that you'll have a nest egg you could rely on. I know you'd feel better about yourself and have a better life!"

Listening to ourselves, experimenting, and being honest with ourselves about what works and what doesn't are part of creating self-care strategies that fit us as individuals. (pp. 15–16)

The questions in Table 15.4 can help clinicians assess their self-care process, recognize barriers to self-care, and develop more effective strategies for self-care.

TABLE **15.4**

Questions for Monitoring One's Professional and Personal Health.

Match between person and clinical role
- Who do you want to be as a person? As a clinician? To what degree are you meeting your goals?
- In what ways is your clinical work different than you had expected before you started?
- How do your emotional, relational, and work styles affect your clinical work? In what ways do the positive aspects of your style sometimes cause problems?
- Are your personal strengths, values, and goals a good match for your work demands? How do you handle limitations and places where there is a poor match?

Stressors and supports
- How stressed are you at work? How does this affect your work? Your relationship with coworkers?
- What challenges have you experienced in your professional life (e.g., mandated reporting of abuse, client suicide, client complaint)? How have you responded to these? What have you learned?
- To what degree is your practice balanced in a way that works for you in terms of number and type of clients, frequency of problems and crises, and degree of progress? To what degree are you able to do the kinds of work that you value and at which you feel competent? What other rewards are you obtaining from your work?
- How are you feeling about your clients? To what degree are you able to be hopeful, respectful, and non-judgmental? To what degree do you see your work with clients as enabling, relevant, effective, or empowering?
- Are you experiencing stressors in your practice as threats of harm? Have you already experienced physical or psychological harm in your practice? How have you responded to this? Instead, are you feeling healthy and growth-promoting challenge in your clinical practice? When?
- How supported do you feel by colleagues at your agency, in your community, or in state and national networks? Are you able to get helpful peer support and consultations when needed? To what degree do you feel that your peers respect you and your work?
- If you have office staff, how supported do you feel by them? Are you getting the kinds of support with managed care and other tasks that you need? Are you avoiding office staff or do you feel supported and respected there?
- How physically and emotionally safe do you feel at work? If you feel unsafe, how has this affected your work? What are you doing to feel safer? Are these accommodations helping you develop as a professional or do they interfere with your personal and professional work?
- How financially safe are you feeling at work? Are you feeling that your financial future is safe and solid or that your client base is contracting and disappearing? Do you have a good retirement plan? A good health care plan?
- What concerns do you have about your future in the profession? What concerns do you have about the future of the profession? How are you handling these?
- If you have considered leaving your current position or the field, how have you handled your concerns?

(continues)

TABLE **15.4**
Questions for Monitoring One's Professional and Personal Health. (Continued)

Self-care
- What messages did you learn from your family of origin about self-care? What messages about self-care do your friends and family give you now?
- What barriers to self-care do you recognize? What makes it especially easy to engage in self-care?
- What have you learned about your self-care needs (e.g., exercise, healthy diet, friendships, family time, religion and spirituality, psychological growth)?
- If you were to identify a place where you are feeling out of balance in your self-care, what would it be?
- To what degree do you feel that you are able to maintain a healthy balance—for you—between work and your personal life?
- How do you take care of yourself as a clinician?
- To what degree do you feel that your life has a sense of meaning and purpose?
- To what degree do you feel that you are able to act within your values both at work and in your personal life?
- To what degree do you feel that you are moving effectively toward your personal goals?

Note: From Baker (2003) and Pope & Vasquez (2005).

My Clients Have Taught Me a Lot
Anonymous

Mistakes can be an opportunity. One of the participants in Jennings and Skovholt's (1999) study of master therapists well-described making mistakes and learning from them:

> My clients have taught me a lot. Early in my career, I saw a couple for a year, and what she complained about was his drinking. What he was basically saying was "I wouldn't be drinking if you didn't bug me so much." And I knew absolutely nothing about alcoholism at that point. They kind of faded out [of therapy], and I don't blame them when I look back on it because we didn't do much. A year later, she called me to make an appointment, came in, sat down, and said, "I just want to tell you face-to-face how destructive you were to us." And that was one of the most powerful things that could have happened. I mean, I am forever grateful. It was incredibly hard to hear, but I had a sense that I had really done a lousy job and there was something about her being strong enough to come back. I was embarrassed.... It made a powerful impression.... I knew it was true and that I had a lot to learn. And I think that the other part was that I was incredibly impressed with the fact that she had the guts to do it. And I thought, you know, if she had the guts to do it, then I've got the guts to learn from it.... It colored my absolute commitment to learn about what I didn't know. (p. 7)

- Although you have little information about this clinician, what do you know about how he or she sees and approaches the world? What influenced you to draw these conclusions?

(continues)

- People often have difficulty transforming their mistakes into something positive, as this master therapist did. If you can, think about a time when you made a mistake and learned from it. What did you learn? How were you able to learn, rather than failing or becoming stuck?
- Perhaps you identified some goals for your own development as a clinician as you read through this section. What are these goals and how are you going to go about meeting them?

SUMMARY

Taking good care of oneself both personally and professionally is important in becoming and remaining an effective clinician. Without good self-care, clinicians may experience boundary blurring, vicarious traumatization, and burnout when working empathically with difficult clients. In addition to client-induced stress, clinicians may experience stress due to the work environment, self-induced internal stress, and stress related to events in one's own personal life.

Coping well with personal and professional stressors and preventing burnout and other dangers of empathic work depend on having effective strategies for recognizing and preventing problems and regularly engaging in good, proactive self-care practice. Self-care and other preventative practices should be increased as stressors increase. These practices can enable clinicians to remain respectful and empathic even in the face of the inevitable stressors that will be experienced in one's work and personal lives.

How Do These Issues Apply to Your Life and Work?

1. With what kinds of people, problems, or situations do you have the most problems? When do you handle these best?
2. What signals help you recognize when you're running into problems in your life (e.g., insomnia, problems concentrating, irritation with clients and coworkers, increased substance use)?
3. What specific things can you do to keep yourself fresh and healthy? What can you do to begin putting these into place right now?
4. What barriers or obstacles might interfere with your ability to regularly engage in self-care? What can you do to begin addressing these barriers and obstacles right now?

Ethics Codes

American Association for Marriage and Family Therapy. (2001). *AAMFT code of ethics.* Retrieved from http://www.aamft.org/resources/lrm_plan/Ethics/ethicscode2001.asp

American Counseling Association. (2005). *ACA code of ethics.* Alexandria, VA: Author. Retrieved from http://www.counseling.org/Resources/CodeOfEthics/TP/Home/CT2.aspx

American Mental Health Counselors Association. (2000). *Code of ethics.* Retrieved from http://www.amhca.org/code/

American Psychological Association. (2002). Ethical principles of psychologists and code of conduct. *American Psychologist, 57,* 1060–1073.

American School Counselors Association. (2004). *Ethical standards for school counselors.* Retrieved from http://www.schoolcounselor.org/content.asp?contentid=173

Canadian Counselling Association. (2007). *Code of ethics.* Retrieved from http://www.ccacc.ca/ECOEJAN07.pdf

Canadian Psychological Association. (2000). *Canadian code of ethics for psychologists.* Retrieved from http://www.cpa.ca/publications/

Commission on Rehabilitation Counselor Certification. (2008). *CRC/CRCC code of ethics.* Retrieved from http://www.crccertification.com/pages/crc_ccrc_code_of_ethics/10.php

National Association of Social Workers. (2008). *Code of ethics of the National Association of Social Workers.* Retrieved from http://www.socialworkers.org/pubs/code/code.asp

GLOSSARY

Abandonment. When treatment is ended in ways that are not ethically or clinically appropriate.

Accommodation. Making radical reconceptualizations in worldview to incorporate new information (as opposed to assimilation).

Accurate empathy. An empathic response by a clinician that neither adds to nor subtracts from the client's meaning.

Action. A stage of change in which clients are committed to changing and willing to accept the costs of change. Change is most rapid for clients in this stage.

Additive empathy. A response that recognizes and shares additional, underlying, often unspoken meanings, thoughts, and feelings.

ADHD. Attention-Deficit/Hyperactivity Disorder, a disorder characterized by problems of hyperactivity, impulsivity, and inattention, generally first seen in childhood.

Advice. A response that involves telling a client what to do, especially how to solve a problem that the client faces.

Affect. Overtly displayed emotion (as opposed to mood, which is more internal and subjective). In a mental status evaluation, discussion of affect includes (a) the overtly displayed mood, (b) the degree of emotional liability, and (c) the congruence between affective expression and verbal content or subjective mood.

Aggression. Statements and behavior that consider the speaker's own needs and feelings rather than those of the other party (as opposed to assertiveness).

Aspirational principles. The ethical principles and goals that clinicians use to guide treatment, although they may never completely meet these in their practice.

Assertiveness. Statements and behavior that consider the needs and feelings of both the speaker and listener equally and that are expressed in a manner that is respectful of both parties.

Assessment. A description of a client in a wide number of realms, based on the findings of a clinical interview and the specific assessment strategies used.

Assessment strategy. The specific strategies clinicians use (e.g., genograms, timelines, mental status evaluation) to draw an overall assessment of a client.

Assimilation. Integration of new information into one's existing worldview (as opposed to accommodation).

Assumption. Underlying, often invisible and untested, beliefs that guide behavior.

Attachment style. The typical pattern of relating to others, especially perceived safety within relationships and how feelings of lack of safety are handled—either by withdrawing or clinging.

Attribution. A belief about the cause of behavior, or a person's quality or trait.

Autonomy. The ability to make decisions for oneself. Promoting autonomy is an aspirational principle guiding ethical decision making.

Barnum statement. A statement that appears to be specifically about one person's characteristics, but in fact applies to almost everyone.

Barriers. Obstacles that get in the way of change, including institutional, financial, environmental, cultural, relational, or intrapsychic factors.

Beneficence. Striving to do good for those with whom one works and society as a whole. An aspirational principle guiding ethical decision making.

Billable hours. Number of hours of clinical service that will be paid by clients and insurance companies.

Biological model. Theoretical perspective that explains problems in terms of biological factors, including neurotransmitters, brain activity, hormone levels, and genetics.

Boundaries. Commonly accepted practice, the "ground rules" supporting the client, clinician, and treatment, generally referring to limits on time, treatment setting, content discussed, and the nature of the relationship.

Boundary crossings. Behaviors deviating from the strictest professional norms, including small self-disclosures. Less inherently risky than boundary violations, but may put clinicians at greater risk of engaging in them.

Boundary violations. Behaviors deviating from professional norms, with high potential for negative consequences for the client (as opposed to boundary crossings).

Burnout. A progressive loss of idealism, energy, and sense of purpose for the work of therapy. Characterized by emotional exhaustion, increased depersonalization of clients, and decreased sense of personal accomplishment. Sometimes called compassion fatigue.

Case conceptualization. An integrated and developed set of hypotheses about the forces driving a person's behavior and the causes and treatment of the presenting problem. Leads to the treatment plan.

Census. Number of clients in a program.

Check-out. A verbal listening skill often taking the form of a closed question, that helps clarify the clinician's understanding of the client. Often used after a paraphrase or a reflection of feeling.

Clinical assessment. Comprehensive conclusions about the causes, maintenance, and treatment of problems and symptoms, which are drawn as a result of the assessment process.

Clinical risk. The risk of disciplinary complaint or legal action during clinical practice.

Closed question. A verbal listening skill. A specific form of question that typically starts with "is," "are," "do," "does," "would," "could" or "have" and can be answered with one or two words (as opposed to open questions).

Cognitive model. Theoretical perspective that explains problems in terms of maladaptive beliefs and interpretations of events.

Cognitive restructuring. The process of identifying negative or irrational thoughts, challenging their accuracy, and developing more balanced and adaptive ways of thinking.

Collectivism. An orientation that emphasizes the needs of the group and family (as opposed to individualism). Group and family obligations are stressed more than self-reliance and independence, or individual wishes, thoughts, and feelings.

Common factors. Agents of change that are shared by all therapies. These include the therapeutic alliance, the clinician's personality, clinician/client match, catharsis, and being provided an acceptable explanation of the problem.

Comorbidity. When two disorders occur at the same time.

Competence. Either (a) relative to ethics, a multidimensional and fluctuating attribute that includes knowledge and skills, as well as the attitudes, values, and judgment necessary to implement them well, or (b) in legal settings, the accused's ability to make important decisions or to assist in his or her own defense in court.

Confidentiality. The ethical principle that a clinician will reveal client information disclosed during treatment only when the client gives permission or when legally required to do so, as with duty to warn (see *Tarasoff*) or mandated reporting of child abuse or neglect.

Confirmatory biases. Tendency to recall behaviors consistent with one's biases and overlook or forget behaviors that are inconsistent with these biases.

Confrontation. Either (a) a verbal influencing skill that identifies a discrepancy within or across realms—for example, between client's behavior and his or her goal, or between behavior and values—and paraphrases these discrepancies, or (b) more colloquially, an angry and aggressive response.

Congruent. (a) When a person's thoughts, feelings, values and behavior are in alignment, (b) referring to the clinician's ability to act in an authentic and genuine manner.

Construct. Either (a) the process of creating individual knowledge and meaning through one's experience with the world, or (b) an abstract idea that is inferred from specific measurements (e.g., love might be inferred by the amount of time a person spends talking about someone).

Constructivist viewpoint. The view that knowledge and meaning are generated through one's experiences with the world (as opposed to the essentialist viewpoint).

Contemplation. A stage of change in which clients are ambivalent about change, recognizing both the costs and benefits of making change and having difficulty choosing either to change or not to change.

Content. The material that is discussed in the course of treatment (as opposed to process).

Context. The broad range of influences on a person, which includes culture, as broadly defined, and also familial, historical, and political influences, trauma, and life events.

Continuing education. Ongoing professional education required to maintain licensure or certification. Often awarded in hourly units referred to as Continuing Education Units or CEUs.

Conversion therapy. Therapies intended to change the sexual orientation of gays, lesbians, and bisexuals. Sometimes referred to as reparative therapy.

Copayments (Copays). The client's responsibility for a portion of the cost of treatment, with the balance paid for by the insurance company.

Corrective experience. An experience in treatment that helps clients feel differently about aspects of their lives, for example, about themselves, their relationships, their past, or their future.

Critical thinking. The purposeful and reflective process of evaluating observations and drawing conclusions about them. It includes identifying assertions, evaluating evidence supporting and contradicting these assertions, identifying other explanations of this evidence, and choosing the most reasonable explanation.

Cultural group. A group that generally has a shared identity, with similar worldviews, patterns of behavior, preferences, values, and norms.

Culture. The shared attitudes, values, beliefs, habits, traditions, norms, arts, history, institutions, and experiences of a group of people that, together, define their general behavior and way of life. Ethnicity, race, gender, class, age cohort, and sexual orientation, among other demographic groups, are frequently identified as cultural groups.

DAP notes. Structured session notes describing the subjective and objective data about the client (D), the clinician's findings and assessment (A), and the plan (P) for subsequent sessions.

Directive. A verbal influencing skill that asks or tells a client to take a specific action. Sometimes it takes the form of a closed question.

Discharge summary. A brief report generally summarizing entering and ending client diagnoses, the course of treatment (e.g., number of sessions and cancellations, interventions used), and factors contributing to the success or failure of treatment.

Discrepancy. Either (a) the gap between where clients are and where they want to be or believe they should be, or (b) the conflict between words and nonverbal behavior, actions, values or goals, which provides the content for a clinician's confrontation.

Discrimination. Unfair treatment of a group based on group membership or the perception of such treatment.

Distraction. The process of doing or thinking about something in order to pull one's attention from something else.

Dual relationship. A second relationship with a client (beyond that of clinician) that has incompatible or competing expectations, goals, or needs with the primary relationship (e.g., being both therapist and friend). Sometimes referred to as multiple relationships.

Dynamic sizing. The ability to know when to generalize from individual experience to a common pattern and to know when an individual situation does not follow the common pattern.

Empathy. The accepting and intuitive understanding of another person from his or her unique point of view.

Employee assistance programs. Employee benefit plans set up by employers, often in association with an insurance plan, to provide assessment, short-term behavioral health treatment, and referrals for follow-up services.

Empowerment. The process of supporting clients to recognize, accept, use, and develop their personal and political power in order to meet their goals.

Encouragers. A verbal listening skill that very briefly paraphrases (in no more than a few words) the most central content or emotion in a client's statement.

Essentialist viewpoint. The view that objects or people have inherent and stable traits (as opposed to constructivist viewpoint).

Ethical standards. Ethical expectations that are part of a profession's code of ethics, violations of which can lead to disciplinary censure.

Evaluation. A formal administration of a number of assessment tools (e.g., interview, projective and objective personality tests, intelligence and achievement tests), to develop a clear response to a referral question.

Expectancy confirmation. Tendency to see behaviors that fit one's expectations and to ignore evidence that would otherwise disconfirm it.

Extrinsic. The value of a behavior or goal that comes not from the behavior or object itself, but through its meeting some other need or value, including belongingness, support, or prestige (as opposed to intrinsic values or goals).

Family genogram. An assessment strategy that visually collects and organizes hypotheses about familial patterns and relationships, which may contribute to the problem or serve as resources for treatment.

Feedback. A verbal influencing skill that is a special case of self-disclosure that shares the clinician's perception of or reaction to the client or client's behavior.

Fidelity. Behaving in a faithful, honest, trustworthy, and responsible manner. An aspirational principle guiding ethical decision making.

Forced terminations. Terminations from treatment that are triggered by a program's or managed care plan's limit on the number of sessions available.

Functional analysis. An assessment procedure in which either the client or clinician observes and records the antecedents to a behavioral problem (a), the behavior itself (b), and the consequences to the behavior (c) in a systematic way in order to identify relationships between internal or environmental stimuli and behaviors.

Fundamental attribution error. The tendency to attribute others' behavior to internal and stable traits, while overlooking unstable, situational factors.

Generalization. The ability to transfer a learned behavior to a similar but different stimulus or setting.

Goal statements. A statement describing the client's short-term and long-term goals.

Goals. Internal representations of desired future processes, events, or outcomes.

Groupthink. The tendency to suppress or resist divergent thought processes or minority opinions when a group is working together to accomplish a task.

Halfway house. Transitional housing and programs that help people reintegrate into society from either a psychiatric hospital or prison while continuing to monitor their status and provide

needed support to stabilize them in the community.

Health Insurance Portability and Accountability Act of 1996 (HIPAA). A federal law giving individuals rights over their health information and setting rules limiting who has access to protected health information.

Here and now. Actively experiencing an issue and understanding it in the context of the therapeutic alliance, the therapy room, or treatment, as opposed to only talking about the problem abstractly.

Hypotheses. A proposed explanation of certain facts or phenomena that may be subject to objective testing.

Implicit biases. Prejudice or stereotypes operating outside of conscious awareness, often measured by the Implicit Bias Test.

Individualism. Emphasizes the needs of the individual over those of the group and family (as opposed to collectivism). Individual wishes, thoughts, and feelings are given priority over group responsibility and obligations.

Inference. Conclusion drawn from observations. Because there is often meaning added to the observations, two parties may disagree about what happened.

Information giving. A verbal influencing skill that provides information to help the client better understand the problem, symptoms, or others.

Informed consent. Both a formal process and an ongoing informal process whereby clinicians provide clients with sufficient information to make informed decisions about their treatment.

Institutionalized discrimination. Unfair treatment of members of a group that has become part of the formal or informal laws, policies, and operating procedures of a company, government, or public institution.

Internalized homophobia. A homosexual or bisexual person's aversion to homosexuals and homosexuality, which might have been internalized from the larger culture's messages, generally without the person's awareness.

Interpretation. A verbal influencing skill that identifies a deeper, underlying meaning to a client's behavior, thoughts, and emotional reactions.

Interventions. The specific strategies that the client and clinician use to meet treatment goals.

Intrinsic. The value of a behavior or goal comes from the behavior or object itself (as opposed to extrinsic values or goals).

Intrusive thoughts. Unwanted, involuntary thoughts, ideas, and images that may become obsessive and ruminative in nature.

Joining. The process of a clinician acting in such a way as to strengthen the therapeutic alliance.

Just world theory. The belief that people get what they deserve and deserve what they get.

Lapse. A return of a problem behavior that the client sees as temporary and as an opportunity to learn about the self and ways to prevent the problem in the future (as opposed to a relapse).

Least restrictive environment. Environment and interventions that allow the client access to the broader environment to the degree possible, while providing only the level of restrictions required to keep the client safe.

Locus of control. The location of a person's perception of control for present and future events, which is either internal and controlled by the person him- or herself, or external and controlled by outside factors including others, the environment, culture, chance, or fate.

Locus of responsibility. The location of a person's perception of responsibility or blame for past events, which is either internal and controlled by the person him- or herself, or external and controlled by outside factors including others, the environment, culture, chance, or fate.

Long-term goal. Primary, superordinate goal of treatment toward which short-term goals are intermediate steps.

Maintenance. A stage of change in which clients have met their goals and are now taking action to maintain those changes. During this stage, clients need to identify and implement strategies to prevent a relapse.

Majority culture. The group in a society that generally possesses greater power and whose language, religion, behavior, values, rituals, and social customs are seen as normative.

Managed care. An insurance plan covering mental and physical health problems, often with a copayment and limits on the number, type, and frequency of services; diagnoses covered; and, sometimes, access to services.

Meditation. Any of a number of internal practices that build calm, awareness, and nonjudgmental self-acceptance, often by turning one's attention to a single focus, such as the breath.

Mental status evaluation. An assessment of the client's functioning in a number of realms (e.g., appearance, relationship with interviewer, affect and mood, speech and language use, cognition and memory, disorders in thinking, and insight and judgment).

Meta-analysis. A statistical process systematically combining the results of research studies addressing a common set of research hypotheses. Normally done by examining effect size across studies.

Microskills. The nonverbal and verbal skills that help clinicians join with clients, develop case conceptualizations, identify problems and change strategies, and help clients change.

Mindfulness. Calm, nonjudgmental awareness of one's body, thoughts, feelings or actions rather than focus on past or future.

Minimal encourager. A verbal listening skill that is an extremely brief paraphrase of the most central content or emotion expressed by the client, including "Uh huh," "Mmm," "Yup," a head nod, or an empathic facial expression.

Mini-Mental State Exam. A standardized assessment of a person's mental state.

Miracle question. A verbal influencing skill that asks clients to imagine that a miracle happened and to identify behaviors that would indicate that their problem had disappeared as a result of this miracle. Usually used to identify treatment goals and to help clients identify when they are already approaching their goals.

Mirroring. Subtly copying someone's breathing, posture and movements in order to build rapport and empathy.

Mood. The client's "emotional atmosphere." As opposed to affect, mood is internal, subjective, and relatively more sustained. Often inferred from the client's verbal tone and subjective report.

Multicultural model. Theoretical perspective that explains problems in terms of oppression, discrimination, and cultural influences that put people at risk or that create strengths and resilience.

Multiple identities. Belonging to or identifying with, and influenced by, multiple cultures (e.g., ethnicity, race, gender, class, religion, sexual orientation, physical ability, etc.).

Nonmaleficence. Avoiding doing harm. An aspirational principle guiding ethical decision making.

Normalization. A verbal influencing skill that frames a behavior that a client has previously perceived negatively as normal, at least under some circumstances.

Normal termination. The manner in which treatment is ended by clinicians using ethical and clinically appropriate processes, including talking ahead of time about how to end treatment.

Observation. Sensory data (things that are seen, heard, felt, tasted, or smelled). Because there is no additional meaning added, two parties who observe it will generally agree that it happened as described (as opposed to inference).

Observer's paradox. Labov's assertion that simply making an observation affects the outcome of a situation; therefore, no one can ever know how a person would behave if the observer were not present.

Open question. A verbal listening skill. A specific form of question that generally starts with "what," "how," "why," or "where" and is often used to encourage discussion (as opposed to closed questions).

Operational definition. A specific statement about how an event or behavior will be measured in order to assess the construct being studied.

Oppression. The process of arbitrarily and unjustly preventing a person from meeting his or her goals or potential (as opposed to privilege). Oppression takes many forms, some of which are overt, others more indirect and subtle.

Paralanguage. The nonverbal aspects of speech that convey important information about meaning (e.g., intonation, cadence, speed, and volume of voice).

Paraphrase. A verbal listening skill that summarizes, in the clinician's own words, what a client said. It is used both to demonstrate the clinician's understanding and to check out that understanding. As opposed to reflections of feeling, paraphrases focus more on facts than emotions.

Person-centered model. Theoretical perspective that explains psychological problems as stemming from conditional self-acceptance, internalized from others' conditional positive regard.

Person First Language. Focuses on the person, rather than the problem. In using Person First Language, the general descriptor is placed first, with the problem identified second (e.g., the woman who has anorexia rather than the anorexic woman).

Placebo. A treatment without an inherent active ingredient. A placebo's action is believed to come from a person's belief that he or she is receiving an effective treatment.

Positive psychology. A field of psychology that focuses on human strengths and behaviors that help people thrive, including gratitude, forgiveness, resiliency, meaning making, and flow.

Positivity. The need to hear positive information about oneself (as opposed to validation).

Post-traumatic growth. Growth following a trauma, including changes such as increased awareness of values, greater spirituality, stronger interpersonal values, greater self-efficacy, etc.

Precontemplation. A stage of change in which clients do not yet recognize that they have a problem and therefore are uncommitted to change.

Prejudice. Negative attitudes about a person based on race, gender, ethnicity, sexual orientation, or other group memberships.

Premature termination. Treatment that is ended before meeting treatment goals and, generally, against the clinician's advice.

Preparation. A stage of change in which clients are preparing to make active change by planning, getting information, getting support, problem solving, and obtaining needed skills.

Private pay clients. Clients who pay for treatment themselves rather than using insurance benefits.

Privilege. Unearned advantages that come solely or primarily from group membership (as opposed to oppression). Group members often assume that privilege is deserved and appropriate.

Pro bono. Literally, "for free." Treatment that is offered without charge.

Problem statement. Statement of a problem from the client's viewpoint and in the client's own words.

Process. The manner in which therapeutic material is presented or talked about (e.g., speed, place of introduction of material, style of interpersonal interaction,

etc.). Often discussed in contrast to content.

Productivity. The number of billable hours performed during a period of time.

Professional identity. One's identity as a professional, including professional values, ethics, goals, and methods.

Progress notes. Brief and informal notes made by a clinician immediately after a session, summarizing the content and process of a session, as well as diagnostic impressions.

Pseudoclient. Research participant asked to respond to a vignette, questionnaire, or experimental intervention as though he or she were a real client.

Psychoanalytic model. Theoretical perspective that explains problems in terms of repressed or unconscious conflicts, impulses, and anxiety, often beginning in childhood, which interfere with more mature ways of relating to the world.

Psychosocial history. An assessment strategy that involves collecting current and historical information about client behavior and functioning in a wide range of realms that have a high potential for impacting treatment, including relative strengths and weaknesses, obstacles to change, available resources and social supports, and client meanings.

QUOID. Sue and Sue's acronym (Quiet, Ugly, Old, Indigent, Dissimilar culturally) used to describe clients for whom traditional therapies are poorly suited (as opposed to YAVIS).

Racial identity. Attitudes and views about self and others based on one's perceptions of one's own and others' races.

Racism. Negative attitudes about a person based on race. A special case of prejudice.

Reactance. An oppositional response style in reaction to rules that are perceived to restrict personal autonomy or freedom.

Referral. The process of recommending that a client receive services from another clinician or program.

Referral question. The specific question leading to a referral for evaluation or treatment.

Reflection of feeling. A verbal listening skill that furthers focus on and discussion of emotions. Like paraphrases, it communicates understanding, but does

so by selectively focusing on the client's feelings.

Reframe. A verbal influencing skill designed to help clients think about an event in a different way, that is, from a new frame of reference.

Relapse. A slip that is perceived as a full-blown return to the problem behavior (as opposed to a lapse).

Relapse prevention. A process of reducing the probability of a relapse by helping clients to think about slips as lapses rather than as relapses, develop coping skills and use them proactively, and recognize triggers to slips and either avoid those triggers or be prepared to handle them more effectively.

Resistance. Overtly or indirectly avoiding or refusing to think about or discuss clinically relevant experiences, generally due to emotions including anxiety, guilt, shame, fear, and embarrassment.

Risk management. Any of a number of strategies used to reduce the clinical risk incurred during evaluations and treatment.

Rumination. Obsessive thought or worry.

Scaling question. A verbal influencing skill where clients are asked to indicate the degree to which a problem is present, often on a scale from 1 to 10. Sometimes used after the miracle question.

Scientific mindedness. The quality of forming tentative hypotheses about observations, recognizing alternative explanations, and testing these before acting.

Self-disclosure. A verbal influencing skill sharing material that is somewhat personal to the clinician, including reactions, memories, dreams, and actions.

Self-efficacy. One's belief in one's own ability to change.

Self-fulfilling prophecy. Predictions, perceptions, and expectations that, by their very nature, shape a person's behavior and influence outcomes.

Session objective. Primary objective or goal for a treatment session.

Short-term goal. The immediate goals that are intermediate steps toward accomplishing long-term goals of treatment.

Situational meaning. The meaning assigned by a person to an event. It includes appraisals of an event as a loss, threat, or challenge, as well as causal attributions for why the event occurred, determination of the extent to which the events are discrepant with one's global system of meaning, and decisions regarding what can be done to cope with the event.

Slip. A return of a problem behavior, which can either be seen as temporary and an opportunity to learn (lapse) or permanent and without eventual positive consequences (relapse).

SOAP notes. Structured session notes describing the client's subjective experience (S), the clinician's observations (O) and assessment (A), as well as the plan (P) for the next session.

Social justice. Being fair and unbiased in treatment and promoting fairness in the community. Applying psychological principles fairly and providing equal access to its products. An aspirational principle guiding ethical decision making.

Solution-focused. Treatment is focused more on solutions than problems, especially attending to the ways that solutions are already occasionally present in part or whole.

Strength-based. Evaluations and treatment that pay attention to strengths, successes, positive intentions and exceptions to problems, in addition to weaknesses, mistakes, problems, and symptoms.

Subtractive empathy. A clinician's response that is off track and misses or subtracts from understanding clients from their own point of view.

Summarization. A verbal influencing skill that pulls together the client's facts and feelings from a relatively longer part of a session or treatment in a way that organizes them and communicates and clarifies understanding. Useful at the beginning and end of a session, as well as at periodic intervals in between.

Tarasoff v. Regents of the University of California. A ruling by the California's Supreme Court that when a clinician knows or should have known that a client is a serious danger to a specific person, an obligation to use reasonable care to protect that person is incurred. This may require that the clinician warn the intended victim, notify the police, or take whatever steps are reasonably necessary under the circumstances.

Therapeutic alliance. The strength of the partnership between client and therapist. About 30% of the variance in therapeutic outcomes is attributable to the client's perceptions of the therapeutic alliance and clinician characteristics, including warmth, genuineness, and empathy.

Therapeutic relationship. See therapeutic alliance.

Timeline. An assessment strategy that records all major events for clients and their immediate family from birth to the present.

Time orientation. Perception of time as either flexible or inelastic. Focus can be primarily on past, present, or future.

Trait. Seeing and describing behavior as a central, unchangeable trait.

Trait negativity bias. Tendency to focus on and give greater meaning to negative rather than positive traits. Negative actions are perceived as more representative of a person than positive ones.

Transfer. Either (a) the ability to use a learned behavior in different settings (e.g., both the clinician's office and at home), or (b) a move from one setting or program to another.

Treatment goals. Either short- or long-term planned objectives for treatment; in the best-case scenario these goals are chosen collaboratively between client and clinician.

Treatment plan. A detailed plan for treatment identifying the clinician's and client's short- and long-term treatment goals, interventions planned for the treatment period, and, sometimes, the anticipated date for when goals will be met.

Triggers. Emotions, settings, and situations that increase the probability of a lapse or relapse of the problem behavior.

Trust. Feelings of interpersonal safety.

Unconditional positive regard. Positive and nonjudgmental feelings toward a client that are not contingent on the client's behavior, values, goals, or cognitions.

Validation. The need to have one's self-perception confirmed by others (as opposed to positivity).

Validity. The extent to which an observation or measurement tool actually measures what it is supposed to measure.

Values. A set of principles concerning the ultimate importance of things that influences a broad range of human behaviors and choices and prescribes modes of conduct.

Verbal underlining. Words that are emphasized by changes in speed or volume, changing the statement's meaning.

Vicarious traumatization. A cumulative process through which clinicians are negatively impacted by listening to and engaging with clients' descriptions of trauma.

Worldview. A person's overarching set of beliefs, values, and goals; used to help a person define, interpret, and navigate reality.

YAVIS. An acronym (Young, Attractive, Verbal, Intelligent, Successful) used to describe clients for whom traditional therapies are well suited (as opposed to QUOID).

REFERENCES

Abelson, R. P., Frey, K. P., & Gregg, A. P. (2004). *Experiments with people: Revelations from social psychology.* Mahwah, NJ: Lawrence Erlbaum.

Abraído-Lanza, A. F., Vásquez, E., & Echeverría, S. E. (2004). En las manos de Dios [in God's hands]: Religious and other forms of coping among Latinos with arthritis. *Journal of Consulting and Clinical Psychology, 72,* 91–102.

Achenbach, T. M., & Rescorla, L. A. (2004). The Achenbach System of Empirically Based Assessment (ASEBA) for ages 1.5 to 18 years. In M. E. Maruish (Ed.), *The use of psychological testing for treatment planning and outcomes assessment. Volume 2: Instruments for children and adolescents* (3rd ed., pp. 179–213). Mahwah, NJ: Lawrence Erlbaum Associates.

Ackerman, S., & Hilsenroth, M. J. (2001). A review of therapist characteristics and techniques negatively impacting the therapeutic alliance. *Psychotherapy: Theory, Research, Practice, Training, 38,* 171–185.

Ai, A. L., & Park, C. L. (2005). Possibilities of the positive following violence and trauma: Informing the coming decade of research. *Journal of Interpersonal Violence, 20,* 242–250.

Ainsworth, M. S., Blehar, M. C., Waters, E., & Wall, S. (1978). *Patterns of attachment: A psychological study of the strange situation.* Oxford, England: Erlbaum.

Alcoholics Anonymous. (2009). *Welcome to Alcoholics Anonymous.* Retrieved from http://www.aa.org/ ?Media=PlayFlash

Aldwin, C. M. (2007). *Stress, coping, and development: An integrative perspective* (2nd ed.). New York, NY: Guilford.

Alexander, F., & French, T. M. (1946). *Psychoanalytic therapy: Principles and applications.* New York, NY: Ronald Press.

Allen, D. M. (2005). The clinical exchange. *Journal of Psychotherapy Integration, 15,* 67–68.

Allport, G. W., & Ross, J. M. (1967). Personal religious orientation and prejudice. *Journal of Personality and Social Psychology, 5,* 432–443.

American Association for Marriage and Family Therapy. (2001). *AAMFT code of ethics.* Retrieved from http://www.aamft.org/resources/lrm_plan/Ethics/ethicscode2001.asp

American Council on Education. (2006, July 11). College enrollment gender gap widens for white and Hispanic students, but race and income disparities still most significant new ACE report finds. *HENA Online News.* Retrieved from http://www.acenet.edu/AM/Template.cfm?Section=HENA&TEMPLATE=/CM/ContentDisplay.cfm&CONTENTID=17251

American Counseling Association. (2005). *ACA code of ethics.* Alexandria, VA: Author. Retrieved from http://www.counseling.org/Resources/CodeOfEthics/TP/Home/CT2.aspx

American Psychological Association. (2002). Ethical principles of psychologists and code of conduct. *American Psychologist, 57,* 1060–1073.

American Psychological Association. (2003). Guidelines on multicultural education, training, research, practice, and organizational change for psychologists. *American Psychologist, 58,* 377–402.

Amrhein, P. C., Miller, W. R., Yahne, C. E., Palmer, M., & Fulcher, L. (2003). Client commitment language during motivational interviewing predicts drug use outcomes. *Journal of Consulting and Clinical Psychology, 71,* 862–878.

Anderson, C. J. (2003). The psychology of doing nothing: Forms of decision avoidance result from reason and emotion. *Psychological Bulletin, 129,* 139–166.

Anderson, S. K., & Kitchener, K. S. (1998). Nonsexual posttherapy relationships: A conceptual framework to assess ethical risks.

Professional Psychology: Research and Practice, 29, 91–99.

Andrea Yates Confession. (2001a, July 14). Clip 7. *Houston Chronicle.* Retrieved from http://media.swagit.com/s/chron/Houston_Chronicle/01062005-8.high.mov.html

Andrea Yates Confession. (2001b, July 14). Clip 8. *Houston Chronicle.* Retrieved from http://media.swagit.com/s/chron/Houston_Chronicle/01062005-10.high.mov.html

Annas, G. J. (2004). Forcible medication for courtroom competence: The case of Charles Sell. *New England Journal of Medicine, 350,* 2297–2301.

Anonymous. (2000, March). Boundaries in therapy: The limits of care. *Pennsylvania Psychologist Update,* pp. 1, 3.

Anonymous. (2008, November 4). Psychotherapist body language. *AllExperts.* Retrieved from http://en.allexperts.com/q/Psychology-2566/2008/11/Psychotherapist-body-language.htm

Asay, T. P., & Lambert, M. J. (1999). The empirical case for the common factors in therapy: Quantitative factors. In M. A. Hubble, B. L. Duncan, & S. D. Miller (Eds.), *The heart & soul of change: What works in therapy* (pp. 23–55). Washington, DC: American Psychological Association.

Associated Press. (2002, February 21). Transcript of Andrea Yates' confession. *Houston Chronicle.* Retrieved from http://www.chron.com/cs/CDA/story.hts/special/drownings/1266294#top

Austin, J. T., & Vancouver, J. B. (1996). Goal constructs in psychology: Structure, process, and content. *Psychological Bulletin, 120,* 338–375.

Axelson, J. (1993). *Counseling and development in a multicultural society.* Belmont, CA: Brooks/Cole.

Baker, E. K. (2003). *Caring for ourselves: A therapist's guide to personal and professional well-being.* Washington, DC: American Psychological Association.

Ball, S. G., Otto, M. W., Pollack, M. H., & Rosenbaum, J. F. (1994). Predicting prospective episodes of depression in patients with panic disorder: A longitudinal study. *Journal of Consulting and Clinical Psychology, 62,* 359–365.

Balsam, K. F., Beauchaine, T. P., Mickey, R. M., & Rothblum, E. D. (2005). Mental health of lesbian, gay, bisexual, and heterosexual siblings: Effects of gender, sexual orientation, and family. *Journal of Abnormal Psychology, 114*(3), 471–476.

Banaji, M. R., Hardin, C., & Rothman, A. J. (1993). Implicit stereotyping in person judgment. *Journal of Personality and Social Psychology, 65,* 272–281.

Bandura, A. (1997). *Self-efficacy: The exercise of control.* New York, NY: W. H. Freeman.

Barnett, J. E., Baker, E. K., Elman, N. S., & Schoener, G. R. (2007). In pursuit of wellness: The self-care imperative. *Professional Psychology: Research and Practice, 38,* 603–612.

Barnett, J. E., Doll, B., Younggren, J. N., & Rubin, N. J. (2007). Clinical competence for practicing psychologists: Clearly a work in progress. *Professional Psychology: Research and Practice, 38,* 510–517.

Barnett, J. E., Lazarus, A. A., Vasquez, M. J. T., Moorehead-Slaughter, O., & Johnson, W. B. (2007). Boundary issues and multiple relationships: Fantasy and reality. *Professional Psychology: Research and Practice, 38,* 401–410.

Barnett, J. E., Wise, E. H., Johnson-Greene, D., & Bucky, S. F. (2007). Informed consent: Too much of a good thing or not enough? *Professional Psychology: Research and Practice, 38,* 179–186.

Barrett, M. S., Chua, W.-J., Crits-Christoph, P., Gibbons, M. B., & Thompson, D. (2008). Early withdrawal from mental health treatment: Implications for psychotherapy practice. *Psychotherapy: Theory, Research, Practice, Training, 45,* 247–267.

Bashe, A., Anderson, S. K., Handelsman, M. M., & Klevansky, R. (2007). An acculturation model for ethics training: The ethics autobiography and beyond. *Professional Psychology: Research and Practice, 38,* 60–67.

Beauchemin, E. (2006, June 20). Dr. Danny Brom: In a traumatized society. *Radio Netherlands.* Retrieved from http://www.radionetherlands.nl/features/dutchhorizons/060620dh

Beck, A. T. (1976). *Cognitive therapy and the emotional disorders.* New York, NY: International Universities Press.

Beck, A. T., Steer, R. A., & Garbin, M. G. (1988). Psychometric properties of the Beck Depression Inventory: Twenty-five years of evaluation. *Clinical Psychology Review, 8,* 77–100.

Becker-Blease, K. A., & Freyd, J. J. (2006). Research participants telling the truth about their lives: The ethics of asking and not asking about abuse. *American Psychologist, 61,* 218–226.

Behnke, S. (2007, February). Adolescents and confidentiality: Letter from a reader. *Monitor on Psychology, 38*(2), 46–47.

Belenky, M. F., Clinchy, B. M., Goldberger, N. R., & Tarule, J. M. (1986). Women's ways of knowing: The development of self, voice, and mind. New York, NY: Basic Books.

Benjet, C., Azar, S. T., & Kuersten-Hogan, R. (2003). Evaluating the parental fitness of psychiatrically diagnosed individuals: Advocating a functional-contextual analysis of parenting. *Journal of Family Psychology, 17,* 238–251.

Bennett, B. E., Bricklin, P. M., Harris, E., Knapp, S., VandeCreek, L., & Younggren, J. N. (2006). *Assessing and managing risk in psychological practice: An individualized approach.* Rockville, MD: The Trust.

Berg, I. K. (1994). *Family-based services: A solution-focused approach.* New York, NY: Norton.

Beutler, L. E., Rocco, F., Moleiro, C. M., & Talebi, H. (2001). Resistance. *Psychotherapy: Theory, Research, Practice, Training, 38,* 431–436.

Bishop, D. R., & Eppolito, J. M. (1992). The clinical management of client dynamics and fees for psychotherapy: Implications for research and practice. *Psychotherapy: Theory, Research, Practice, Training, 29,* 545–553.

Blair, I. V., & Banaji, M. R. (1996). Automatic and controlled processes in stereotype priming. *Journal of Personality and Social Psychology, 70,* 1142–1163.

Blake, P. (Writer), & Yaitanes, G. (Director). (2008). The itch [Television series episode]. In P. Attanasio, K. Jacobs, D. Shore, & B. Singer (Executive Producers), *House, M.D.* Santa Monica, CA: Heel & Toe Films.

Blatner, A. (2002). *Using role playing in teaching empathy.* Retrieved from http://www.blatner.com/adam/pdntbk/tchempathy.htm

Bloom, B. S. (1984). *Taxonomy of educational objectives: Book 1. Cognitive domain.* Boston, MA: Allyn & Bacon.

Bohart, A. C. (2001). The evolution of an integrative experiential therapist. In M. R. Goldfried (Ed.), *How therapists change: Personal and professional reflections* (pp. 221–246). Washington, DC: American Psychological Association.

Bolter, K., Levenson, H., & Alvarez, W. F. (1990). Differences in values between short-term and long-term therapists. *Professional Psychology: Research and Practice, 21,* 285–290.

Borckardt, J. J., Nash, M. R., Murphy, M. D., Moore, M., Shaw, D., & O'Neil, P. (2008). Clinical practice as natural laboratory for psychotherapy research: A guide to case-based time-series analysis. *American Psychologist, 63*(2), 77–95.

Bornstein, B. F. (2005). The dependent patient: Diagnosis, assessment, and treatment. *Professional Psychology: Research and Practice, 36,* 82–89.

Boyd-Franklin, N., Franklin, A. J., & Toussaint, P. (2000). *Boys into men: Raising our African American teenage sons.* New York, NY: Dutton.

Bozza, A. (2002, July 4). Eminem: The Rolling Stone interview. *Rolling Stone.* Retrieved from http://www.rollingstone.com/news/story/5938445/ eminem_the_rolling_stone_interview

Brabeck, M., & Brown, L. (1997). Feminist theory and psychological practice. In J. Worell & N. G. Johnson (Eds.), *Shaping the future of feminist psychology: Education, research, and practice* (pp. 15–35). Washington, DC: American Psychological Association.

Brennan, J. (2001). Adjustment to cancer—Coping or personal transition? *Psycho-Oncology, 10,* 1–18.

Briñol, P., Petty, R. E., & Wheeler, S. C. (2006). Discrepancies between explicit and implicit self-concepts: Consequences for information processing. *Journal of Personality and Social Psychology, 91,* 154–170.

Brogan, M. M., Prochaska, J. O., & Prochaska, J. M. (1999). Predicting termination and continuation status in psychotherapy using the transtheoretical model. *Psychotherapy: Theory, Research, Practice, Training, 36*(2), 105–113.

Brown, G. K., Jeglic, E., Henriques, G. R., & Beck, A. T. (2006). Cognitive therapy, cognition, and suicidal behavior. In T. E. Ellis (Ed), *Cognition and suicide Theory, research, and therapy* (pp. 53–74).

Washington, DC: American Psychological Association.

Brown, L. M. (1998). *Raising their voices: The politics of girls' anger.* Cambridge, MA: Harvard University Press.

Brown, L. S. (2004). Feminist paradigms of trauma treatment. *Psychotherapy: Theory, Research, Practice, Training, 41,* 464–471.

Brown, N. R., Lee, P. J., Krslak, M., Conrad, F. G., Hansen, T. G. B., Havelka, J., et al. (2009). Living in history: How war, terrorism, and natural disaster affect the organization of autobiographical memory. *Psychological Science, 20,* 399–405.

Buhs, E. S., Ladd, G. W., & Herald, S. L. (2006). Peer exclusion and victimization: Processes that mediate the relation between peer group rejection and children's classroom engagement and achievement? *Journal of Educational Psychology, 98,* 1–13.

Bureau of Justice Statistics. (2006a). *Homicide trends in the United States.* Retrieved from http://www.ojp.usdoj.gov/bjs/homicide/tables/kidstab.htm

Bureau of Justice Statistics. (2006b). *Prison statistics.* Retrieved from http://www.ojp.usdoj.gov/bjs/prisons.htm

Caldwell, L. D. (2009). Counseling with the poor, underserved, and underrepresented. In C. M. Ellis & J. Carlson (Eds.), *Cross cultural awareness and social justice in counseling* (pp. 283–300). New York, NY: Routledge/Taylor & Francis.

Canadian Psychological Association. (2000). *Canadian code of ethics for psychologists.* Retrieved from http://www.cpa.ca/publications/

Candib, L. M. (2002). Truth telling and advance planning at the end of life: Problems with autonomy in a multicultural world. *Families, Systems, & Health, 20,* 213–228.

Cantor, D. W. (1998). Achieving a mental health bill of rights. *Professional Psychology: Research and Practice, 29,* 315–316.

Cantor, D. W., & Fuentes, M. A. (2008). Psychology's response to managed care. *Professional Psychology: Research and Practice, 39,* 638–645.

Carew, J. (1998). Malcolm X's mother in Montreal: A pioneering educator. In V. R. D'Oyley (Ed.). *Re/visioning:*

Canadian perspectives on the education of Africans in the late 20th century (pp. 18–24). North York, Ontario: Captus Press.

Carkhuff, R. R. (1969). *Helping and human relations: A primer for lay and professional helpers.* New York, NY: Holt, Rinehart, & Winston.

Carlson, J., & Kjos, D. (Producers). (1998). *Psychotherapy with the experts: Person Centered Therapy with Dr. Natalie Rogers.* Boston, MA: Allyn & Bacon.

Carluccio, S. (2009, March 7). Taking care of the caretaker x 2. Message posted to Pennsylvania Psychological Association electronic mailing list.

Carroll, L., Gilroy, P. J., & Murra, J. (1999). The moral imperative: Self-care for women psychotherapists. *Women and Therapy, 22,* 133–143.

Celenza, A. (1995). Love and hate in the countertransference supervisory concerns. *Psychotherapy: Theory, Research, Practice, Training, 32,* 301–307.

Centers for Disease Control and Prevention. (2004, December 3). Diagnoses of HIV/AIDS – 32 States, 2000–2003. *MMWR Weekly, 53,* 1106–1110. [Electronic version] Retrieved from http://www.cdc.gov/mmwr/preview/mmwrhtml/mm5347a3.htm#tab2

Centers for Disease Control and Prevention. (2006). *CDC Wonder.* Retrieved from http://wonder.cdc.gov/

Chaney, J. M., Mullins, L. L., Wagner, J. L., Hommel, K. A., Page, M. C., & Doppler, M. J. (2004). A longitudinal examination of causal attributions and depression symptomatology in rheumatoid arthritis. *Rehabilitation Psychology, 49,* 126–133.

Chang, J., Chan, M., & Stern, O. (2008, February 2). To drink or not to drink: Pregnancy and alcohol. *Good Morning America.* Retrieved from http://abcnews.go.com/video/playerindex?id=4232465

Chasin, R., Grunebaum, M., & Herzig, M. (Eds.), (1990). *One couple/Four realities.* New York, NY: Guilford.

Chavez, A. F., & Guido-DiBrito, F. (1999, Winter). Racial and ethnic identity and development. In M. C. Clark & R. S. Caffarella (Eds.), *An update on adult development theory: New ways of thinking about the life course. New Directions for Adult and Continuing Education, 84* (pp. 39–47). San Francisco, CA: Jossey-Bass.

Chen, S. W.-H., & Davenport, D. S. (2005). Cognitive–behavioral therapy with Chinese American clients: Cautions and modifications. *Psychotherapy: Theory, Research, Practice, Training, 42*, 101–110.

Cheng, S.-T. (2004). Age and subjective well-being revisited: A discrepancy perspective. *Psychology and Aging, 19*, 409–415.

Cohen, A. B. (2009). Many forms of culture. *American Psychologist, 64*, 194–204.

Cokley, K. O. (2002). Testing Cross's revised racial identity model: An examination of the relationship between racial identity and internalized racialism. *Journal of Counseling Psychology, 49*, 476–483.

Cokley, K. O. (2005). Racial(ized) identity, ethnic identity, and Afrocentric values: Conceptual and methodological challenges in understanding African American identity. *Journal of Counseling Psychology, 52*, 517–526.

Contemporary Authors Online. (2003). Anna Michener. *Gale.* PEN: 0000131492

Cooper, A. (2006, January 3). One man found dead in West Virginia mine; Search continues for remaining 12 miners. *Anderson Cooper 360 Degrees.* Retrieved from http://transcripts.cnn.com/TRANSCRIPTS/0601/03/acd.01.html

Cooper, C., & Costas, L. (1994, Spring). Ethical challenges when working with Hispanic/Latino families: Personalismo. *The Family Psychologist, 10*(2), 32–34.

Coster, J. S., & Schwebel, M. (1997). Well-functioning in professional psychologists. *Professional Psychology: Research and Practice, 28*(1), 5–13.

Craig, M. (2002). *The pocket Dalai Lama.* Boston, MA: Shambhala Publications.

Csikszentmihalyi, M. (1990). *Flow: The psychology of optimal experience.* New York, NY: HarperPerennial.

Cullen, D. (2009). *Columbine.* New York, NY: Hatchett Book Group.

Curtis, R. (2002). Termination from a psychoanalytic perspective. *Journal of Psychotherapy Integration, 12*(3), 350–357.

Dalai Lama. (2009). *The Dalai Lama's little book of inner peace: The essential life and teachings.* Charlottesville, VA: Hampton Roads Publishing.

Dalgleish, T., & Power, M. J. (2004). Emotion-specific and emotion-non-specific components of posttraumatic stress disorder (PTSD): Implications for a taxonomy of related psychopathology. *Behaviour Research and Therapy, 42*, 1069–1088.

Dau, J. B., & Sweeney, M. S. (2007). *God grew tired of us: A memoir.* Washington, DC: National Geographic Society.

de Shazer, S. (1988). *Clues: Investigating solutions in brief therapy.* New York, NY: W. W. Norton.

Denno, D. W. (2003). Appendix 1. Time line of Andrea Yates' life and trial. *Duke Journal of Gender Law and Policy, 10*, 61–84. Retrieved from http://www.law.duke.edu/journals/journaltoc?journal=djglp&toc=gentoc10n1.htm

Doherty-Sneddon, G., & Phelps, F. G. (2005). Gaze aversion: A response to cognitive or social difficulty? *Memory and Cognition, 33*, 727–733.

Dumont, F., & Corsini, R. J. (2011). Introduction to twenty-first psychotherapies. In D. Wedding & R. J. Corsini (Eds.), *Case studies in psychotherapy* (9th ed.). Belmont, CA: Cengage.

Dunkley, J., & Whelan, T. A. (2006). Vicarious traumatisation: Current status and future directions. *British Journal of Guidance and Counselling, 34*, 107–116.

Dunn, D. S., & Dougherty, S. B. (2005). Prospects for a positive psychology of rehabilitation. *Rehabilitation Psychology, 50*, 305–311.

Eberlein, L. (1987). Introducing ethics to beginning psychologists: A problem-solving approach. *Professional Psychology: Research and Practice, 18*, 353–359.

Emmons, R. A. (2005). Emotion and religion. In R. F. Paloutzian & C. L. Park (Eds.), *Handbook of the psychology of religion and spirituality* (pp. 235–252). New York, NY: Guilford Press.

Epstein, R. S., & Simon, R. I. (1990). The Exploitation Index: An early warning indicator of boundary violations in psychotherapy. *Bulletin of the Menninger Clinic, 54*, 450–465.

Epston, D., & White, M. (1995). Termination as a rite of passage: Questioning strategies for a therapy of inclusion. In R. A. Neimeyer, & M. J. Mahoney (Eds.), *Constructivism in psychotherapy* (pp. 339–354). Washington, DC: American Psychological Association.

Evans, I. M. (1993). Constructional perspectives in clinical assessment. *Psychological Assessment, 5*, 264–272.

Ewing, C. P. (2005). Judicial Notebook: Tarasoff reconsidered. *Monitor on Psychology, 36*(7), 112.

Faderman, L. (1998). *I begin my life all over: The Hmong and the American immigrant experience.* Boston, MA: Beacon Press.

Fadiman, A. (1997). *The spirit catches you and you fall down.* New York, NY: Farrar, Straus and Giroux.

Farber, B. A., Berano, K. C., & Capobianco, J. A. (2004). Clients' perceptions of the process and consequences of self-disclosure in psychotherapy. *Journal of Counseling Psychology, 51*, 340–346.

Faunce, P. S. (1990). Self-care and wellness of feminist therapists. In H. Lerman & N. Porter (Eds.), *Feminist ethics in psychotherapy* (pp.123–130). New York, NY: Springer.

Faust, J., & Katchen, L. B. (2004). Treatment of children with complicated posttraumatic stress reactions. *Psychotherapy: Theory, Research, Practice, Training, 41*, 426–437.

Fehr, B. (2004). Intimacy expectations in same-sex friendships: a prototype interaction-pattern model. *Journal of Personality and Social Psychology, 86*, 265–284.

Finn, S. E., & Tonsager, M. E. (1997). Information-gathering and therapeutic models of assessment: Complementary paradigms. *Psychological Assessment, 9*, 374–385.

Folkins, J. (1992). Resource on Person-First Language: The language used to describe individuals with disabilities. *American Speech-Language-Hearing Association.* Retrieved from http://www.asha.org/publications/journals/submissions/person_first.htm

Folkman, S., & Moskowitz, J. T. (2004). Coping: Pitfalls and promise. *Annual Review of Psychology, 55*, 745–774.

Folstein, M. F., Folstein, S. E., & McHugh, P. R. (1975). Mini-mental state: A practical method for grading the cognitive state of patients for the clinician. *Journal of Psychiatric Research, 125*, 189–198.

Ford, M. P., & Hendrick, S. S. (2003). Therapists' sexual values for self and clients: Implications for practice and training. *Professional Psychology: Research and Practice, 34*, 80–87.

Fowers, B. J., & Davidov, B. J. (2006). The virtue of multiculturalism: Personal transformation, character, and openness to the other. *American Psychologist, 61,* 581–594.

Frank, J. D., & Frank, J. B. (1993). *Persuasion and healing: A comparative study of psychotherapy* (3rd ed.). Baltimore: Johns Hopkins Paperbacks.

Frankl, V. E. (1946/1984). *Man's search for meaning* (rev. ed.). New York: NY: Washington Square Press.

Fraser, J. S., & Solovey, A. D. (2007). *Second-order change in psychotherapy: The golden thread that unifies effective treatments.* Washington, DC: American Psychological Association.

Frazier, P. A., Mortensen, H., & Steward, J. (2005). Coping strategies as mediators of the relations among perceived control and distress in sexual assault survivors. *Journal of Counseling Psychology, 52,* 267–278.

Friedlander, M. L., Escudero, V., & Heatherington, L. (2006). *Therapeutic alliances in couple and family therapy: An empirically informed guide to practice.* Washington, DC: American Psychological Association.

Friedlander, M. L., Thibodeau, J. R., & Ward, L. G. (1985). Discriminating the "good" from the "bad" therapy hour: A study of dyadic interaction. *Psychotherapy: Theory, Research, Practice, Training, 22,* 631–642.

Fukuyama, M. (1990). Taking a universal approach to multicultural counseling. *Counselor Education and Supervisor, 30,* 6–17.

Fukuyama, M. A., & Sevig, T. D. (1999). *Integrating spirituality into multicultural counseling.* Thousand Oaks, CA: Sage.

Gabriella. (2001, February). Interview with Eminem: It's lonely at the top. *NY Rock.* Retrieved from http://www.nyrock.com/interviews/2001/eminem_int.asp

Gandy, K. (2002, March 13). Yates verdict can serve as warning to prevent future tragedies. *National Organization for Women.* Retrieved from http://www.now.org/press/03-02/03-13a.html

Garcia, J. A., & Weisz, J. R. (2002). When youth mental health care stops: Therapeutic relationship problems and other reasons for ending youth outpatient treatment. *Journal of Consulting and Clinical Psychology, 70,* 439–443.

Gately, G. (2006, January 7). Miner's wife hopes prayers and Metallica will help him pull through. *New York Times.* Retrieved from http://www.nytimes.com/2006/01/07/national/07survivor.html?_r=1&n=Top%2fNews%2fNational%2fU.S.%20States%2c%20Territories%20and%20Possessions%2fWest%20Virginia

Gawthrop, J. C., & Uhlemann, M. R. (1992). Effects of the problem-solving approach in ethics training. *Professional Psychology: Research and Practice, 23,* 38–42.

Gesn, P. R., & Ickes, W. (1999). The development of meaning contexts for empathic accuracy: Channel and sequence effects. *Journal of Personality and Social Psychology, 7,* 746–761.

Getzinger, A. (1993). Informed consent and systems consultation: A description of the process and a prescription for change. *Family Systems Medicine, 11,* 235–245.

Gilbert, D. T., & Malone, P. S. (1995). The correspondence bias. *Psychological Bulletin, 117,* 21–38.

Gilligan, C. (1982). *In a different voice: Psychological theory and women's development.* Cambridge, MA: Harvard University Press.

Gilroy, P. J., Carroll, L., & Murra, J. (2002). A preliminary survey of counseling psychologists' personal experiences with depression and treatment. *Professional Psychology: Research and Practice, 33,* 402–407.

Gilstrap, L. L. (2004). A missing link in suggestibility research: What is known about the behavior of field interviewers in unstructured interviews with young children? *Journal of Experimental Psychology: Applied, 10,* 13–24.

Ginzburg, K. (2004). PTSD and world assumptions following myocardial infarction: A longitudinal study. *American Journal of Orthopsychiatry, 74,* 286–292.

Glick, D., Keene-Osborn, S., Gegax, T. T., Bai, M., Clemetson, L., Gordon, D., et al. (1999, May 3). Anatomy of a massacre. *Newsweek, 153,* 24–30.

Glosoff, H. L., & Kocet, M. M. (2005). Highlights of the 2005 ACA Code of Ethics. In G. R. Walz, J. C. Bleuer, & R. K. Yep (Eds.), *Vistas: Compelling perspectives on counseling 2006* (pp. 5–9). Alexandria, VA: American Counseling Association.

Goerke, M., Möller, J., Schulz-Hardt, S., Napiersky, U., & Frey, D. (2004). "It's not my fault—but only I can change it": Counterfactual and prefactual thoughts of managers. *Journal of Applied Psychology, 89,* 279–292.

Goldfried, M. R. (2002). A cognitive-behavioral perspective on termination. *Journal of Psychotherapy Integration, 12*(3), 364–372.

Goldfried, M. R. (2004). Integrating integratively oriented brief psychotherapy. *Journal of Psychotherapy Integration, 14,* 93–105.

Goldfried, M. R. (2007). What has psychotherapy inherited from Carl Rogers? *Psychotherapy: Theory, Research, Practice, Training, 44,* 249–252.

Goldfried, M. R., & Davila, J. (2005). The role of relationship and technique in therapeutic change. *Psychotherapy: Theory, Research, Practice, Training, 42,* 421–430.

Gollan, T., & Witte, E. H. (2008). "It was right to do it, because …" Understanding justifications of actions as prescriptive attributions. *Social Psychology, 39,* 189–196.

Gonzalez, J. S., Safren, S. A., Cagliero, E., Wexler, D. J., Delahanty, L., Wittenberg, E., et al. (2009). Depression, self-care, and medication adherence in Type 2 Diabetes: Relationships across the full range of symptom severity. *Diabetes Care, 30,* 2222–2227.

Gray, M. J., Maguen, S., & Litz, B. T. (2007). Schema constructs and cognitive models of posttraumatic stress disorder. In L. P. Riso, P. L. du Toit, D. J. Stein, & J. E. Young, (Eds.), *Cognitive schemas and core beliefs in psychological problems: A scientist-practitioner guide* (pp. 59–92). Washington, DC: American Psychological Association.

Greenberg, D., & Wiesner, I. S. (2004). Jews. In A. M. Josephson & J. R. Peteet (Eds.), *Handbook of spirituality and worldview in clinical practice* (pp. 91–109). Arlington, VA: American Psychiatric Association.

Greenberg, L. (2008). Emotion and cognition in psychotherapy: The transforming power of affect. *Canadian Psychology/Psychologie canadienne, 49,* 49–59.

Greenberg, L. S. (2002). Termination of experiential therapy. *Journal of*

Psychotherapy Integration, 12(3), 358–363.

Greenberg, L. S., Elliot, R., Watson, J. C., & Bohart, A. C. (2001). Empathy. *Psychotherapy: Theory, Research, Practice, Training, 38,* 380–384.

Greenberg, L. S., & Safran, J. D. (1987). *Emotion in psychotherapy: Affect, cognition, and the process of change.* New York, NY: Guilford Press.

Greene, B. A. (1985). Considerations in the treatment of Black patients by White therapists. *Psychotherapy, 22,* 389–393.

Greenfield, P. M., Trumbull, E., Keller, H., Rothstein-Fisch, C., Suzuki, L., & Quiroz, B. (2006). Cultural conceptions of learning and development. In P. A. Alexander & P. H. Winne (Eds.), *Handbook of educational psychology* (pp. 675–692). Mahwah, NJ: Lawrence Erlbaum.

Grigsby, N., & Hartman, B. R. (1997). The Barriers Model: An integrated strategy for intervention with battered women. *Psychotherapy: Theory, Research, Practice, Training, 34,* 485–497.

Guthiel, T., & Gabbard, G. (1993). The concept of boundaries in clinical practice: Theoretical and risk management dimensions. *American Journal of Psychiatry, 150,* 188–196.

Guy, J. D. (2000). Self-care corner: Holding the holding environment together: Self-psychology and psychotherapist care. *Professional Psychology: Research and Practice, 31*(3), 351–352.

Haldeman, D. C. (2002). Gay rights, patient rights: The implications of sexual orientation conversion therapy. *Professional Psychology: Research and Practice, 33,* 260–264.

Hall, J. A., & Schmid Mast, M. (2007). Sources of accuracy in the empathic accuracy paradigm. *Emotion, 7,* 438–446.

Hampton-Robb, S., Qualls, R. C., & Compton, W. C. (2003). Predicting first-session attendance: The influence of referral source and client income. *Psychotherapy Research, 13,* 223–233.

Handelsman, M. M., Gottlieb, M. C., & Knapp, S. (2005). Training ethical psychologists: An acculturation model. *Professional Psychology: Research and Practice, 36,* 59–65.

Handelsman, M. M., Knapp, S., & Gottlieb, M. C. (2002). Positive ethics. In C. R. Snyder & S. Lopez (Eds.), *Handbook of positive psychology* (pp. 731–744). New York, NY: Oxford University Press.

Handelsman, M. M., & Martin, W. L. (1992). Effects of readability on the impact and recall of written informed consent material. *Professional Psychology: Research and Practice, 23,* 500–503.

Hardin, E. E., Weigold, I. K., Robitschek, C., & Nixon, A. E. (2007). Self-discrepancy and distress: The role of personal growth initiative. *Journal of Counseling Psychology, 54,* 86–92.

Hart, J., Shaver, P. R., & Goldenberg, J. L. (2005). Attachment, self-esteem, worldviews, and terror management: Evidence for a tripartite security system. *Journal of Personality and Social Psychology, 88,* 999–1013.

Hatchett, G. T., & Park, H. L. (2003). Comparison of four operational definitions of premature termination. *Psychotherapy: Theory, Research, Practice, Training, 40*(3), 226–231.

Hawley, K. M., & Weisz, J. R. (2003). Child, parent and therapist (dis)agreement on target problems in outpatient therapy: The therapist's dilemma and its implications. *Journal of Consulting and Clinical Psychology, 71,* 62–70.

Hays, J. R. (2002, May/June). State of Texas v. Andrea Yates. *National Psychologist, 11*(3). Retrieved from http://nationalpsychologist.com/articles/art_v11n3_3.htm

Hazan, C., & Shaver, P. (1987). Romantic love conceptualized as an attachment process. *Journal of Personality and Social Psychology, 52,* 511–524.

Heilbrun, K., & Kramer, G. M. (2005). Involuntary medication, trial competence, and clinical dilemmas: Implications of Sell v. United States for psychological practice. *Professional Psychology: Research and Practice, 36,* 459–466.

Helms, J. E., & Cook, D. A. (1999). *Using race and culture in counseling and psychotherapy: Theory and process.* Boston, MA: Allyn & Bacon.

Hinrichsen, G. A., & Pollack, S. (1997). Expressed emotion and the course of late-life depression. *Journal of Abnormal Psychology, 106,* 336–340.

Hirt, E. R., McDonald, H. E., & Erikson, G. A. (1995). How do I remember thee? The role of encoding set and delay in reconstructive memory processes. *Journal of Experimental Social Psychology, 63,* 724–738.

Hodges, K., Doucette-Gates, A., & Liao, Q. (1999). The relationship between the Child and Adolescent Functional Assessment Scale (CAFAS) and indicators of functioning. *Journal of Child and Family Studies, 8,* 109–122.

Holmes, T. H., & Rahe, R. H. (1967). The Social Readjustment Rating Scale. *Journal of Psychosomatic Research, 11,* 213–218.

Hooley, J. M., & Hiller, J. B. (2000). Personality and expressed emotion. *Journal of Abnormal Psychology, 109,* 40–44.

Hooley, J. M., & Teasdale, J. D. (1989). Predictors of relapse in unipolar depressives: Expressed emotion, marital distress, and perceived criticism. *Journal of Abnormal Psychology, 98*(3), 229–235.

Hubble, M. A., Duncan, B. L., & Miller, S. D. (Eds.). (1999). *The heart & soul of change: What works in therapy.* Washington, DC: American Psychological Association.

Ibrahim, F. A. (1985). Effective cross-cultural counseling and psychotherapy: A framework. *Counseling Psychologist, 13,* 625–638.

Ito, T. A., Larsen, J. T., Smith, N. K., & Cacioppo, J. T. (1998). Negative information weighs more heavily on the brain: The negativity bias in evaluative categorizations. *Journal of Personality and Social Psychology, 75,* 887–900.

Ivey, A. E., & Ivey, M. B. (2003). *Intentional interviewing and counseling: Facilitating client development in a multicultural society* (5th ed.). Pacific Grove, CA: Brooks/Cole.

Ivey, A. E., Ivey, M. B., & Simek-Morgan, L. (1997). *Counseling and psychotherapy: A multicultural perspective.* Boston, MA: Allyn & Bacon.

Janis, I. L. (1997). Groupthink. In W. A. Lesko (Ed.), *Readings in social psychology* (3rd ed., pp. 333–337). Boston, MA: Allyn & Bacon.

Janoff-Bulman, R. (1989). Assumptive worlds and the stress of traumatic events: Applications of the schema construct. *Social Cognition, 7,* 113–136.

Jenaro, C., Flores, N., & Arias, B. (2007). Burnout and coping in human service practitioners.

Professional Psychology: Research and Practice, 38(1), 80–87.

Jennings, L., & Skovholt, T. M. (2001). The cognitive, emotional, and relational characteristics of master therapists. *Journal of Counseling Psychology, 46*, 3–11.

Jennings, L., Sovereign, A., Botorff, N., Mussell, M. P., & Vye, C. (2005). Nine ethical values of master therapists. *Journal of Mental Health Counseling, 27*, 32–47.

John, E. (2005, April 21). Eminem. *Rolling Stone, 972*, 90.

Jones, E. E. (1979). The rocky road from acts to dispositions. *American Psychologist, 34*, 107–117.

Jones, G. C., Rovner, B. W., Crews, J. E., & Danielson, M. L. (2009). Effects of depressive symptoms on health behavior practices among older adults with vision loss. *Rehabilitation Psychology, 54*, 164–172.

Kabacoff, R. I., Miller, I. W., Bishop, D. S., Epstein, N. B., & Keitner, G. (1990). A psychometric study of the McMaster Family Assessment Device in psychiatric, medical, and non-clinical samples. *Journal of Family Psychology, 3*, 431–439.

Kahana, B., Hurel, Z., & Kahana, E. (1988). Predictors of psychological well-being among survivors of the Holocaust. In J. Wilson, Z. Harel, & B. Kahana (Eds.), *Human adaptation to extreme stress* (pp. 171–192). New York, NY: Plenum.

Karno, M. P., & Longabaugh, R. (2005). Less directiveness by therapists improves drinking outcomes of reactant clients in alcoholism treatment. *Journal of Consulting and Clinical Psychology, 73*, 262–267.

Kerwin, C., Ponterotto, J. G., Jackson, B. L., & Harris, A. (1993). Racial iden-tity in biracial children: A qualitative investigation. *Journal of Counseling Psychology, 40*, 221–231.

Keyes, C. L. M., & Haidt, J. (2003). *Flourishing: Positive psychology and the life well-lived.* Washington, DC: American Psychological Association.

Kidd, S. M. (2006). *When the heart waits: Spiritual direction for life's sacred questions.* New York, NY: HarperOne.

Kids Count Data Center. (2009). Data book. *Annie E. Casey Foundation.* Retrieved from http://datacenter.kidscount.org/databook/2009/Default.aspx

Kim, B. S. K., Ng, G. F., & Ahn, A. J. (2005). Effects of client expectation for counseling success, client–counselor worldview match, and client adherence to Asian and European American cultural values on counseling process with Asian Americans. *Journal of Counseling Psychology, 52*, 67–76.

Kirsch, I., Deacon, B. J., Huedo-Medina, T. B., Scoboria, A., Moore, T. J., & Johnson, B. T. (2008). Initial severity and antidepressant benefits: A meta-analysis of data submitted to the FDA. *PLoS Medicine, 5*, 260–268.

Kitchener, K. S. (1984). Intuition, critical evaluation and ethical principles: The foundation for ethical decisions in counseling psychology. *Counseling Psychologist, 12*, 43–55.

Kitchener, K. S. (1986). Teaching applied ethics in counselor education: An integration of psychological processes and philosophical analysis. *Journal of Counseling and Development, 64*, 306–310.

Knapp, S., & Slattery, J. M. (2004). Professional boundaries in non-traditional settings. *Professional Psychology: Research and Practice, 35*, 553–558.

Knapp, S. J., & Vandecreek, L. D. (2006). *Practical ethics for psychologists: A positive approach.* Washington, DC: American Psychological Association.

Knapp, S., & Vandecreek, L. (2007). Balancing respect for autonomy with competing values with the use of principle-based ethics. *Psychotherapy: Theory, Research, Practice, Training, 44*, 397–404.

Kohlberg, L. (1966). Moral education in the schools: A developmental view. *School Review, 74*, 1–30.

Koltko-Rivera, M. E. (2004). The psychology of worldviews. *Review of General Psychology, 8*, 3–58.

Kottler, J. A. (2004). *Introduction to therapeutic counseling: Voices from the field* (5th ed.). Pacific Grove, CA: Brooks/Cole.

Kramen-Kahn, B., & Hansen, N. D. (1998). Rafting the rapids: Occupational hazards, rewards, and coping strategies of psychotherapists. *Professional Psychology: Research and Practice, 29*, 130–134.

Labov, W. (1997). Some further steps in narrative analysis. *The Journal of Narrative and Life History, 7*, 395–415.

Lakin, J. L., & Chartrand, T. L. (2003). Using nonconscious behavioral mimicry to create affiliation and rapport. *Psychological Science, 14*, 334–339.

Lam, A. G., & Sue, S. (2001). Client diversity. *Psychotherapy: Theory, Research, Practice, Training, 38*, 479–486.

Lamb, D. H., & Catanzaro, S. J. (1998). Sexual and nonsexual boundary violations involving psychologists, clients, supervisees, and students: Implications for professional practice. *Professional Psychology: Research and Practice, 29*, 498–503.

Lambert, M. J. (1992). Implications of outcome research for psychotherapy integration. In J. C. Norcross & M. R. Goldstein (Eds.), *Handbook of psychotherapy integration* (pp. 94–129). New York, NY: Basic Books.

Lambert, M. J., & Archer, A. (2006). Research findings on the effects of psychotherapy and their implications for practice. In C. D. Goodheart, A. E. Kazdin, & R. J. Sternberg (Eds.), *Evidence-based psychotherapy: Where practice and research meet* (pp. 111–130). Washington, DC: American Psychological Association.

Lambert, M. J., & Barley, D. E. (2001). Research summary on the therapeutic relationship and psychotherapy outcome. *Psychotherapy: Theory, Research, Practice, Training, 38*, 357–361.

Lambert, M. J., Gregersen, A. T., & Burlingame, G. M. (2004). The Outcome Questionnaire-45. In M. E. Maruish (Ed.), *The use of psychological testing for treatment planning and outcome assessment* (3rd ed., pp. 191–234). Mahwah, NJ: Erlbaum.

Lane, S. (2004). *Eminem.* New York, NY: Gale.

Langton, S. R. H., O'Malley, C., & Bruce, V. (1996). Actions speak no louder than words: Symmetrical cross-modal interference effects in the processing of verbal and gestural information. *Journal of Experimental Psychology: Human Perception and Performance, 22*(6), 1357–1375.

Lao Family Community of Minnesota, Inc. (1997). *Hmong history and culture.* Retrieved from http://www.laofamily.org/hmong-history-culture.htm

Larsen, D. L., Atkisson, C. C., Hargreaves, W. A., & Nguyen, T.D.

(1979). Assessment of client/patient satisfaction: Development of a general scale. *Evaluation and Program Planning, 2,* 197–207.

LaTorre, R. A. (1977). Pretherapy role induction procedures. *Canadian Psychological Review, 18,* 308–321.

Laudet, A. B., Magura, S., Vogel, H. S., & Knight, E. L. (2004). Perceived reasons for substance misuse among persons with a psychiatric disorder. *American Journal of Orthopsychiatry, 74,* 365–375.

Lazarus, A. A. (1993). Tailoring the therapeutic relationship, or being an authentic chameleon. *Psychotherapy: Theory, Research, Practice, Training, 30,* 404–407.

Leahy, R. L. (2002). A model of emotional schemas. *Cognitive and Behavioral Practice, 9,* 177–190.

Lee, D. Y., Uhlemann, M. R., & Haase, R. F. (1985). Counselor verbal and nonverbal responses and perceived expertness, trustworthiness, and attractiveness. *Journal of Counseling Psychology, 32,* 181–187.

Lee, R. E. (2009). "If you build it, they may not come": Lessons from a funded project. *Research on Social Work Practice, 1,* 251–260.

Lent, R. W. (2004). Toward a unifying theoretical and practical perspective on well-being and psychosocial adjustment. *Journal of Counseling Psychology, 51,* 482–509.

Lerner, M. J. (1970). The desire for justice and reactions to victims: Social psychological studies of some antecedents and consequences. In J. Macaulay & L. Berkowitz (Eds.), *Altruism and helping behavior.* New York, NY: Academic Press.

Liberman, A., & Chaiken, S. (1991). Value conflict and thought-induced attitude change. *Journal of Experimental Social Psychology, 27,* 203–216.

Lilliengren, P., & Werbart, A. (2005). A model of therapeutic action grounded in the patients' view of curative and hindering factors in psychoanalytic psychotherapy. *Psychotherapy: Theory, Research, Practice, Training, 42,* 324–339.

Linehan, M. M. (1993). *Cognitive-behavioral treatment of borderline personality disorder.* New York, NY: Guilford.

Liszcz, A. M., & Yarhouse, M. A. (2005). Same-sex attraction: A survey regarding client-directed

treatment goals. *Psychotherapy: Theory, Research, Practice, Training, 42,* 111–115.

Lopez, S. J., & Snyder, C. R. (2003). The future of positive psychological assessment: Making a difference. In S. J. Lopez & V. R. Snyder (Eds.), *Positive psychological assessment: A handbook of models and measures* (pp. 461–468). Washington, DC: American Psychological Association.

Lopez, S. J., Snyder, C. R., & Rasmussen, H. N. (2003). Striking a vital balance: Developing a complementary focus on human weakness and strength through positive psychological assessment. In S. J. Lopez & V. R. Snyder (Eds.), *Positive psychological assessment: A handbook of models and measures* (pp. 3–20). Washington, DC: American Psychological Association.

López, S. R., Nelson Hipke, K., Polo, A. J., Jenkins, J. H., Karno, M., Vaughn, C., et al. (2004). Ethnicity, expressed emotion, attributions, and course of schizophrenia: Family warmth matters. *Journal of Abnormal Psychology, 113,* 428–439.

Luster, T., Qin, D., Bates, L., Johnson, D., & Rana, M. (2009). The Lost Boys of Sudan: Coping with ambiguous loss and separation from parents. *American Journal of Orthopsychiatry, 79,* 203–211.

Maio, G., & Olson, J. M. (1998). Values as truisms: Evidence and implications. *Journal of Personality and Social Psychology, 74,* 294–311.

Malcolm X, & Haley, A. (1964/1999). *The autobiography of Malcolm X.* New York, NY: Ballantine Books.

Martin, D. J., Garske, J. P., & Davis, M. K. (2000). Relation of the therapeutic alliance with outcome and other variables: A meta-analytic review. *Journal of Consulting and Clinical Psychology, 68*(3), 438–450.

Mathews, T. J., & MacDorman, M. F. (2006). Infant mortality statistics from the 2003 period linked birth/infant death data set. *National Vital Statistics Reports.* Retrieved from http://www.cdc.gov/nchs/data/nvsr/nvsr54/nvsr54_16.pdf

Mattlin, J. A., Wethington, E., & Kessler, R. (1990). Situational determinants of coping and coping effectiveness. *Journal of Health and Social Behavior, 31,* 103–122.

May, R. (1967). *The art of counseling.* Nashville, TN: Abingdon.

McCabe, G. H. (2007). The healing path: A culture and community-derived indigenous therapy model. *Psychotherapy: Theory, Research, Practice, Training, 44,* 148–160.

McGoldrick, M. (1999). Explaining genogram symbols. *Multicultural Family Institute.* Retrieved from http://www.multiculturalfamily.org/genograms/genogram_symbols.html

McGoldrick, M., Gerson, R., & Shellenberger, S. (1999). *Genograms: Assessment and intervention* (2nd ed.). New York, NY: W. W. Norton.

McIntosh, P. (1989, July/August). White privilege: Unpacking the invisible knapsack. *Peace and Freedom,* pp. 10–12.

McKinnon, J. (2003). *The Black Population in the United States: March 2002.* U.S. Census Bureau, Current Population Reports, Series P20-541. Washington, DC. Retrieved from http://www.census.gov/prod/2003pubs/p20-541.pdf

McLellan, A. T., Alterman, A. I., Metzger, D. S., Grissom, G. R., Woody, G. E., Luborsky, L., et al. (1994). Similarity of outcome predictors across opiate, cocaine, and alcohol treatments: Role of treatment services. *Journal of Consulting and Clinical Psychology, 62,* 1141–1158.

Meehl, P. E. (1954). *Clinical versus statistical prediction.* Minneapolis, MN: University of Minnesota Press.

Meichenbaum, D. (2005). 35 years of working with suicidal patients: Lessons learned. *Canadian Psychology, 46,* 64–72.

Merton, R. K. (1948). The self-fulfilling prophecy. *Antioch Review, 8,* 193–210.

Michener, A. J. (1998). *Becoming Anna: The autobiography of a sixteen-year-old.* Chicago, IL: University of Chicago Press.

Mikulincer, M. (1998). Adult attachment style and affect regulation: Strategic variations in self-appraisals. *Journal of Personality and Social Psychology, 75,* 420–435.

Miller, R. B. (2005). Suffering in psychology: The demoralization of psychotherapeutic practice. *Journal of Psychotherapy Integration, 15,* 299–336.

Moline, M. E., Williams, G. T., & Austin, K. M. (1998). *Documenting psychotherapy: Essentials for mental health practitioners.* Thousand Oaks, CA: Sage.

Moos, R. H. (2003). Addictive disorders in context: Principles and puzzles of effective treatment and recovery. *Psychology of Addictive Behaviors, 17,* 3–12.

Mordecai, E. M. (1991). A classification of empathic failures for psychotherapists and supervisors. *Psychoanalytic Psychology, 8,* 251–262.

Mozdrzierz, G. J., Peluso, P. R., & Lisiecki, J. (2009). *Principles of counseling and psychotherapy: Learning the essential domains and nonlinear thinking of master practitioners.* New York, NY: Routledge.

Muder, D. (2007, Fall). Not my father's religion: Unitarian Universalism and the working class. *UU World, 21*(3), pp. 33–37.

Mulvey, E. P., & Cauffman, E. (2001). The inherent limits of predicting school violence. *American Psychologist, 56,* 797–802.

Murphy, B. C., & Dillon, C. (2003). *Interviewing in action: Relationship, process, and change.* Pacific Grove, CA: Brooks/Cole.

Murphy, H., Dickens, C., Creed, F., & Bernstein, R. (1999). Depression, illness perception and coping in rheumatoid arthritis. *Journal of Psychosomatic Research, 46,* 155–164.

National Association of Social Workers. (2008). *Code of ethics of the National Association of Social Workers.* Retrieved from http://www.social workers.org/pubs/code/code.asp

Neimeyer, R. A., & Stewart, A. E. (2000). Constructivist and narrative psychotherapies. In C. R. Snyder & R. E. Ingram (Eds.), *Handbook of psychotherapy* (pp. 337–357). New York, NY: Wiley.

Nelson, M. L., Englar-Carlson, M., Tierney, S. C., & Hau, J. M. (2006). Class jumping into academia: Multiple identities for counseling academics. *Journal of Counseling Psychology, 53,* 1–14.

Neugebauer, A., Katz, P. P., & Pasch, L. A. (2003). Effect of valued activity disability, social comparisons, and satisfaction with ability on depressive symptoms in rheumatoid arthritis. *Health Psychology, 22,* 253–262.

News conference with EO of International Coal Group. (2006, January 4).

New York Times. Retrieved from http://www.nytimes.com/2006/01/04/national/04text-hatfield.html?emc=eta1

Nolen-Hoeksema, S., Wisco, B. E., & Lyubomirsky, S. (2008). Rethinking rumination. *Perspectives on Psychological Science, 3,* 400–424.

Norcross, J. C. (2000). Psychotherapist self-care: Practitioner-tested, research-informed strategies. *Professional Psychology: Research and Practice, 31,* 710–713.

Norcross, J. C., & Wogan, M. (1987). Values in psychotherapy: A survey of practitioners' beliefs. *Professional Psychology: Research and Practice, 18,* 5–7.

Nowell, D., & Spruill, J. (1993). If it's not absolutely confidential, will information be disclosed? *Professional Psychology: Research and Practice, 24,* 367–369.

Noy-Sharav, D. (1998). Who is afraid of STDP? Termination in STDP and therapist's personality. *Psychotherapy: Theory, Research, Practice, Training, 35,* 69–77.

O'Connor, K. (2005). Addressing diversity issues in play therapy. *Professional Psychology: Research and Practice, 36,* 566–573.

O'Farrell, T. J., Hooley, J., Fals-Stewart, W., & Cutter, H. S. G. (1998). Expressed emotion and relapse in alcoholic patients. *Journal of Consulting and Clinical Psychology, 66,* 744–752.

O'Hanlon, W. H., & Weiner-Davis, M. (1989). *In search of solutions: A new direction in psychotherapy.* New York, NY: W. W. Norton.

Olopade, D. (2009, July 21). Skip Gates speaks. *The Root.* Retrieved from http://www.theroot.com/views/skip-gates-speaks?page=0,0

O'Malley, S. (2004). *"Are you there alone?": The unspeakable crime of Andrea Yates.* New York, NY: Simon & Schuster.

Orlinsky, D. E., & Ronnestad, M. H. (2005a). Aspects of professional development. In D. E. Orlinsky & M. H. Ronnestad (Eds.), *How psychotherapists develop: A study of therapeutic work and professional growth* (pp. 103–116). Washington, DC: American Psychological Association.

Orlinsky, D. E., & Ronnestad, M. H. (2005b). Career development: Correlates of evolving expertise. In D. E. Orlinsky & M. H. Ronnestad

(Eds.), *How psychotherapists develop: A study of therapeutic work and professional growth* (pp. 131–142). Washington, DC: American Psychological Association.

Orlinsky, D. E., Ronnestad, M. H., Gerin, P., Davis, J. D., Ambühl, H., Davis, M. L., et al. (2005). The development of psychotherapists. In D. E. Orlinsky & M. H. Ronnestad (Eds.), *How psychotherapists develop: A study of therapeutic work and professional growth* (pp. 3–13). Washington, DC: American Psychological Association.

Oyserman, D. (1993). The lens of personhood: Viewing the self and others in a multicultural society. *Journal of Personality and Social Psychology, 65,* 993–1009.

Oyserman, D., Coon, H. M., & Kemmelmeier, M. (2002). Rethinking individualism and collectivism: Evaluation of theoretical assumptions and meta-analyses. *Psychological Bulletin, 128,* 3–72.

Paniagua, F. A. (1998). *Assessing and treating culturally diverse clients: A practical guide* (2nd ed.). Thousand Oaks, CA: Sage.

Park, C. L. (2004). The notion of stress-related growth: Problems and prospects. *Psychological Inquiry, 15,* 69–76.

Park, C. L. (2005). Religion and meaning. In R. F. Paloutzian & C. L. Park (Eds.), *Handbook of the psychology of religion and spirituality* (pp. 295–314). New York, NY: Guilford Press.

Park, C. L., Aldwin, C. M., Fenster, J. R., & Snyder, L. B. (2008). Pathways to posttraumatic growth versus posttraumatic stress: Coping and emotional reactions following the September 11, 2001, terrorist attacks. *American Journal of Orthopsychiatry, 78,* 300–312.

Park, C. L., Edmondson, D., & Mills, M. A. (in press). Reciprocal influences of religiousness and global meaning in the stress process. In T. Miller (Ed.), *Coping with life transitions.* Mahwah, NJ: Erlbaum.

Park, C. L., & Folkman, S. (1997). Meaning in the context of stress and coping. *Review of General Psychology, 1,* 115–144.

Park, C. L., Folkman, S., & Bostrom, A. (2001). Appraisals of controllability and coping in caregivers and HIV+ men: Testing the goodness-of-fit hypothesis. *Journal of Consulting and Clinical Psychology, 69,* 481–488.

Park, C. L., Lechner, S. C., Antoni, M. H., & Stanton, A. L. (Eds.). (2009). *Medical illness and positive life change: Can crisis lead to personal transformation?* Washington, DC: American Psychological Association.

Park, C. L., & Slattery, J. M. (2009). Including spirituality in case conceptualizations: A meaning system approach. In J. Aten & M. Leach (Eds.), *Spirituality and the therapeutic practice: A guide for mental health professionals* (pp. 121–142). Washington, DC: American Psychological Association.

Park, J., & Banaji, M. R. (2000). Mood and heuristics: The influence of happy and sad states on sensitivity and bias in stereotyping. *Journal of Personality and Social Psychology, 78,* 1005–1023.

Partie, M. (2005, October). Flying back over the cuckoo's nest. *Therapeutic Options.* Retrieved from http://therops.net/node/26

Pearlman, L. A., & Mac Ian, P. S. (1995). Vicarious traumatization: An empirical study of the effects of trauma work on trauma therapists. *Professional Psychology: Research and Practice, 26*(6), 558–565.

Pedersen, P. B., Crethar, H. C., & Carlson, J. (2008). *Inclusive cultural empathy: Making relationships central in counseling and psychotherapy.* Washington, DC: American Psychological Association.

Petty, S. C., Sachs-Ericsson, N., & Joiner, T. E. (2004). Interpersonal functioning deficits: Temporary or stable characteristics of depressed individuals? *Journal of Affective Disorders, 81,* 115–122.

Piaget, J. (1929/1960). *The child's conception of the world.* Oxford, England: Littlefield, Adams.

Pinel, E. C., & Constantinou, M. J. (2003). Putting self psychology to good use: When social and clinical psychologists unite. *Journal of Psychotherapy Integration, 13,* 9–32.

Pipes, R. B., Blevins, T., & Kluck, A. (2008). Confidentiality, ethics, and informed consent. *American Psychologist, 63,* 623–624.

Pitts, G., & Wallace, P. A. (2003). Cultural awareness in the diagnosis of Attention Deficit/Hyperactivity Disorder. *Primary Psychiatry, 10,* 84–88.

Pomerantz, A. M., & Handelsman, M. M. (2004). Informed consent revisited: An updated written question format. *Professional Psychology: Research and Practice, 35,* 201–205.

Pope, K. S., & Brown, L. S. (1996). *Recovered memories of abuse: Assessment, therapy, forensics.* Washington, DC: American Psychological Association.

Pope, K. S., Keith-Spiegel, P., & Tabachnick, B. G. (1986). Sexual attraction to clients: The human therapist and the (sometimes) inhuman training system. *American Psychologist, 41*(2), 147–158.

Pope, K. S., & Keith-Spiegel, P. (2008). A practical approach to boundaries in psychotherapy: Making decisions, bypassing blunders, and mending fences. *Journal of Clinical Psychology: In Session, 64,* 638–652.

Pope, K. S., Sonne, J. L., & Holroyd, J. (1993). *Sexual feelings in psychotherapy: Explorations for therapists and therapists-in-training.* Washington, DC: American Psychological Association.

Pope, K. S., & Tabachnick, B. G. (1993). Therapists' anger, hate, fear, and sexual feelings: National survey of therapist responses, client characteristics, critical events, formal complaints, and training. *Professional Psychology: Research and Practice, 24,* 142–152.

Pope, K. S., Tabachnick, B. G., & Keith-Spiegel, P. (1988). Good and poor practices in psychotherapy: National survey of beliefs of psychologists. *Professional Psychology: Research and Practice, 19,* 547–552.

Pope, K. S., & Vasquez, M. T. (1998). *Ethics in psychotherapy and counseling* (2nd ed.). San Francisco, CA: Jossey-Bass.

Pope, K. S., & Vasquez, M. T. (2005). *How to survive and thrive as a therapist: Information, ideas, and resources for psychologists in practice.* Washington, DC: American Psychological Association.

Prager, E., & Solomon, Z. (1995). Perceptions of world benevolence, meaningfulness, and self-worth among elderly Israeli Holocaust survivors and non-survivors. *Anxiety, Stress, and Coping, 8,* 265–277.

Pretzer, J. L., & Walsh, C. A. (2001). Optimism, pessimism, and psychotherapy: Implications for clinical practice. In E. C. Chang (Ed.), *Optimism & pessimism: Implications for theory, research, and practice* (pp. 321–346). Washington, DC: American Psychological Association.

Prochaska, J. O. (1999). How do people change, and how can we change to help many more people? In M. A. Hubble, B. L. Duncan, & S. D. Miller (Eds.), *The heart & soul of change: What works in therapy* (pp. 227–255). Washington, DC: American Psychological Association.

Prochaska, J. O., & DiClemente, C. C. (1982). Transtheoretical therapy: Toward a more integrative model of change. *Psychotherapy: Theory, Research & Practice, 19,* 276–288.

Prochaska, J. O., & Norcross, J. C. (2001). Stages of change. *Psychotherapy: Theory, Research, Practice, Training, 38,* 443–448.

Radeke, J. T., & Mahoney, M. J. (2000). Comparing the personal lives of psychotherapists and research psychologists. *Professional Psychology: Research and Practice, 31,* 82–84.

Raphaely, D. (1991). Informed consent near death: Myth and actuality. *Family Systems Medicine, 9,* 343–370.

Religious Tracts by Michael Woroniecki. (2008, November 13). Retrieved from http://www.flickr.com/photos/86593188@N00/3028898336/sizes/l/in/set-72157609022093567/

Reust, C. E., Thomlinson, R. P., & Lattie, D. (1999). Keeping or missing the initial behavioral health appointment: A qualitative study of referrals in a primary care setting. *Families, Systems and Health, 17,* 399–411.

Reyes, C. J., Kokotovic, A. M., & Cosden, M. A. (1996). Sexually abused children's perceptions: How they may change treatment focus. *Professional Psychology: Research and Practice, 27,* 588–591.

Rigazio-DiGilio, S. A., Ivey, A. E., Kunkler-Peck, K. P., & Grady, L. T. (2005). *Community genograms: Using individual, family and cultural narratives with clients.* New York, NY: Teachers College Press.

Robin, K. (Writer), & Garcia, R. (Director). (2001). A private life [Television series episode]. In A. Ball (Executive Producer), *Six feet under.* HBO Home Video.

Robinson, K. (2002). *A single square picture*. New York, NY: Berkley.

Roche, T. (2002a, March 18). Andrea Yates: More to the story. *Time*. Retrieved from http://www.time.com/time/nation/article/0,8599,218445,00.html

Roche, T. (2002b, January 20). The Yates odyssey. *Time*, 42–50.

Rogers, A. (2001, Winter). Alphabets of the night: Toward a poetics of trauma. *Radcliffe Quarterly*, pp. 20–23.

Rogers, A. G. (1995). *A shining affliction: A story of harm and healing in psychotherapy*. New York, NY: Penguin Books.

Rogers, A. G. (2006). *The unsayable: The hidden language of trauma*. New York, NY: Random House.

Rogers, A. G., Casey, M. E., Ekert, J., Holland, J., Nakkula, V., & Sheinberg, N. (1999). An interpretive poetics of languages of the unsayable. In R. Josselson & A. Lieblich (Eds.), *Making meaning of narratives* (pp. 77–106). Thousand Oaks, CA: Sage.

Rogers, C. R. (1980). *A way of being*. Boston, MA: Houghton Mifflin.

Rogers, C. R. (1957/1992). The necessary and sufficient conditions of therapeutic personality change. *Journal of Consulting and Clinical Psychology, 60*, 827–832.

Rokeach, M., & Ball-Rokeach, S. J. (1989). Stability and change in American value priorities, 1968–1981. *American Psychologist, 44*, 775–784.

Ronnestad, M. H., & Orlinsky, D. E. (2005). Clinical implications: Training, supervision, and practice. In D. E. Orlinsky & M. H. Ronnestad (Eds.), *How psychotherapists develop: A study of therapeutic work and professional growth* (pp. 103–116). Washington, DC: American Psychological Association.

Rosenthal, R. (2002). Covert communication in classrooms, clinics, courtrooms, and cubicles. *American Psychologist, 57*, 839–849.

Rosenzweig, S. (1936). Some implicit common factors in diverse methods of psychotherapy. *American Journal of Orthopsychiatry, 6*, 412–415.

Ross, L. (1977). The intuitive psychologist and his shortcomings: Distortions in the attribution process. In L. Berkowitz (Ed.), *Advances in zexperimental social psychology*

(Vol. 10, pp. 174–221). New York, NY: Academic Press.

Rothschild, B. (2004, September/October). Mirror, mirror. *Psychotherapy Networker, 28*(5), 46–50, 69.

Rowe, M., Frey, J., Bailey, M., Fisk, D., & Davidson, L. (2001). Clinical responsibility and client autonomy: Dilemmas in mental health work at the margins. *American Journal of Orthopsychiatry, 71*, 400–407.

Rupert, P. A., & Baird, K. A. (2004). Managed care and the independent practice of psychology. *Professional Psychology: Research and Practice, 35*, 185–193.

Rupert, P. A., & Kent, J. S. (2007). Gender and work setting differences in career-sustaining behaviors and burnout among professional psychologists. *Professional Psychology: Research and Practice, 38*, 88–96.

Sabin-Farrell, R., & Turpin, G. (2003). Vicarious traumatization: Implications for the mental health of health workers? *Clinical Psychology Review, 23*, 449–480.

Saks, E. R. (2007). *The center cannot hold: My journey through madness*. New York, NY: Hyperion.

Saltzman, N., & Norcross, J. C. (Eds.). (1990). *Therapy wars: Contention and convergence in different clinical approaches*. San Francisco, CA: Jossey-Bass.

Samson, S. (2006, January). KY miners comment about WV mine explosion. *WFIE.COM*. Retrieved from http://www.14wfie.com/global/story.asp?s=4313743

Sanchez, R. (2000). *My bloody life: The making of a Latin King*. Chicago, IL: Chicago Review Press.

Sanchez, R. (2003). *Once a king, always a king: The unmaking of a Latin King*. Chicago, IL: Chicago

Santrock, J. W. (2006). *Human adjustment*. Boston, MA: McGraw-Hill.

Schafer, R. (2002). Experiencing termination: Authentic and false depressive positions. *Psychoanalytic Psychology, 19*, 235–253.

Schopp, R. F. (2001). *Competence, condemnation, and commitment: An integrated theory of mental health law*. Washington, DC: American Psychological Association.

Schure, M. B., Christopher, J., & Christopher, S. (2008). Mind-body medicine and the art of self-care: Teaching mindfulness to counseling students through yoga, meditation,

and qigong. *Journal of Counseling and Development, 86*, 47–56.

Schwarzer, R. (2001). Stress, resources, and proactive coping. *Applied Psychology: An International Review, 50*, 400–407.

Schwebel, M., & Coster, J. (1998). Well-functioning in professional psychologists: As program heads see it. *Professional Psychology: Research and Practice, 29*(3), 284–292.

Seelye, K. Q. (2009, July 23). Obama wades into a volatile racial issue. *New York Times*. Retrieved from http://www.nytimes.com/2009/07/23/us/23race.html?_r=2&hp

Seligman, L. (2004). *Technical and conceptual skills for mental health professionals*. Upper Saddle River, NJ: Pearson.

Seligman, L. (2006). *Theories of counseling and psychotherapy: Systems, strategies and skills* (2nd ed.). Upper Saddle River, NJ: Pearson.

Seligman, M. E. P. (1995). The effectiveness of psychotherapy: The Consumer Reports study. *American Psychologist, 50*, 965–974.

Seligman, M. E. P., Walker, E. F., & Rosenhan, D. L. (2001). *Abnormal psychology* (4th ed.). New York, NY: W. W. Norton.

Senior, J. (2009, April 16). The end of the Trench Coat Mafia. *New York Times*. Retrieved from http://www.nytimes.com/2009/04/19/books/review/Senior-t.html

Serran, G., Fernandez, Y., Marshall, W. L., & Mann, R. E. (2003). Process issues in treatment: Application to sexual offender programs. *Professional Psychology: Research and Practice, 34*, 368–374.

Shafranske, E. P. (2005). The psychology of religion in clinical and counseling psychology. In R. F. Paloutzian & C. L. Park (Eds.), *Handbook of the psychology of religion and spirituality* (pp. 496–514). New York, NY: Guilford Press.

Shapiro, J. P. (1989). Self-blame versus helplessness in sexually abused children: An attributional analysis with treatment recommendations. *Journal of Social and Clinical Psychology, 8*, 442–455.

Shapiro, J. P. (1995). Attribution-based treatment of self-blame and helplessness in sexually abused children. *Psychotherapy, 32*, 581–591.

Sharkansky, E. J., Brief, D. J., Peirce, J. M., Meehan, J. C., & Mannix, L. M. (1999). Substance abuse patients with posttraumatic stress disorder (PTSD): Identifying specific triggers of substance use and their associations with PTSD symptoms. *Psychology of Addictive Behaviors, 13,* 89–97.

Sheeran, P., Aubrey, R., & Kellett, S. (2007). Increasing attendance for psychotherapy: Implementation intentions and the self-regulation of attendance-related negative affect. *Journal of Consulting and Clinical Psychology, 75,* 853–863.

Sherby, L. B. (2009). Considerations on countertransference love. *Contemporary Psychoanalysis, 45,* 65–81.

Sherman, M. D., & Thelen, M. H. (1998). Distress and professional impairment among psychologists in clinical practice. *Professional Psychology: Research and Practice, 29,* 79–85.

Shiffman, S., Hickcox, M., Paty, J. A., Gnys, M., Kassel, J. D., & Richards, T. J. (1996). Progression from a smoking lapse to relapse: Prediction from abstinence violation effects, nicotine dependence, and lapse characteristics. *Journal of Consulting and Clinical Psychology, 64,* 993–1002.

Simmons, T., & Dye, J. L. (2003). Grandparents living with grandchildren: 2000. *US Census Bureau.* Retrieved from http://www.census.gov/prod/2003pubs/c2kbr-31.pdf

Slattery, J. M. (2004). *Counseling diverse clients: Bringing context into therapy.* Belmont, CA: Brooks/Cole.

Slattery, J. M. (2005). Preventing role slippage during work in the community: Guidelines for new psychologists and supervisees. *Psychotherapy: Theory, Research, Practice, Training, 42,* 384–394.

Slattery, J. M., & Park, C. L. (in press a). Clinical approaches to discrepancies in meaning: Conceptualization, assessment, and treatment. In P. Wong (Ed.), *Human quest for meaning* (2nd ed.). New York, NY: Lawrence Erlbaum.

Slattery, J. M., & Park, C. L. (in press b). Meaning making and spiritually oriented interventions. In J. Aten, M. R. McMinn, & E. V. Worthington (Eds.), *Spiritually oriented interventions for counseling and psychotherapy.* Washington, DC: American Psychological Association.

Smith, D., & Fitzpatrick, M. (1995). Patient-therapist boundary issues: An integrative review of theory and research. *Professional Psychology: Research and Practice, 26,* 499–506.

Snibbe, A. C., & Markus, H. R. (2005). You can't always get what you want: Educational attainment, agency, and choice. *Journal of Personality and Social Psychology, 88,* 703–720.

Snyder, C. R., Michael, S. T., & Cheavens, J. S. (1999). Hope as a psychotherapeutic foundation of common factors, placebos, and expectancies. In M. A. Hubble, B. L. Duncan, & S. D. Miller (Eds.), *The heart & soul of change: What works in therapy* (pp. 179–200). Washington, DC: American Psychological Association.

Snyder, T. A., & Barnett, J. E. (2006). Informed consent and the process of psychotherapy. *Psychotherapy Bulletin, 41,* 37–42.

Starbranch, E. K. (1999). Psychiatric assessment of Andrea Yates. *Court TV.* Retrieved from http://www.courttv.com/trials/yates/docs/psychiatric1.html

Steele, C. M. (1997). A threat in the air: How stereotypes shape intellectual identity and performance. *American Psychologist, 52,* 613–629.

Steinberg, L. (2001). We know some things: Parent-adolescent relations in retrospect and prospect. *Journal of Research on Adolescence, 11,* 1–20.

Strupp, H. H. (1996). Some salient lessons from research and practice. *Psychotherapy: Theory, Research, Practice, Training, 33,* 135–138.

Stuart, R. B. (2004). Multiculturalism: Questions, not answers. *Professional Psychology: Research and Practice, 36,* 576–578.

Stuentzner-Gibson, D., Koren, P. E., & DeChillo, N. (1995). The Youth Satisfaction Questionnaire: What kids think of services. *Families in Society, 76,* 616–624.

Sue, D. W. (1992). The challenge of multiculturalism: The road less traveled. *American Counselor, 1,* 7–14.

Sue, D. W. (2004). Whiteness and ethnocentric monoculturalism: Making the "invisible" visible. *American Psychologist, 59,* 761–769.

Sue, D. W., Bingham, R. P., Porché-Burke, L., & Vasquez, M. (1999). The diversification of psychology: A multicultural revolution. *American Psychologist, 54,* 1070–1077.

Sue, D. W., & Sue, S. (2003). *Counseling the culturally diverse: Theory and practice* (4th ed.). New York, NY: John Wiley & Sons.

Sue, S. (1998). In search of cultural competence in psychotherapy and counseling. *American Psychologist, 53,* 440–448.

Sullivan, J. R., Ramirez, E., Rae, W. A., Razo, N. R., & George, C. A. (2002). Factors contributing to breaking confidentiality with adolescent clients: A survey of pediatric psychologists. *Professional Psychology: Research and Practice, 33,* 396–401.

Sullivan, T., Martin, W. L., & Handelsman, M. M. (1993). Practical benefits of an informed-consent procedure: An empirical investigation. *Professional Psychology: Research and Practice, 24,* 160–163.

Swann, W. B. Jr., Chang-Schneider, C., & Larsen McClarty, K. (2007). Do people's self-views matter? Self-concept and self-esteem in everyday life. *American Psychologist, 62,* 84–94.

Taft, C. T., Murphy, C. M., Musser, P. H., & Remington, N. A. (2004). Personality, interpersonal, and motivational predictors of the working alliance in group cognitive-behavioral therapy for partner violent men. *Journal of Consulting and Clinical Psychology, 72,* 349–354.

Teasdale, J. D., Segal, Z. V., Williams, J. M. G., Ridgeway, V. A., Soulsby, J. M., & Lau, M. A. (2000). Prevention of relapse/recurrence in major depression by mindfulness-based cognitive therapy. *Journal of Consulting and Clinical Psychology, 68,* 615–623.

Thomas, P. M. (2005). Dissociation and internal models of protection: Psycho-therapy with child abuse survivors. *Psychotherapy: Theory, Research, Practice, Training, 42,* 20–36.

Thompson, C. E., & Jenal, S. T. (1994). Interracial and intraracial quasi-counseling interactions when counselors avoid discussing race. *Journal of Counseling Psychology, 41,* 484–491.

Thompson, J. P. (1999). *Psychiatric assessment of Andrea Yates.* Retrieved from http://www.courttv.com/trials/yates/docs/psychiatric6.html

Thompson, K., & Thompson, C. W. (2009, July 24). Officer tells his side of the story in Gates arrest. *Washington Post.* Retrieved from http://www.washingtonpost.com/ wp-dyn/content/article/2009/07/23/ AR2009072301073.html

Tinsley-Jones, H. A. (2001). Racism in our midst: Listening to psychologists of color. *Professional Psychology: Research and Practice, 32,* 573–580.

Tinsley-Jones, H. (2003). Racism: Calling a spade a spade. *Psychotherapy: Theory, Research, Practice, Training, 40,* 179–186.

Triandis, H. C., & Gelfand, M. J. (1998). Converging measurement of horizontal and vertical individualism and collectivism. *Journal of Personality and Social Psychology, 74,* 118–128.

Trope, Y., & Thompson, E. P. (1997). Looking for truth in all the wrong places? Asymmetric search of individuating information about stereotyped group members. *Journal of Personality and Social Psychology, 73,* 229–241.

Turchik, J. A., Karpenko, V., Hammers, D., & McNamara, J. R. (2007). Practical and ethical assessment issues in rural, impoverished, and managed care settings. *Professional Psychology: Research and Practice, 38,* 158–168.

Twenty-first Century Books. (2008). *Malcolm X: A research site.* Retrieved from http://www.broth ermalcolm.net/

Uffelman, R. A., & Hardin, S. I. (2002). Session limits at university counseling centers: Effects on help-seeking attitudes. *Journal of Counseling Psychology, 49,* 127–132.

U.S. Census Bureau. (2006). *Statistical abstract of the United States: 2006.* Retrieved from http://www.census .gov/prod/2005pubs/06statab/ pop.pdf

Vallacher, R. R., & Wegner, D. M. (1987). What do people think they're doing? Action identification and human behavior. *Psychological Review, 94,* 3–15.

van Baaren, R. B., Holland, R. W., Kawakami, K., & van Knippenberg, A. (2004). Mimicry and prosocial behavior. *Psychological Science, 15,* 71–74.

Wachtel, P. L. (2002). Termination of therapy: An effort at integration. *Journal of Psychotherapy Integration, 12*(3), 373–383.

Wade, N. G., Vogel, D. L., Liao, K. Y., & Goldman, D. B. (2008). Measuring state-specific rumination: Development of the Rumination About an Interpersonal Offense Scale. *Journal of Counseling Psychology, 55,* 419–426.

Walker, M., Jacobs, M. (Producers), & Crisp, D. (Director). (1992). *The clumsy counselor: Loaded remarks from the client's perspective* [Motion picture]. (Available from University of Leicester, P. O. Box 138, Maurice Shock Building, University Road, Leicester LE1 9HN)

Walter, J. L., & Peller, J. E. (1992). *Becoming solution-focused in brief therapy.* New York, NY: Brunner/ Mazel.

Ward, S., Donovan, H., Gunnarsdottir, S., Serlin, R. C., Shapiro, G. R., & Hughes, S. (2008). A randomized trial of a representational intervention to decrease cancer pain (RIDCancerPain). *Health Psychology, 27,* 59–67.

Watson, J. C. (2007). Reassessing Rogers' necessary and sufficient conditions of change. *Psychotherapy: Theory, Research, Practice, Training, 44,* 268–273.

Watzlawick, P., Weakland, J. H., & Fisch, R. (1974). *Change: Principles of problem formation and problem resolution.* New York, NY: Norton.

Weiss, L. (2004). *Therapist's guide to self-care.* New York, NY: Brunner-Routledge.

Weisz, J. R., & Hawley, K. M. (2002). Developmental factors in the treatment of adolescents. *Journal of Consulting and Clinical Psychology, 70,* 21–43.

Weltner, J. (1998, May/June). Different strokes: A pragmatist's guide to intervention. *Family Therapy Networker,* pp. 53–57.

Wicks, R. J. (2008). *The resilient clinician.* New York, NY: Oxford University Press.

Wright, M. A. (1998). *I'm chocolate, you're vanilla: Raising healthy black and biracial children in a race-conscious world.* San Francisco, CA: Jossey-Bass.

Yalom, I. D. (2003). *The gift of therapy: An open letter to a new generation of therapists and their patients.* New York, NY: HarperCollins.

Yates, R. (2004, January 18). *Are you there alone? A review.* Retrieved from http://www.yateskids.org/ are_you_there_alone.php

Yates, R. (n.d.). *Welcome.* Retrieved from http://www.yateskids.org/

Young, M. E. (2005). *Learning the art of helping: Building blocks and techniques* (3rd ed.). Upper Saddle River, NH: Pearson.

Younggren, J. N., & Gottlieb, M. C. (2008). Termination and abandonment: History, risk, and risk management. *Professional Psychology: Research and Practice, 39*(5), 498–504.

Zaki, J., Bolger, N., & Ochsner, K. (2008). It takes two: The interpersonal nature of empathic accuracy. *Psychological Science, 19,* 399–404.

Zimbardo, P. G., & Boyd, J. N. (1999). Putting time in perspective: A valid, reliable individual-differences metric. *Journal of Personality and Social Psychology, 77,* 1271–1288.

Zimmerman, G. L., Olsen, C. G., & Bosworth, M. F. (2000). A stages of change' approach to helping patients change behavior. *American Family Physician, 61,* 1409–1416.

Zuckerman, E. (2000). *Clinician's thesaurus: The guide for writing psychological reports* (5th ed.). New York, NY: Guilford.

Zur, O. (2001, Spring). Out-of-office experience: When crossing office boundaries and engaging in dual relationships are clinically beneficial and ethically sound. *Independent Practitioner, 21*(1), 96–100. Retrieved from http://www.zurinsti tute.com/outofoffice.html

AUTHOR INDEX

Aapro, N., 284, 293
Abelson, R. P., 101
Abraído-Lanza, A. F., 174
Achenbach, T. M., 126
Ackerman, S., 194
Ahn, A. J., 44
Ai, A. L., 45, 50
Ainsworth, M. S., 46
Alcoholics Anonymous, 144
Aldwin, C. M., 236, 246, 308, 309
Alexander, F., 236
Allen, D. M., 169
Allport, G. W., 55
Alterman, A. I., 154
Alvarez, W. F., 92
Ambühl, H., 284, 293
American Association for Marriage and Family Therapy, 24, 134, 314
American Council on Education, 68
American Counseling Association, 24, 36, 314
American Mental Health Counselors Association, 314
American Psychological Association, 22, 134, 314
American School Counselors Association, 314
Amrhein, P. C., 52, 151
Anderson, C. J., 52
Anderson, S. K., 52
Andrea Yates Confession, 5, 127, 220–221
Annas, G. J., 31
Anonymous, 22, 23, 38, 144, 198, 240
Antoni, M. H., 236, 238, 239, 240, 241, 242, 243, 245
Archer, A., 10, 11, 12, 15

Arias, B., 302
Asay, T. P., 12, 13, 164
Associated Press, 127, 220, 221
Atkisson, C. C., 184
Aubrey, R., 207
Austin, J. T., 45
Austin, K. M., 134
Axelson, J., 53
Azar, S. T., 99

Bai, M., 101
Bailey, M., 31
Baird, K. A., 289
Baker, E. K., 295, 300, 302, 303, 304, 306, 307, 309, 312
Ball, S. G., 246
Ball-Rokeach, S. J., 45
Balsam, K. F., 68
Banaji, M. R., 93
Bandura, A., 44, 52, 53, 150
Barley, D. E., 12, 13, 235
Barnett, J. E., 24, 25, 27, 28, 39, 291, 300, 302, 307
Barrett, M. S., 207
Bashe, A., 40, 294, 297, 300
Bates, L., 253
Beauchaine, T. P., 68
Beauchemin, E., 69
Beck, A. T., 10, 184, 252
Becker-Blease, K. A., 293
Behnke, S., 31
Belenky, M. F., 77
Benjet, C., 99
Bennett, B. E., 26, 27, 30, 31, 34, 35, 36, 39, 142, 260, 262, 269, 271, 272, 279, 282, 284, 285, 294, 297, 300, 301, 302, 305, 307, 308

Berano, K. C., 36
Berg, I. K., 177, 245, 249, 255
Bernstein, R., 174
Beutler, L. E., 10, 151, 194, 202, 237, 252, 255
Bingham, R. P., 69
Bishop, D. R., 288
Bishop, D. S., 184
Blair, I. V., 93
Blais, M. A., 246
Blake, P., 206
Blatner, A., 193
Blehar, M. C., 46
Blevins, T., 207
Bloom, B. S., 179
Bohart, A. C., 62, 151, 202, 241, 255
Bolger, N., 193
Bolter, K., 92
Borckardt, J. J., 184
Bornstein, B. F., 47
Bostrom, A., 244
Bosworth, M. F., 151
Botermans, J-F., 284, 293
Botorff, N., 280
Boyd, J. N., 52, 53, 54, 55
Boyd-Franklin, N., 68
Bozza, A., 90
Brabeck, M., 310
Brennan, J., 45, 46, 50, 52
Brief, D. J., 154
Briñol, P., 250
Brogan, M. M., 261
Brown, G. K., 10, 238, 245
Brown, L., 310
Brown, L. M., 91, 224
Brown, L. S., 47, 74

SUBJECT INDEX

Note: page numbers followed by f or t refer to Figures or Tables

339